Proteolysis in the Interstitial Space

PROTEIN SCIENCE SERIES

SERIES EDITOR

Roger L. Lundblad
Lundblad Biotechnology
Chapel Hill, North Carolina, U.S.A.

PUBLISHED TITLES

Proteolysis in the Interstitial Space
Salvatore V. Pizzo, Roger L. Lundblad, and Monte S. Willis

Biotechnology of Plasma Proteins
Roger L. Lundblad

Chemical Modification of Biological Polymers
Roger L. Lundblad

Development and Application of Biomarkers
Roger L. Lundblad

Approaches to the Conformational Analysis of Biopharmaceuticals
Roger L. Lundblad

Application of Solution Protein Chemistry to Biotechnology
Roger L. Lundblad

Proteolysis in the Interstitial Space

Salvatore V. Pizzo
Roger L. Lundblad
Monte S. Willis

PROTEIN SCIENCE SERIES

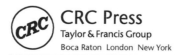

CRC Press
Taylor & Francis Group
Boca Raton London New York

CRC Press is an imprint of the
Taylor & Francis Group, an **informa** business

CRC Press
Taylor & Francis Group
6000 Broken Sound Parkway NW, Suite 300
Boca Raton, FL 33487-2742

First isued in paperback 2020

© 2017 by Taylor & Francis Group, LLC
CRC Press is an imprint of Taylor & Francis Group, an Informa business

No claim to original U.S. Government works

ISBN-13: 978-1-4665-7207-2 (hbk)
ISBN-13: 978-0-367-73698-9 (pbk)

Visit the Taylor & Francis Web site at
http://www.taylorandfrancis.com

and the CRC Press Web site at
http://www.crcpress.com

Dedication

Salvatore V. Pizzo dedicates this work to Susan Pizzo, an author in her own right.

Roger L. Lundblad dedicates this work to Sharon Mason, the flame of the class of '57 that refuses to dim.

Monte S. Willis dedicates this book to Tina, Connor, and Declan, and their devious plots to make him happy.

Contents

Preface

The emergence of biotechnologies to foster discoveries in genomics, proteomics, and other branches of molecular biosciences has provided the potential for greater precision in medical care, from diagnostics to therapies. However, their successful application to patients has been slow for multiple reasons. The complexity of regulatory frameworks that clinical laboratory tests must adhere to and the sheer complexity of the protein and macromolecules identified as diagnostic and/or prognostic biomarkers in experimental systems account for some of these barriers. Understanding the environments in which these proteins may be assayed will be crucial, particularly where precision medicine is concerned. Thus, the concept of human extravascular fluids and bodily secretions, or more broadly *interstitial fluids*, is something we have grappled with for some time with increasing application in biotechnology.

Conceptually, interstitial fluids may not be as foreign as they first appear. For example, both urine and saliva are interstitial fluids commonly assayed in clinical laboratory tests. While assays for urine (a plasma ultrafiltration) and saliva (derived from glandular secretion and plasma proteins) are simple and quite basic, our further understanding of their makeup and relationship to disease in expanding biosignatures will have commercial importance in therapeutics and diagnostics. Their dynamic properties, currently viewed as static processes, are surprising. With 60% of serum albumin in the extravascular space, the dynamic movement of fluid between the intravascular and extravascular space, exchanging one entire plasma volume every 9 hours, brings to light a context in which understanding biomarkers and biomarker signatures will be needed. Similarly, understanding the dynamics of extravascular spaces derived from sources other than plasma, such as cerebral spinal fluid, will bring to light how biomarkers for specific diseases (e.g., multiple myeloma) can be created with diagnostic/therapeutic value.

This book has been organized into broad biologically relevant categories in the context of interstitial fluids. In the first half of the book, we cover the fundamental concepts of interstitial fluid. We begin by defining its composition and function (Chapter 1), then discuss the extracellular matrices, which are responsible for regulating the composition of interstitial fluids (Chapter 2). We then focus our attention on the biochemistry of the large carbohydrate heteropolymer hyaluronan, as it is a major constituent of the interstitial space and is critically important in understanding synovial fluid (Chapter 3). Lastly, we discuss the factors that regulate proteolysis in the interstitial space, including the possible effects of extracellular matrix components such as collagen and hyaluronan (Chapter 4).

The coagulation system has been studied extensively in terms of diagnostics, primarily by assaying vascular spaces. However, a disconnect with this approach has always been that many of the components exist in the interstitial spaces, notably tissue factor, matrix metalloproteinases, serine protease inhibitors, and coagulation factors. The second part of this book investigates the fibrinolytic system (Chapter 5), kallikreins (Chapter 6), matrix metalloproteinases (Chapter 7), coagulation factors (Chapter 8), and protease inhibitors (e.g., serpins; Chapter 9) in the interstitial space.

With increasing recognition that the interstitial environment is where many of the primary reactions of the coagulation system are playing out in the pathogenesis of disease, future assays will depend on understanding how each of these major systems contributes to the interstitial environment.

By covering a unique array of topics with a broad application to biomedical workers, including physicians and scientists in industrial and academic pursuits of biotechnology, we hope this book expands the understanding of those creating greater precision in medical care. We extend our gratitude to the many scientists that we called upon that have made substantial contributions to the literature. We hope you find our synthesis of their work a useful and valuable resource.

Acknowledgments

We wish to thank Jill Jurgensen, Barbara Norwitz, and Chuck Crumly at CRC Press/ Taylor & Francis Group for their support of this work. We also acknowledge the valuable support of Ashley Rivenbark, PhD (a paid independent contractor) and Steve Conlon (Duke PhotoPath) with editing and creating, respectively, the original figures used throughout this textbook.

Authors

Roger L. Lundblad is a native of San Francisco, California. He received his undergraduate education at Pacific Lutheran University and his PhD in biochemistry at the University of Washington. After his postdoctoral work in the laboratories of Stanford Moore and William Stein at the Rockefeller University, he joined the faculty of the University of North Carolina at Chapel Hill. He joined the Hyland division of Baxter Healthcare in 1990. Currently, Dr. Lundblad works as an independent consultant at Chapel Hill, North Carolina, and writes on biotechnological issues. He is an adjunct professor of pathology at the University of North Carolina at Chapel Hill.

Salvatore V. Pizzo is distinguished professor of pathology in the School of Medicine at Duke University in Durham, North Carolina. Dr. Pizzo received his MD and PhD from Duke University and has spent his entire academic career at this institution. He served as chair of the Department of Pathology at Duke from 1991 to 2015 and has also been the director of several interdisciplinary research programs. Dr. Pizzo is a fellow of the American Association for the Advancement of Science and has served in an editorial capacity for several biomedical journals. His current research focuses on the function of GRP-78, a molecular chaperone.

Monte S. Willis lives and runs in Chapel Hill, North Carolina, with his family. He received his MD/PhD from the University of Nebraska Medical Center in biochemistry and pathology. He completed his medical residency in pathology and postdoctoral fellowship training program in burns, trauma, and critical care at the University of Texas Southwestern in Dallas, Texas. He then joined the Department of Pathology and Laboratory Medicine and the McAllister Heart Institute at the University of North Carolina at Chapel Hill, where he currently is a National Institutes of Health and Leducq Foundation–supported translational researcher, investigating the role of the ubiquitin proteasome system and protein misfolding as therapeutic targets in heart failure. He recently completed his MBA from the Kenan–Flagler School of Business. He routinely writes and edits textbooks in cardiology and cardiovascular pathology and is involved in training MDs, PhDs, postdocs, and undergraduates interested in the heart. He is an adjunct professor of pharmacology at the University of North Carolina.

1 Composition and Function of the Interstitial Fluid

1.1 DEFINITION OF INTERSTITIAL FLUID

Body water is divided between intracellular and extracellular fluid, with the great bulk being intracellular fluid and approximately 30% extracellular fluid. The latter is divided between extravascular and intravascular fluid (blood plasma).[1] Extravascular fluid can be further demarcated into interstitial fluid and specialized fluids found in the cerebrospinal, synovial, and ocular compartments (aqueous humor of the eye). The peritoneal transudate, synovial fluid, and interstitial fluid share some characteristics related to their formation from plasma. There is evidence for connectivity between brain interstitial fluid and cerebrospinal fluid.[2-5] Abbott[2] presents evidence for brain interstitial flow into the cerebrospinal fluid and the possibility of cerebrospinal fluid flow into the brain. Iliff and coworkers[3] showed that cerebrospinal fluid exchange with brain interstitial fluid provides a mechanism for the removal of brain interstitial solutes. This group[3,4] have designated this exchange between brain interstitial fluid and cerebrospinal fluid as the glymphatic system and suggested that an imbalance in this system could be responsible for brain edema. The term *glymphatic* is defined as a paravascular fluid exchange pathway that enables brain interstitial and cerebrospinal fluid turnover and is facilitated by glial cells.[4] Stukas and coworkers[5] have shown that apolipoprotein A-1 passes into the brain via cerebrospinal fluid. These investigators suggest that apolipoprotein A-1 passes from the vascular system into cerebrospinal fluid by specific cellular transport (transcytosis). The exchange between brain interstitial fluid and cerebrospinal fluid would be confined to the brain and associated nervous tissue with little systemic consequence. That said, there is the curious issue of prothrombin expression in the brain[6] and the importance of PAR-1 receptors in neurobiology.[7] Some characteristics of several human body fluids are shown in Table 1.1.

The concept of the interstitial space dates at least to the work of William Harvey in the sixteenth century on the circulation of blood.[8] Although we could not find a direct mention of the interstitium, it follows from the description of the circulation that there is a process for transport from the circulation to tissue and return. Early work by Claude Bernard and others[9] defined the interstitial space (*milieu intérieur*) as the space between the cells, and that space is between the circulatory system and the lymphatics. A more recent definition defines the interstitial space as the space outside the blood vessels and lymphatic vessels that consists of interstitial fluid and the extracellular matrix (ECM).[10] A substantial portion of a number of plasma

TABLE 1.1
Protein Content of Various Human Body Fluids and Secretions

Fluid	Protein (mg/mL)[a]	Comment	Refs.
Extracellular fluid	N/A	The body fluid can be divided into two major components: the intracellular fluid and the extracellular fluid. Between 60% and 70% of the body fluid is intracellular in nature, while the remainder is extracellular in nature. The extracellular fluid, in turn, consists of two primary components: intravascular fluid (blood plasma; approximately 25%) and extravascular fluid (approximately 75%). The extravascular fluid consists mostly of interstitial fluid with small specialized fluids in various spaces; specialized fluids include cerebrospinal fluid, synovial fluid, and ocular fluid.	1–5
Blood plasma	78.9 ± 0.5[b]	A protein-rich fluid defined by being confined within the vascular system and representing one-quarter to one-fifth of the total extracellular fluid. It is in equilibrium with the interstitial fluid, which feeds into the lymphatic system and is returned to the venous system. Other areas of extracellular fluid include the peritoneal fluid, ocular fluid, and cerebrospinal fluid. Plasma is also defined as the protein-rich fluid obtained by the removal of the cellular elements of whole blood collected with an anticoagulant.	6–8
Blood serum	72.9 ± 0.5[b]	A protein-rich fluid derived from the clotting of plasma or whole blood. Most frequently collected by the clotting of whole blood collected without the addition of an anticoagulant. The protein concentration of serum is usually less that of corresponding plasma, reflecting the loss of fibrinogen and other plasma proteins. Serum may also contain products secreted by platelets and other cellular elements during the process of coagulation.	6–8
Interstitial fluid[c]	50.9[d]	The concentration of protein in interstitial fluid is 40–60% of that in plasma. The volume of interstitial fluid is two to three times larger than plasma volume and the concentration of a given protein in the interstitial fluid depends on the excluded interstitial volume for a specific protein and the size of the protein. Albumin is the most common protein in interstitial fluid, with lower concentrations of larger proteins such as IgG.	9–11
Interstitial fluid	29.8	Plasma protein concentration was given at 70.0 mg/mL; the interstitial volume was 8.4 L, with an excluded interstitial volume of 2.1 L.	12
Interstitial fluid	27.2	Wick fluid.[e]	13
	18.3	Blister technique.[e]	

Interstitial fluid	37[f]	Perivascular.	14
	24	Peribronchial.	
Lymph	26–51[e]	Lymph is derived from plasma via interstitial fluid. There is tissue variability in lymph flow rate and regional composition. In this study, as with others, albumin was the major protein. This study also referred to other proteins as members of the classical globulin fractions.	15
Lymph	17–25[f]	Protein concentration increased to 44 mg/mL in skin lymph but not muscle lymph after thermal injury.	16
Lymph[g]	42	The lymph/plasma ratio was 0.71 for total protein, 0.70 for albumin, and 0.25 for immunoglobulin.	17
Lymph[h]	25–27	The protein concentration of lymph was slightly less than that of interstitial fluid. The concentration of lactic dehydrogenase was much higher in interstitial fluid than in lymph; the concentration in lymph in turn is much higher than that in plasma.	18
Lymph[i]	27	The protein concentration of lymph was slightly less than that obtained for interstitial fluid (25 mg/mL). Albumin is the major protein (18 mg/mL), with smaller quantities of globulin[j] (8.2 mg/mL).	19
Peritoneal fluid	25	Peritoneal fluid is usually obtained only the in the case of ascites; it is labeled a transudate if the protein concentration is less than 25 mg/mL and an exudate if the protein concentration is greater than 25 mg/mL.[k] A transudate can result from increased hydrostatic pressure, while an exudate can result from decreased capillary permeability.	20–22
Peritoneal fluid	42.2 ± 6	Peritoneal fluid obtained from normal women over the course of a menstrual cycle.	23
Peritoneal fluid	43.2 ± 0.8	The concentration of protein in peritoneal fluid is 68% of that in plasma; the relationship of plasma transcortin and peritoneal fluid is similar (71%). Luteinizing hormone (LH) and follicle-stimulating hormone (FSH) are also found in peritoneal fluid but correlated with plasma concentrations are lower (LH, 42%; FSH, 63%). The concentration of steroid hormones such as 17β-estradiol and androstanedione are equal or higher in peritoneal fluid than in plasma, while the concentration of cortisol is lower in peritoneal fluid than in plasma.	24
Cerebrospinal fluid	0.21[b]	Protein in cerebrospinal fluid is derived from brain and plasma. Albumin is the major protein in cerebrospinal fluid; the ratio of serum albumin concentration to CSF albumin concentration (Q_{Alb}) is used as a diagnostic tool for determination of blood–brain barrier integrity. There are tight barriers between blood and cerebrospinal fluid; the brain is suggested to be an immunologically privileged area.	25–35

(Continued)

TABLE 1.1 (CONTINUED)
Protein Content of Various Human Body Fluids and Secretions

Fluid	Protein (mg/mL)[a]	Comment	Refs.
Cerebrospinal fluid	0.21–2.74 (median, 0.49; n=62) 0.21–2.6 (median, 0.49; n=62)	Pyrogallol red–molybdate method. Coomassie brilliant blue dye binding.[1]	36
Cerebrospinal fluid	0.78[m]	Coomassie brilliant blue in the presence of sodium dodecyl sulfate.	37
Cerebrospinal fluid	0.149–1.07	Pediatric population ranging in age from 0.1 to 210 months. Protein concentration changes with age. Albumin is the major protein. It is suggested that 80% of cerebrospinal proteins are derived from blood plasma by a transcellular or paracellular process.	38
Ocular fluid	0.26–0.28[n] 0.15–0.48[o]	MRI signals from Gd show the presence of Gd in ocular fluid after IV administration. Concentrations of albumin, IgG, and α_1-antitrypsin aqueous humor are similar to those in cerebrospinal fluid and have been suggested to show circadian variation. There are tight barriers to the ocular space and the eye is an immunologically privileged region.	39–43
Perilymph	2.75[b]	Inner-ear fluid, similar in composition to interstitial fluid. There are connections to cerebrospinal fluid.	25,43,44
Endolymph	0.38[b]	Inner-ear fluid, thought to be derived from the perilymph.	25
Synovial fluid	10.9[p] 20–35[q] 0.718±0.705[r]	Synovial fluid is a viscous fluid with non-Newtonian behavior found within various joints in the body, such as the knee and temporomandibular joints. Synovial fluid has a lubricating function within the joint. The high concentration of hyaluronic acid is thought to provide the basis of the viscosity as well as providing some of the lubrication characteristics. The interaction of hyaluronic acid with plasma proteins such as fibrinogen may be responsible for the non-Newtonian behavior of synovial fluid. The composition does change with inflammation, with a decrease in viscosity possibly reflecting the degradation of hyaluronic acid. There is some evidence that injection of hyaluronic acid into osteoarthritic joints has a positive therapeutic effect.	45–52

Gingival crevicular fluid	0.022–0.060[s]	Gingival crevicular fluid is largely supplied by an ultrafiltrate of plasma entering the oral cavity via the gingival crevice (between the tooth and the epithelial integument). Flow rate is increased with gingival inflammation. Gingival crevicular fluid is the source of most of the plasma proteins found in saliva.	53–56
Saliva		Saliva is composed of contributions from several glandular sources including the parotid gland, submaxillary (submandibular) gland, and sublingual glands, as well as minor volume contributions from gingival crevicular fluid. Saliva serves a variety of functions including digestive and antibacterial. There are factors in saliva that promote wound healing inside and outside the oral cavity. The determination of protein concentration of saliva is dependent on method and standard.	57–62
Saliva	1.4–6.4[t] 1.8–4.2[u]	Mixed human saliva (also referred to as whole saliva) refers to saliva obtained from all salivary secretions. Mixed saliva represents the combined glandular secretions with gingival crevicular fluid, which is mixed with food during mastication. The collection of mixed saliva is considered a noninvasive process and saliva is receiving increased attention for diagnostic purposes. Unstimulated saliva is collected by "drooling," while stimulated saliva is collected after some stimulation of the salivary glands, as by chewing. Stimulation influences the quality of the salivary secretion, and so *gleeking*, the process of forcibly ejecting saliva from the submandibular gland by application of pressure with the tongue, can be used to collect a stimulated salivary sample (see Chapter 2).	63–69
Parotid saliva	2.35±3.87[t] 1.64±0.51[u]	Parotid saliva is a serous secretion considerably less viscous than either submandibular or sublingual saliva. There is considerable homology between the parotid gland and the pancreas. Several enzymes show an inverse level of expression in the parotid or pancreas. For example, mouse parotid glands express a high level of DNAse I, while there is a low level of expression in the mouse pancreas.	63,70–74
Submandibular fluid	1.14±0.58[t] 0.77±0.36[u]	Submandibular saliva is a mucous secretion more viscous that parotid saliva. The viscosity is a property of the mucins present in submandibular saliva. Submaxillary secretion composes approximately two-thirds of the total volume of unstimulated human saliva and one-third of the volume of stimulated human saliva. The remaining volume of saliva is primarily provided by parotid saliva, with minor volume contributions from other glandular sources and gingival crevicular fluid. On stimulation, the relative volume contribution of submaxillary secretion decreases, while that of parotid secretion increases.	63,75–77

(Continued)

TABLE 1.1 (CONTINUED)

Protein Content of Various Human Body Fluids and Secretions

Fluid	Protein (mg/ mL)[a]	Comment	Refs.
Digestive secretions		There are a variety of digestive secretions, including the secretion of pepsinogen by the chief cells in the stomach and a variety of proenzymes, such as chymotrypsinogen and trypsinogen, by the pancreas. The secretion of the proenzymes is exocrine. The pancreas is an example of separation between exocrine function and endocrine function, with insulin produced by the endocrine side and secretion of pancreatic proenzymes and enzymes produced by the exocrine side.	78–81
Seminal fluid	55	Seminal fluid is secreted by the gonads and other male sexual accessory glands and may contain spermatozoa. It also contains a variety of proteins and other organic compounds.	82–88
Cervico-vaginal secretions		Vaginal fluid is composed of transudate and contributions from leukocytes and other cellular materials. Proteomic analysis suggests that 50% of the proteins are of plasma origin, although composition does depend on the sampling process. Samples obtained via colposcopy are more complex than those obtained by vaginal fluid lavage. As with other transudates, albumin is a major component of vaginal fluid. There may be contributions from cervical mucus, leading to the use of the terms *cervical-vaginal fluid* and *cervico-vaginal fluid* to describe this material. Cervical secretion is thought to be distinct from vaginal secretion. Much of the work used a mixture of fluids obtained from the cervix, vaginal secretion, and other sources such as amniotic fluids. Cervical secretion is much more viscous than the other fluids, reflecting the high concentration of mucins.	89–93
Tear fluid	5.77 ± 1.32[m]	Coomassie brilliant blue/bovine serum albumin standard.	94–98
	11.09 ± 1.94	Coomassie brilliant blue/IgG standard.	
	9.59 ± 1.32	Lowry/bovine serum albumin standard.	
	7.47 ± 1.28	Lowry/IgG standard.	

Note: Information is for human fluids unless otherwise indicated.

[a] There are a number methods for protein determination that can yield different results for the same biological fluid. (From Sapan, C.V., et al., *Biotechnol. Appl. Biochem.* 29, 99–108, 1999.)

[b] Biuret method; the plasma was collected with heparin as the anticoagulant.[6]

c Rat, Folin–Lowry.

d Also referred to as extracellular fluid in some publications. The strict definition of extracellular fluid is all fluid outside of the cell, which includes blood plasma and interstitial fluid as the constituents. Movement of protein in the interstitial space depends on protein charge, leading to the concept of excluded interstitial space. (From Gyenge, C.C., et al., *J. Physiol.* 552, 907–916, 2003.)

e Sampling of interstitial fluid is a technical challenge and is discussed in Chapter 6.

f Rabbit, protein concentration determined by bicinchoninic acid method.

g Rat tail lymph, protein determined by Lowry method.

h Rabbit, protein concentration estimated from graphical data.

i Rabbit.

j Individual protein concentrations estimated from electrophoretic analysis.

k Transudates and exudates are also seen with pleural effusions. (From Lee, Y.C., et al., *Chest* 131, 942–943, 2007; Porcel, J.M., *Clin. Chest Med.* 34, 27–37, 2013.)

l There have been some issues with the use of Coomassie brilliant blue for estimation of total protein for other biological fluids.[61]

m Somewhat different values were obtained by the other protein assay methods (Lowry, turbidimetric), which also varied by protein standard used. The value was obtained with Coomassie brilliant blue in the presence of sodium dodecyl sulfate. (From Macart, M. and Gerbaut, L., *Clin. Chim. Acta* 122, 93–101, 1982.)

n Rabbit vitreous humor, determined by Coomassie blue dye binding; value estimated from graphical representation of values determined over a 24-hour cycle. There was no significant circadian variation.

o Rabbit aqueous humor, determined by Coomassie blue dye binding; values estimated from graphical representation of values determined over a 24-hour cycle. Unlike the data obtained from the vitreous humor, the aqueous humor showed circadian variation.

p Mean value (equine; n = 15)[45] determined by Coomassie blue dye binding.

q Equine determined by refractometry; shown to increase on injection with pentosan polysulfate/N-acetylglucoseamine.[46]

r Human temporomandibular.

s The protein concentration increased with increasing sample time. Electrophoretic analysis also showed that the composition of gingival crevicular fluid increasingly resembled serum with increasing sample time.

t Unstimulated saliva, determined by the Lowry method.

u Stimulated saliva, determined by the Lowry method.

v Unfortunately, no other term exists to describe this process. The aim is to collect the saliva as passively as possible. (From Durdiaková, J., et al., *Steroids* 78, 1325–1331, 2013.)

w There is variance in the values obtained for tear fluid, dependent on assay method and standard. Similar variance was observed for saliva.[61]

REFERENCES TO TABLE 1.1

1. Jaffrin, M.Y. and Morel, H., Body fluid volumes measurements by impedance: A review of bioimpedance spectroscopy (BIS) and bioimpedance analysis (BIA) methods, *Med. Eng. Phys.* 30, 1257–1269, 2008.
2. Sircar, S., Body fluids and blood, in *Principles of Medical Physiology*, Chapter 22, Thieme, Stuttgart, Germany, 2008.
3. Schoeller, D.A., Changes in total body water with age, *Am. J. Clin. Nutr.* 50(5 Suppl.), 1176–1181, 1989.
4. Altman, P.L. and Dittmer, D.S., eds., *Blood and Other Biological Fluids Federation of American Societies for Experimental Biology*, Washington, DC, 1961.
5. Elhassan, E.A. and Schrier, R.W., Disorders of extracellular volume, in *Comprehensive Clinical Neurology*, eds. J. Floege, R.J. Johnson, and J. Feehally, Chapter 7, pp. 85–99, Elsevier/Saunders, St. Louis, MI, 2010.
6. Laderson, J.H., Tsai, L.B., Michael, J.M., et al., Serum versus heparinized plasma for eighteen common chemistry tests: Is serum the appropriate specimen? *Am. J. Pathol.* 62, 545–552, 1974.
7. Tammen, H., Schulte, I., Hess, R., et al., Peptidomic analysis of human blood specimens: Comparison between plasma specimens and serum by differential peptide display, *Proteomics* 5, 3414–3422, 2005.
8. Luque-Garcia, J.L. and Neubert, T.A., Sample preparation for serum/plasma profiling and biomarker identification by mass spectrometry, *J. Chromatog. A* 1153, 259–276, 2007.
9. Starling, E.H., On the absorption of fluids from the connective tissue spaces, *J. Physiol.* 19, 312–326, 1896.
10. Rasmussen, P., The concentration of calcium, inorganic phosphate and protein in the interstitial fluid of rats, *Calcif. Tis. Res.* 6, 197–203, 1970.
11. Wiig, H. and Tenstad, O., Interstitial exclusion of positively and negatively charged IgG in rat skin and muscle, *Am. J. Physiol. Heart Circ. Physiol.* 280, H1505–1512, 2001.
12. Tatara, T. and Tashino, C., Quantitative analysis of fluid balance during abdominal surgery, *Anesth. Analg.* 104, 347–354, 2007.
13. Haaverstad, R., Romslo, I., Larsen, S., and Myhre, H.O., Protein concentration of subcutaneous interstitial fluid in the human leg: A comparison between the wick technique and the blister suction technique, *Int. J. Microcirc. Clin. Exp.* 16, 111–117, 1996.
14. Negrini, D., Passi, A., Bertin, K., et al., Isolation of pulmonary interstitial fluid in rabbits by a modified wick technique, *Am. J. Physiol. Lung Cell Mol. Physiol.* 280, L1057–1065, 2001.
15. Altman, P.L. and Dittmer, D.S., *Blood and Other Body Fluids*, FASEB, Washington, DC, 1961.
16. Bach, C. and Lewis, G.P., Lymph flow and lymph protein concentration in the skin and muscle of the rabbit hind limb, *J. Physiol.* 235, 477–492, 1973.
17. Aukland, K., Kramer, G.C., and Renkin, E.M., Protein concentration of lymph and interstitial fluid in the rat tail, *Am. J. Physiol.* 247, H74–H79, 1984.
18. Szabó, G., Enzymes in tissue fluid and peripheral lymph, *Lymphology* 11, 147–155, 1978.
19. Rutili, G. and Arfors, K.-E., Protein concentration in interstitial and lymphatic fluids from the subcutaneous tissue, *Acta Physiol. Scand.* 99, 1–8, 1977.
20. Runyon, B.A., Montano, A.A., Akrividis, E.A., et al., The serum-ascites albumin gradient is superior to the exudate-transudate concept in the differential diagnosis of ascites, *Ann. Intern. Med.* 117, 215–220, 1992.
21. Tarri, A.G. and Lapworth, R., Biochemical analysis of ascitic (peritoneal) fluid: What should we measure? *Ann. Clin. Biochem.* 47, 397–407, 2010.

22. Brunsel, N.A., Pleural, pericardial, and peritoneal fluid analysis, in *Fundamentals of Urine and Body Fluid Analysis*, Chapter 15, W.B. Saunders, Philadelphia, PA, 1994.

23. Maathuis, J.B., Van Look, P.F.A., and Michie, E.A., Changes in volume total protein and ovarian steroid concentrations of peritoneal fluid throughout the menstrual cycle, *J. Endocrinol.* 76, 123–133, 1978.

24. Koninckx, P.R., Heyns, W., Verhoeven, G., et al., Biochemical characterization of peritoneal fluid in women during the menstrual cycle, *J. Clin. Endocrinol. Metab.* 51, 1239–1244, 1980.

25. Reiber, H., Dynamics of brain-derived proteins in cerebrospinal fluid, *Clin. Chim. Acta* 310, 173–186, 2001.

26. Seyfert, S., Faulstich, A., and Marx, P., What determines the CSF concentrations of albumin and plasma-derived IgG? *J. Neurol. Sci.* 219, 31–33, 2004.

27. Mangin, P., Lugnier, A.-A., Chaumont, A.-J., et al., Forensic significance of postmortem estimation of the blood cerebrospinal fluid barrier permeability, *Forensic Sci. Intern.* 22, 143–149, 1983.

28. Ganrot-Norlin, K., Relative concentrations of albumin and IgG in cerebrospinal fluid in health and acute meningitis, *Scand. J. Infect. Dis.* 10, 57–60, 1978.

29. Vatassery, G.T., Krezowski, A.M., and Sheridan, M.A., Comparison of manual methods of determination of albumin in human cerebrospinal fluid by the bromcresol green and immuno-precipitation methods, *Clin. Biochem.* 13, 78–80, 1980.

30. Wood, J.H., Physiology, pharmacology, and dynamics of cerebrospinal fluid, in *Neurobiology of Cerebrospinal Fluid*, ed. J.H. Wood, pp. 1–16, Plenum Press, New York, 1980.

31. Livrea, P., Trojano, M., and Simons, I.L., Heterologous models for blood-cerebrospinal fluid barrier permeability to serum proteins in normal and abnormal cerebrospinal fluid/serum protein concentration gradients, *J. Neurol. Sci.* 64, 245–258, 1984.

32. Wada, H., Blood–brain barrier permeability of the demented elderly as studied by cerebrospinal fluid–serum albumin ratio, *Intern. Med.* 37, 509–513, 1998.

33. Lenzlinger, P.M., Hans, V.H.J., Joller-Jemelka, H.I., et al., Markers for cell-mediated immune response are elevated in cerebrospinal fluid and serum after severe traumatic brain injury in humans, *J. Neurotrauma* 18, 479–489, 2001.

34. Pisani, V., Stefani, A., Pierantrozzi, M., et al., Increased blood–cerebrospinal fluid transfer of albumin in advanced Parkinson's disease, *J. Neuroinflammation* 9, 188, 2012.

35. Ringsrud, K.M. and Linne, J.J., *Urinalysis and Body Fluids: A Color Text and Atlas*, Mosby, St. Louis, MI, 1995.

36. Williams, K.M. and Marshall, T., Protein concentration of cerebrospinal fluid by precipitation with Pyrogallol Red prior to sodium dodecyl sulphate–polyacrylamide gel electrophoresis, *J. Biochem. Biophys. Methods* 47, 197–207, 2001.

37. Gerbaut, L. and Macart, M., Is standardization more important than methodology for assay of total protein in cerebrospinal fluid? *Clin. Chem.* 32, 353–355, 1986.

38. Barnard, K., Herold, R., Siemes, H., and Siegert, M., Quantification of cerebrospinal fluid proteins in children by high-resolution agarose gel electrophoresis, *J. Child. Neurol.* 13, 51–58, 1998.

39. Grabner, G., Zehetbauer, G., Bettelheim, H., et al., The blood–aqueous barrier and its permeability for proteins of different molecular weight, *Albrecht v. Graefe Arch. Klin. Exp. Ophthalmol.* 207, 137–148, 1978.

40. Liu, J.H.K., Lindsey, J.D., and Weinreb, R.N., Physiological factors in the circadian rhythm of protein concentration in aqueous humor, *Invest. Ophthalmol. Vis. Sci.* 39, 553–558, 1998.

41. Hornof, M., Toropaninen, E., and Urtti, A., Cell culture models of the ocular barriers, *Eur. J. Pharm. Biopharm.* 60, 207–225, 2005.

42. Zhou, R., Horai, R., Mattapallil, M.J., and Caspi, R.R., A new look at immune privilege of the eye: Dual role for the vision-related molecule retinoic acid, *J. Immunol.* 187, 4170–4177, 2011.

43. Nakashima, T., Sone, M., Teranishi, M., et al., A perspective from magnetic resonance imaging findings of the inner ear: Relationships among cerebrospinal, ocular and inner ear fluids, *Auris Nasus Larynx* 39, 345–355, 2012.

44. Ferrary, E. and Sterkers, O., Mechanisms of endolymph secretion, *Kidney Int. Suppl.* 65, S98–S103, 1998.

45. Korenek, N.L., Andrews, F.M., Maddux, J.M., et al., Determination of the total protein concentration and viscosity of synovial fluid from the tibiotarsal joints of horses, *Am. J. Vet. Res.* 53, 781–784, 1992.

46. Kwan, C., Bell, R., Koenig, T., et al., Effects of intra-articular sodium pentosan polysulfate and glucosamine on the cytology, total protein concentration and viscosity of synovial fluid in horses, *Aust. Vet. J.* 90, 315–320, 2012.

47. Fan, J., Myant, C., Underwood, R., and Cann, P., Synovial fluid lubrication of artificial joints: Protein film formation and composition, *Faraday Discuss.* 156, 69–85, 2012.

48. Barton, K.I., Ludwig, T.W., and Archari, Y., Characterization of proteoglycan 4 and hyaluronan composition of ovine synovial fluid following knee surgery, *J. Orthop. Res.* 31, 1549–1554, 2013.

49. Rinaudo, M., Rheological investigation on hyaluronan–fibrinogen interaction, *Int. J. Biol. Macromol.* 43, 444–450, 2008.

50. Greenwald, R.A. and Moak, S.A., Degradation of hyaluronic acid by polymorphonuclear leukocytes, *Inflammation* 10, 15–30, 1986.

51. Brunzel, N.A., Synovial fluid analysis, in *Fundamentals of Urine and Body Fluid Analysis*, Chapter 14, W.B. Saunders, Philadelphia, PA, 1994.

52. Arden, N.K., Akermark, C., Andersson, M., et al., A randomized saline-controlled trial of NASHA hyaluronic acid for osteoarthritis, *Curr. Med. Res. Opin.* 30, 279–286, 2014.

53. Griffiths, G.S., Formation, collection and significance of gingival crevice fluid, *Periodontology* 31, 32–42, 2000.

54. Curtis, M.A., Griffiths, G.S., Price, S.J., et al., The total protein concentration of gingival crevicular fluid, *J. Clin. Periodontol.* 15, 628–632, 1988.

55. Carneiro, L.G., Venuleo, C., Oppenheim, F.G., and Salih, E., Proteome data set of human gingival crevicular fluid from healthy periodontium sites by multidimensional protein separation and mass spectrometry, *J. Periodontal Res.* 47, 248–262, 2012.

56. Siqueira, W.L. and Dawes, C., The salivary proteome: Challenges and perspectives, *Proteomics Clin. Appl.* 5, 575–579, 2011.

57. Amado, F.M., Ferreira, R.P., and Vitorino, R., One decade of salivary proteomics: Current approaches and outstanding challenges, *Clin. Biochem.* 46, 506–517, 2013.

58. Carpenter, G.H., The secretion, components, and properties of saliva, *Annu. Rev. Food Sci. Technol.* 4, 267–276, 2013.

59. Sun, X., Salih, E., Oppenheim, F.G., and Helmerhorst, E.J., Kinetics of histatin proteolysis in whole saliva and the effect on bioactive domains with metal-binding, antifungal, and wound-healing properties, *FASEB J.* 23, 2691–2701, 2009.

60. Oudhoff, M.J., van den Keijbus, P.A., Kroeze, K.L., et al., Histatins enhance wound closure with oral and non-oral cells, *J. Dent. Res.* 88, 846–850, 2009.

61. Jenzano, J.W., Hogan, S.L., Noyes. C.M., et al., Comparison of five techniques for the determination of protein content in mixed human saliva, *Anal. Biochem.* 159, 370–376, 1986.

62. Rayman, S.A., Liu, B., Soares, R.V., et al., The effects of duration and intensity of stimulation on total protein and mucin concentrations in resting and stimulated whole saliva, *J. Dent. Res.* 80, 1584–1587, 2001.

63. Mason, D.K. and Chisholm, D.M., Saliva, in *Salivary Glands in Health and Disease*, Chapter 3, pp. 37–69, W.B. Saunders, Philadelphia, PA, 1975.
64. Lee, S.R., MacCullough, C., Chan, M.M., et al., Salivary diagnostics: A new industry; Perspectives from business development, government, regulatory, and payers, *Adv. Dent. Res.* 23, 369–374, 2011.
65. Gough, H., Luke, G.A., Beeley, J.A., and Geddes, D.A., Human salivary glucose analysis by high-performance ion-exchange chromatography and pulsed amperometric detection, *Arch. Oral Biol.* 41, 141–145, 1996.
66. Beltzer, E.K., Fortunato, C.K., Guaderrama, M.M., et al., Salivary flow rate and alpha-amylase: Collection technique, duration, and oral fluid type, *Physiol. Behav.* 101, 289–296, 2010.
67. Mohamed, R., Campbell, J.L., Cooper-White, J., et al., The impact of saliva collection and processing methods on CRP, IgE, and myoglobin immunoassays, *Clin. Transl. Med.* 1, 19, 2012.
68. Allgrove, J.E., Oliveira, M., and Gleeson, M., Stimulating whole saliva affects the response of antimicrobial proteins to exercise, *Scand. J. Med. Sci. Sports* 24, 649–655, 2014.
69. Veeregowda, D.H., Bussher, H.J., Vissink, A., et al., Role of structure and glycosylation of adsorbed protein films in biolubrication, *PLoS One* 7(8), e42600, 2012.
70. Percival, R.S., Challacombe, S.J., and Marsh, P.D., Flow rates of resting whole and stimulated parotid saliva in relation to age and gender, *J. Dent. Res.* 73, 1416–1420, 1994.
71. Samuelson, L.C., Wiebauer, K., Snow, C.M., and Meisler, M.H., Retroviral and pseudogene insertion sites reveal the linage of human salivary and pancreatic amylase genes from a single gene during primate evolution, *Mol. Cell. Biol.* 10, 2513–2520, 1990.
72. Won, J.H., Cottrell, W.J., Foster, T.H., and Yule, D.I., Ca^{2+} release dynamics in parotid and pancreatic exocrine acinar cells evoked by spatially limited flash photolysis, *Am. J. Physiol. Gastrointest. Liver Physiol.* 293, G1166–G1177, 2007.
73. Novak, I., Jans, I.M., and Wohlfahrt, L., Effect of $P2X_7$ receptor knockout on exocrine secretion of pancreas, salivary glands and lacrimal glands, *J. Physiol.* 588, 3615–3627, 2010.
74. Ball, W.D. and Rutter, W.J., The DNase activities of the mouse, *J. Exp. Zool.* 176, 1–14, 1971.
75. Hanning, S., Motoi, L., Medlicott, N., and Swindells, S., A device for the collection of submandibular saliva, *N. Z. Dent. J.* 108, 4–8, 2012.
76. Levine, M.J., Reddy, M.S., Tabak, L.A., et al., Structural aspects of salivary glycoproteins, *J. Dent. Res.* 66, 436–441, 1987.
77. Song, B., Zhang, L., Liu, X.J., et al., Proteomic analysis of secretion from human transplanted submandibular gland replacing lacrimal gland with severe keratoconjunctivitis sicca, *Biochim. Biophys. Acta* 1824, 550–560, 2012.
78. Gritti, I., Banfi, G., and Roi, G.S., Pepsinogens: Physiology, pharmacology pathophysiology and exercise, *Pharmacol. Res.* 41, 265–281, 2000.
79. Schapiro, H., Rosato, F.E., Jackson, H.J., and Dreiling, D.A., Effect of gastrin on the exocrine pancreas: A review, *Am. J. Gastroenterol.* 71, 53–60, 1979.
80. Kapica, M., Puzio, I., Kato, I., et al., Role of feed-regulating peptides on pancreatic exocrine secretion, *J. Physiol. Pharmacol.* 59(Suppl. 2), 145–159, 2008.
81. Schubert, M.L., Gastric exocrine and endocrine secretion, *Curr. Opin. Gastroenterol.* 25, 529–536, 2009.
82. Shivaji, S., Scheit, K.-H., and Bhargava, P.M., *Proteins of Seminal Plasma*, John Wiley, New York, 1990.
83. Lilja, H., Structure, function, and regulation of the enzyme activity of prostate-specific antigen, *World J. Urology* 11, 188–191, 1993.
84. Sitaram, N. and Nagaraj, R., Seminal plasmin, *Bioessays* 17, 415–422, 1995.

85. Weinberg, E.D., The therapeutic potential of lactoferrin, *Expert Opin. Invest. Drugs* 12, 841–851, 2003.
86. Veveris-Lowe, T.L., Kruger, S.J., Walsh, T., et al., Seminal fluid characterization for male fertility and prostate cancer: Kallikrein-related serine proteases and whole proteome approaches, *Semin. Thromb. Hemost.* 33, 87–99, 2007.
87. Rodríguez-Martínez, H., Kvist, H., Ernerudh, J., et al., Seminal plasma proteins: What role do they play? *Am. J. Reprod. Immunol.* 66(Suppl. 1), 11–22, 2011.
88. Laflamme, B.A. and Wolfner, M.F., Identification and function of proteolysis regulators in seminal fluid, *Mol. Reprod. Dev.* 80, 80–101, 2013.
89. Raffi. R.O., Moghissi, K.S., and Sacco, A.G., Proteins of human vaginal fluid, *Fertil. Steril.* 28, 1345–1348, 1972.
90. Usala, S.J., Usala, F.O., Haciski, R., et al., IgG and IgA content of vaginal fluid during the menstrual cycle, *J. Reprod. Med.* 34, 292–294, 1989.
91. Tang, L.-J., De Seta, F., Odreman, F., et al., Proteomic analysis of human cervical-vaginal fluid, *J. Proteome Res.* 6, 2874–2883, 2007.
92. Zegels, G., Van Raemdonck, G.A.A., Coen, E.P., et al., Comprehensive proteomic analysis of human cervical-vaginal fluid using colposcopy samples, *Proteome Sci.* 7, 17, 2009.
93. Shaw, J.L., Smith, C.R., and Diamandis, E.P., Proteomic analysis of human cervico-vaginal fluid, *J. Proteome Res.* 6, 2859–2865, 2007.
94. Ng, V. and Cho, P., The relationship between total tear protein concentrations determined by different methods and standards, *Graefe's Arch. Clin. Exp. Ophthalmol.* 238, 571–576, 2000.
95. Mann, A.M. and Tighe, B.J., Tear analysis and lens-tear interactions: Part I. Protein fingerprinting with microfluidic technology, *Cont. Lens Anterior Eye* 30, 163–173, 2007.
96. Filik, J. and Stone, N., Analysis of human tear fluid by Raman spectroscopy, *Anal. Chim. Acta* 616, 177–184, 2008.
97. Zhou, L., and Beuerman, R.W., Quantitative proteomic analysis of N-linked glycoproteins in human tear fluid, *Methods Mol. Biol.* 951, 297–306, 2013.
98. Ihnatko, R., Edén, U., Lagali, N., et al., Analysis of protein composition and protein expression in the tear fluid of patients with congenital aniridia, *J. Proteomics* 94, 78–88, 2013.

proteins can be found in the interstitial space as the volume of interstitial fluid is two to three times the size of the plasma volume.[11,12] For example, approximately 60% of total body albumin is in the extravascular space.[13] The use of the term *interstitial fluid* is not exclusive to biology, which can lead to some confusion. It is derived from the Latin *interstitium*, meaning a space between,[14] so it has been used considerably to describe spaces in geological studies.[15–17] Interstitial fluid has poroelastic qualities resulting from its composition, including the maintenance of connective tissue function.[18,19] But this space and its fluid content also play a role in disease. The interstitial space is a dynamic environment where an interplay of proteases, polysaccharides, cytokines, and inflammatory cells dictates the pathophysiological responses to tissue injury. In the subsequent chapters, we will consider the various compartments of this fluid, their components, and their regulation.

1.2 EXTRAVASATION

The primary source of interstitial fluid, water, and solutes is the capillary network of the vascular system; the process by which fluid and solutes are transported through the vascular wall is referred to as *extravasation* (transcapillary transport/escape). The phenomenology of fluid and solute transfer across the capillary wall was formalized by Starling in papers published in 1894[20] and 1896.[21] The *Starling principle* or *hypothesis* states that transport across the capillary wall is dependent on the difference in hydrostatic and oncotic pressure between the intravascular and interstitial space.* Starling[21] did not actually say as much, but the data in the two papers provided the impetus for the identification of the forces responsible for net transvascular fluid flow. Starling[21] did make the critical observation that colored materials (various dyes) were absorbed into the vascular system from serous cavities. Starling also observed that *proteids* (proteins, glycoproteins)[22] were absorbed by the lymphatic system and not directly by the vascular system.[21] Starling's hypothesis on the forces responsible for transvascular transport was validated by further work, most notably by Landis in 1927.[23] However, although the work of Starling[20,21] provided a framework for both research and the use of resuscitation fluids, it was considered too simple to account for the considerable complexity in the microcirculation.[24] While capillaries are short in length (0.4–0.7 mm), with an average diameter of 5–20 μm, the estimated surface area of the capillary wall is 300–600 m[2†] and not all capillaries are open at the same time.[25] Thus, a large number of small individual capillaries have a potentially large surface area available for fluid transport.

The classical Starling equation (Figure 1.1)[26] has been instrumental as a starting point in understanding the movements of interstitial fluids. This equation represents transcapillary flow across a continuous membrane and includes a capillary permeability coefficient, which is a function of the capillary membrane.[27] The transport of solutes across a membrane is also affected by the reflection constant (δ), which is unique to given solutes, water, and membrane, reflecting the interaction between a specific solute and a specific membrane.[28–32] Kongstad and coworkers[27] showed that the reflection coefficient for albumin and capillary hydraulic conductance (the capillary permeability coefficient) both changed in response to traumatic muscle injury.

Subsequent work by Lundblad and coworkers[33] showed that inhibition of Rho kinase decreased the capillary permeability coefficient and increased the reflection coefficient for albumin. Improvements in knowledge of vasculature microstructure and physiology have led to a revision of the Starling hypothesis. The major change is in the understanding of the role of the endothelial glycocalyx and variability in capillary permeability resulting from heterogeneity in capillary wall structure. The term *glycocalyx* was introduced by H. Stanley Bennett in 1963[34] to describe the extracellular polysaccharide that coats the plasma membrane of cells; it is derived from the Greek word for sweet and translates as "sweet husk." The early work on the characterization of the glycocalyx has been summarized by Ito.[35] While the term *glycocalyx* is a general term to describe cellular polysaccharides, including the mucin that coats epithelial cells,[36,37] its use in the literature is predominantly applied to the endothelial glycocalyx.[38] The thickness and continuity of the glycocalyx can vary depending on the nature of the vascular bed and tissue, resulting in changes in

---

* Starling was also responsible for Starling's law, which related the strength of ventricular contraction to muscle fiber length in the heart.
† Estimates vary from 300 to 1000 m^2.

$J_v = K_f(P_c - P_i) + \sigma(\Pi_c - \Pi_i)$

J_v, = net transcapillary flux

P_c = capillary pressure

P_i = intersitial pressure

Π_i = average interstitial oncotic pressure

Π_p = average plasma oncotic pressure

σ = reflection coefficient

K_f = capillary permeability coefficient

Adapted from Civetta, J.M., A new look at the Starling equation, *Crit.Care Med.* 7, 84–91, 1979.

$J_v = K_f(P_c - P_g) + \sigma(\Pi_c - \Pi_g)$

J_v, = net transcapillary flux

P_c = capillary hydrostatic pressure

P_g = subglycocalyx hydrostatic pressure

Π_p = plasma oncotic pressure

Π_g = subglycocalyx oncotic pressure

σ = reflection coefficient

K_f = capillary permeability coefficient

Adapted from Levick, J.R., Revision of the Starling principle: new views of tissue fluid balance, *J. Physiol.* 557, 704, 2004.

FIGURE 1.1 The classic and revised Starling equation for transvascular transport. (Adapted from Civetta, J.M., *Crit. Care Med.* 7, 84–91, 1979; Levick, J.R., *J. Physiol.* 557, 704, 2004.)

the glycocalyx and influencing capillary permeability.[39–43] The other factor was the recognition that there is insufficient oncotic pressure in the interstitial space to cause fluid flow back into the circulation.[44] Adamson and coworkers[44] showed that the osmotic pressures opposing filtration in nonfenestrated capillaries[45] are developed across the endothelial glycocalyx and that the oncotic pressures in interstitial fluid do not affect net filtration (J_v). This is important for fluid balance but not relevant for protein transport through large pores in fenestrated capillaries.[45,46] The observations of Adamson and coworkers[44] with other work in this field led Levick[46] to propose a revised Starling equation (Figure 1.1).

In the past decade, there has been substantial improvement in our understanding of capillary permeability and the mechanisms involved in protein extravasation beyond molecular weight, size, and concentration. The two-pore model of capillary filtration, a hypothesis used for some time, provides a basic process for intravascular protein passage to the extravascular space.[45,47–50] However, it struggles to predict what is seen in reality. Nakamura and coworkers[51] demonstrated a relationship between molecular size and distribution between the intravascular (plasma) and extravascular (thoracic lymph) spaces, based on experimental distribution of several iodinated proteins in rabbits. They identified a [lymph]/[plasma] ratio of 0.66 for bovine and rabbit serum albumin, a ratio of 0.50 for human immunoglobulin G (IgG), and a ratio of 0.18 for rabbit fibrinogen. The fibrinogen [lymph]/[plasma] ratio is lower than expected based on the ratio determined for other proteins of a similar or larger molecular weight. This reflects the asymmetry of the fibrinogen molecule, which results in a larger hydrodynamic radius. More recent work[52] studying the distribution of human protein concentrations in plasma and peripheral lymph has identified that the albumin and IgG [lymph]/[plasma] ratios were 0.35 and 0.19, respectively.[52] These values are somewhat less than those determined by Nakamura and coworkers in the rabbit model. There is some reason to think that the concentration of plasma protein would be less in peripheral lymph than in thoracic lymph. Brinkhous and Walker[53] reported that the concentrations of prothrombin and fibrinogen were much higher in portal (thoracic) lymph than in peripheral lymph. Woodcock and Woodcook[45] estimated that 50% of total body lymph production is derived from the liver and suggested that this is a major site of extravasation of plasma proteins. In their study[52] on the distribution of proteins between plasma and lymph, Michel and coworkers[52] also showed that the extravasation of low-density lipoprotein (LDL) and high-density lipoprotein (HDL) is consistent with a two-pore model for vascular permeability and does not involve an active transport process. These investigators do state that this conclusion is valid for capillaries and venules with a continuous endothelial surface; fenestrated endothelium, such as that found, for example, in the spleen and liver, may be more permeable. These investigators do note that the two-pore hypothesis has not been validated and likely is a function of the glycocalyx rather than the endothelium. Stukas and coworkers[5] did suggest a transcellular mechanism for apolipoprotein A-1 transport from the vascular bed to the cerebrospinal fluid. Worm[54] determined that the ratio of albumin concentration in skin blister fluid to the albumin concentration in plasma was 0.57, consistent with skin blister fluid being a measure of "average" interstitial fluid.

There is regional heterogeneity in capillary structure, resulting in differences in permeability to proteins and other large molecules. Woodcock and Woodcock[45] have reviewed the structure and function of three capillary phenotypes, including sinusoidal capillary, fenestrated capillary, and nonfenestrated capillary. The distribution of these capillary subtypes is tissue specific. Sinusoidal capillaries, which do not possess a glycocalyx, can be found in the liver and spleen, fenestrated capillaries in the endocrine and gut mucosa, and nonfenestrated capillaries in the nervous system and muscles. As such, there is local variation in the distribution of the various capillary types, which results in altered permeability from tissue to tissue and within tissues.[55,56] Bar and coworkers[55] observed that insulin stimulated movement of insulin-like growth factor binding protein-1 (IGFBP-1) from the vascular space to tissue in an isolated beating rat heart, while there was no effect on IGFBP-2 but a decrease in endothelial cell IGFBP. Areskog and coworkers[56] used dextrans of various molecular sizes to measure capillary permeability in the heart, suggesting that heart capillaries had "large" pores (120–300 Å) compared with leg or cervical capillaries. Lastly, the fenestrated capillaries in the glomerulus are different from fenestrated capillaries in other tissues[45] in that capillaries in the glomerulus are the only capillaries in the body that are not surrounded by interstitial space.[57] Rather, the glomerular capillaries with fenestrated epithelium (70–100 nm in diameter) are surrounded by a basement membrane (BM) composed of structural proteins, such as collagen IV, laminin, and proteoglycans, which is in turn surrounded by cells, including podocytes (visceral epithelial cells) and mesangial cells.[34,58]

Systemic effects, such as trauma[27,33] and inflammation,[50] affect protein transport across the capillary wall. Juweld and coworkers[56] studied the effect of a focal inflammation (*Escherichia coli* implanted in rodent thigh muscle) on the capillary permeability of ^{111}In-labeled IgG and ^{111}In-labeled albumin. There was an approximate threefold increase in IgG at the site of infection compared with control muscle, while there was a twofold increase in albumin. Juweld and coworkers[59] observed that while the concentration of albumin is higher than IgG in control muscle, the ratio approaches unity in infected muscle. These investigators concluded that an increase in vascular permeability results in increased extravasation of both fluid and protein. However, the transport of protein showed some selectivity in that there was preferential transport of IgG. Reed and Rubin[60] suggested that the edema response in inflammation is of functional significance in promoting the diffusion of plasma protein into the inflamed tissue. The transcapillary escape rate (transport from intravascular space to extravascular space) of albumin, IgG, and IgM increased in angiotensin-II-induced hypertension; the relative increase was much higher for IgG and immunoglobulin M (IgM) than for albumin.[61] Other factors can influence capillary permeability, such as ε-aminocaproic acid (EACA; 0.3 g/kg body weight), which has been reported to decrease or eliminate the radiation-induced (x-ray; 500 R) increase in capillary permeability in a rabbit skin model.[62] This is the description of an exudate and would contain inflammatory cells that release cytokines and so on, which would impact on the process and on fluid composition.

1.3   CELL SECRETION IN INTERSTITIAL SPACE

Cell secretion includes substances derived from fibroblasts as well as basolateral secretion from endothelial cells and epithelial cells.[63–66] The term *secretome* has been advanced to describe the proteins secreted by a tissue at a certain time.[67–70] There has been considerable interest in the identification of biomarkers in the cancer secretome[71,72] (Section 1.9).

The basolateral surface of the endothelial cell can be considered to line the interstitial space in a manner similar to the apical surface of the endothelial cell lining the vascular space. Likewise, the basolateral surface of the epithelial cell can be considered to line the interstitial space. Pillai and coworkers[66] advanced the concept of directional secretome in the analysis of polarity-specific secretion and identified proteins unique to either apical or basolateral secretion. These investigators used human bronchial epithelial cells in culture to study apical (external) and basolateral (subepithelial) secretion. Proteomic technology was used to identify proteins in apical and basolateral conditioned media. Cells obtained from three donors were used and 243 proteins of a total of 377 were identified in all three cultures; 69 proteins were consistently observed in apical cultures, while 13 proteins were consistently observed in basolateral cultures. This work clearly showed that there is polarity of secretion in epithelial cells.

The polarity of protein secretion can be influenced by agonists[73] and local physiology, such as inflammation.[74,75] Venkatesh and coworkers[73] reported that isoproterenol increased basolateral secretion of amylase and parotid secretory protein, with a resulting increase in the concentration of proteins in blood. Fiorentino and coworkers[75] reported on the effect of *Helicobacter pylori* on a monolayer of human gastric epithelial cells. While cell viability was unaffected, there was a markedly increased permeability of the monolayer; live bacteria were more effective than heat-killed bacteria in causing an increase in permeability. These investigators also evaluated the effect of *H. pylori* on the secretion of cytokines (e.g., IL-12, TNF-α, IL-10) by the epithelial monolayer. There was a marked increase in basolateral secretion of the cytokines in response to the *H. pylori* with much less apical secretion; in contrast to the permeability studies, heat-killed *H. pylori* were more effective in stimulating basolateral cytokine secretion.

The large multimeric glycoprotein von Willebrand factor (vWF) plays an important role in hemostasis, particularly in the vasculature. vWF secretion from endothelial cells can occur at both the apical (luminal) surface and the basolateral (subluminal, subendothelial) surface. van Buul-Wortelboer and coworkers[76] observed polarity in the secretion of vWF in human umbilical vein endothelial cells cultured on a collagen lattice. Constitutive secretion of vWF occurs in both basolateral and apical (luminal) compartments, with preferential secretion in the basolateral compartment. Stimulated (regulated) secretion of vWF stored in Weible–Palade bodies preferentially occurs at the apical or luminal surface. Differing results were obtained by Sporn and coworkers,[77] who used human umbilical vein endothelial cells cultured on a polycarbonate membrane. Their results differed from those of van Buul-Wortelboer and coworkers[76] in that they observed equal amounts of constitutive basolateral secretion and apical secretion of vWF, whereas stimulation (calcium ionophore, phorbol ester) provided preferential basolateral secretion.[76,77] It is possible that the use of collagen as a matrix influenced the polarity of endothelial cell secretion, as previously observed,[78] underlying the differences in results. However, there is limited work to draw on studying the effect of the ECM on the polarity of cell secretion.

1.4 CONNECTIVITY OF INTERSTITIAL FLUID AND OTHER EXTRAVASCULAR FLUIDS

There are discrete fluid compartments that vary with respect to "connection" with interstitial fluid and blood plasma, including the synovial fluid and cerebrospinal fluids. Synovial fluid is found in joints and is an ultrafiltrate of plasma, which contains hyaluronan.[79] Proteins such as complement can be found in synovial fluid and may be involved in the etiology of rheumatoid arthritis.[80] Cerebrospinal fluid is contained within the ventricles of the brain and is discussed briefly in Section 1.1. Cerebrospinal fluid is produced by choroid plexus epithelial cells[81,82] and is subject to continual secretion/resorption.[83,84] Cerebrospinal fluid drains to the lymphatic system and is suggested to be fully exchanged every six hours. Cerebrospinal fluid is contained within an immunologically privileged region and the entry of immune cells is restricted.[85,86] Ocular fluid is also contained within an immunologically privileged area.[87,88] The blood–brain barrier is a highly restrictive membrane separating the interstitial fluid/vascular bed from the cerebrospinal fluid/brain.[89–91]

The ratio of IgG in cerebrospinal fluid to plasma is 0.003, while it is 0.80 for urea, demonstrating the relative impermeability of the cerebrospinal barrier.[92] For comparison, the ratio of IgG concentration between interstitial fluid and plasma is 0.52, while albumin is 0.62. The bulk of the fluid and solute composition of the interstitial fluid and lymphatic system is contributed by the *ultrafiltration* of plasma. However, this process of ultrafiltration is selective with respect to the size of protein and other macromolecular solutes, as well as there being regional differences in capillary permeability.

1.5 RELATIONSHIP OF INTERSTITIAL FLUID TO LYMPH

There is fluid and solute exchange between the various compartments of the extravascular fluid, but the exchange is variable depending on the compartment. The bulk of the fluid in lymph is derived from interstitial fluid and returned to the circulatory system. The composition of lymph is largely dependent on the selective ultrafiltration of plasma based on capillary pressure[93] and the molecular processes of the glycocalyx, resulting in selective ultrafiltration[94] and substances derived from the various tissues.[95]

Thus, plasma proteins, excluding extravascular synthesis, would be derived from the intravascular space into the interstitial fluid by extravasation[96] and then via lymph returning to the circulation.[97] Analytes in lymph may be degraded and at a lower concentration than in the parent interstitial fluid; it should be noted that we could not find data to either substantiate or negate this assumption. It may be easier to obtain reasonable samples of peripheral lymph than interstitial fluid.[98] On occasion, we will be using lymph as a surrogate for interstitial fluid in later discussions in this book. Much of our understanding of the composition of interstitial fluid is based on results obtained with lymph. However, just as interstitial fluid is not an ultrafiltrate of blood, lymph also is not an ultrafiltrate of plasma.[99] Regional differences complicate the use of lymph as a surrogate.

1.6 STRUCTURE OF INTERSTITIUM

The *interstitium* (also known as the *interstitial space*) is complex,[100,101] containing fixed elements and amorphous material originally described as "ground substance."[102] While the majority of interest is directed toward proteins, such as collagen, and complex proteins, such as proteoglycans, macromolecules, such as hyaluronan and other glycosaminoglycans[103] (ground substance),[102] are also found in the interstitial space and other extravascular spaces. The presence of fibroblasts,[104] smooth muscle cells,[105] and other interstitial cells[106,107] add a degree of complexity to the interstitium by serving as targets for agonists and antagonists secreted by endothelial cells and epithelial cells. The BM is considered to be a loose connective tissue supporting the capillaries and providing the matrix for the interstitium.[108–110] Collagen IV is a unique component of the BM and is known for the specific binding of some proteins.[111–114] Collagen VI is also a component of the BM.[104] There is a discussion in Chapter 2 of the various collagen species present in the interstitial space.

1.6.1 Heterogeneity in Interstitium

The interstitial space is not a homogeneous space, but the quality varies from organ to organ and within an organ. This is a reflection of differences in capillary permeability and local synthesis. The presence of components such as collagen and hyaluronan influence the distribution of solutes within the interstitial space, contributing to the three-compartment model of drug distribution.[116] Wiig and coworkers[117,118] have made extensive contributions to our understanding of factors impacting protein drug distribution in the interstitium. Hyaluronidase (Chapter 3) and collagenase (Chapter 4) have been used to enhance protein drug distribution in the interstitial space.[119–121] Collagenase appears to be more effective than hyaluronidase within tumors, but collagenase is less acceptable, reflecting regulatory considerations. Hyaluronidase[122] has seen increasing therapeutic use for the subcutaneous (SC) administration of proteins.[186] The amount of hyaluronan can differ from organ to organ and within an organ, as observed in the kidney, where large amounts are present in the medulla (papilla) and small amounts in the cortex,[123,124] where it is suggested to participate in water processing (diuresis/antidiuresis).[125] This is an example of differences in the distribution of hyaluronan and other glycosaminoglycans within an organ and there are differences in tissue distribution.[126] Plante[126] described skin as having the highest hyaluronan concentration (weight of hyaluronan/weight of dry tissue) and kidney cortex as having the lowest concentration. Skeletal muscle was intermediate. The amount of hyaluronan in tissues appears to increase with age, based on measurements in the kidney.

Reust and coworkers[127,128] studied the interstitial distribution of EACA in a porcine model following intravenous (IV) infusion. These investigators used implanted microdialysis chambers[129] to measure interstitial concentration of EACA in liver, kidney, heart, and quadriceps muscle. The infusion of a fluorogenic substrate for plasmin through the microdialysis chamber permitted the determination of the effect of EACA on plasmin activity in the interstitial space. The peak concentration of EACA in each of the tissues occurred 30 minutes after infusion. The highest concentrations occurred in kidney, with somewhat lower concentration in heart (approximately 85% of that in kidney). Concentration in liver was lower (approximately 40% of that in kidney) and in quadriceps the lowest (approximately 23% of that in kidney). The effect on plasmin activity as measured with the fluorogenic substrate varied among the tissues tested, with consistent inhibition only observed in liver.

Local factors such as inflammation can be expected to influence local capillary permeability and thus influence the local composition of interstitial fluid. Haaverstad and coworkers[130] compared interstitial fluid composition in the ipsilateral and contralateral legs of patients following reconstructive surgery for lower-limb atherosclerosis. These investigators used the blister fluid technique, having previously established that it was equivalent to the wick technique for obtaining interstitial fluid.[131] Haaverstad and coworkers[130] showed that concentrations of albumin, transferrin, immunoglobulin, and α_2-macroglobulin were higher in the ipsilateral leg compared with the contralateral leg. It should be emphasized that each subject was able to serve his/her own control. In another study, Anvar[132] measured the concentration of α_2-macroglobulin in patients with critical leg ischemia and compared the values with an age-matched control population with a proximal femur fracture. These investigators did not observe a difference in α_2-macroglobulin concentration between the two populations, while the concentration of albumin, IgG, and transferrin were all lower in the blister fluid from the patient group than that of the control group. While it could be argued that opposite results were obtained by the two groups, the control population was different in the two studies. We could not find any further studies in this area, which is unfortunate as such data would be most useful.

A consideration of this information leads to the following conclusions:

- There is heterogeneity in the interstitium.
- Heterogeneity in the interstitium can be based on permanent or transient differences in capillary permeability.
- Heterogeneity in the interstitium can be based on physical exclusion within the interstitium.
- Heterogeneity in the interstitium has consequences for drug distribution.

1.7 METHODS FOR OBTAINING INTERSTITIAL FLUID AND SOME DIAGNOSTIC APPLICATIONS

There are challenges in obtaining interstitial fluid in quantities sufficient for research or diagnostic applications. Advances in spectroscopy[133,134] and proteomics[135–138] have, however, provided new approaches to the study of interstitial fluid. The major work on the use of spectroscopy to study interstitial fluid has focused on the measurement of glucose for continuous monitoring of diabetes. The bulk of proteomic investigation has focused on the study of tumor interstitial fluid (Section 1.9).

There has been considerable work on the use of near-infrared (NIR) spectroscopy for measurement of glucose concentration in interstitial fluid.[139–141] Rebrin and Steil[142] showed that it was possible to use glucose concentration in interstitial fluid as an index of the concentration of glucose in blood and, as such, as a method for measuring glucose concentration for the management of diabetes. There is a time delay between blood glucose and interstitial glucose (5–12 minutes), a correction for which has been developed to improve the accuracy of continuous glucose measurement in interstitial fluid.[143] There has been somewhat less use of Raman spectroscopy for the determination of glucose concentration in interstitial fluid.[144,145] Raman spectroscopy has been used to determine the concentration of carotenoids in skin as a measure of the dietary intake of fruits and vegetables.[146] Another study showed a decrease in skin carotenoids in individuals with metabolic syndrome.[147] Other studies have used Raman spectroscopy to study drug penetration into the skin[148,149] and for the diagnosis of skin cancer.[150–152]

Advances in electrophoresis, ultrahigh-performance chromatography (UHPLC), and mass spectrometry, together with bioinformatics, have made it possible to garner large amounts of information from small samples. These advances make it practical to study the qualitative protein composition of interstitial fluid. Magistroni and coworkers[153] have explored the possibility of using interstitial fluid from kidney biopsies as renal biomarkers using proteomic technology. Interstitial fluid was collected from the biopsy samples by low-speed centrifugation in a column with a glass fiber filter. The material collected was distinct from serum (albumin and IgG were removed from both serum and interstitial fluid by immunoaffinity depletion). The biopsy sample can be used for histology after the extraction procedure. The authors describe the harvested fluid as being conceptually similar to secretomes described for other tissues.[67–70] Magistroni and coworkers[153] demonstrated the presence of proteins derived from kidney at a higher concentration than that derived from other renal fluids. Oveland and coworkers[135] used proteomic methods (liquid chromatography–mass spectrometry [LC–MS] of tryptic peptides with protein identification using the SwissProt *Rattus norvegicus* database) to identify proteins in lymph and interstitial fluid from rat spleens following lipopolysaccharide (LPS)-induced sepsis. The presence of proteins identified by LC–MS was confirmed through the use of enzyme-linked immunosorbent assays (ELISAs). Lymph was collected by cannulation and interstitial fluid (proximal fluid) was collected by low-speed centrifugation of intact spleens; 3–10 μL quantities were collected. Elevated levels of cytokines were observed in interstitial fluid and lymph following LPS-induced sepsis; the increase in interstitial fluid was considerably higher than that observed in lymph. A number of proteins were seen in lymph and interstitial fluid only following LPS. A large increase in the level of ADAMTS-1 was seen in serum, lymph, and interstitial fluid following LPS. Earlier work from this group[154] reported on the secretion of cytokines into rat trachea interstitial fluid subsequent to LPS-induced systemic inflammatory response syndrome. Interstitial fluid was collected from isolated rat trachea by low-speed centrifugation through a nylon mesh. The protein concentration of rat trachea interstitial fluid was only slightly less (83%) than that of plasma. There were higher interstitial fluid concentrations of high-molecular proteins, such as IgM (interstitial fluid/plasma, 6.9), α_2-macroglobulin (interstitial fluid/plasma, 0.5), and fibrinogen (interstitial fluid/plasma, 0.6). The markedly high concentration of IgM suggests local production; plasminogen was also present at a higher concentration in interstitial fluid than that reported for plasma. LPS induced marked increases of IL-1β and IL-6 in interstitial fluid compared with plasma, while increases of IL-10 and TNF-α in plasma were higher than those observed in interstitial fluid. There was no significant change in cytokine concentrations in bronchoalveolar lavage. Olausson and coworkers[155] used an implanted microdialysis catheter to collect interstitial fluid from trapezius muscle. They were able to identify several proteins elevated in subjects with chronic myalgia compared with a control group.

　　　Celis and coworkers[156,157] used the passive extraction of excised tissues to obtain tissue interstitial fluid. The assumption underlying this technical approach was that a tissue, in particular a tumor, would secrete proteins into the interstitium at a much higher concentration than that which would be later found in the circulation. The observations of Semaevo and coworkers[154] support this concept based on their work on normal rat trachea, where higher than expected levels of proteins were obtained in harvested interstitial fluid. Semaevo and coworkers[154] obtained tissue interstitial fluid by low-speed centrifugation of tissue without the addition of solvent, while the approach developed by Celis and coworkers[156] involved the incubation of a tissue sample with buffer under CO_2 at 37°C for various periods of time. The supernatant fraction is obtained by low-speed centrifugation and used for proteomic analysis. Teng and coworkers[158] evaluated various solvents for the incubation of tissue samples in the preparation of tissue interstitial fluid. Teng and coworkers found that phosphate-buffered saline (PBS) was the best of five fluids that they evaluated for the incubation of the tissue samples. This evaluation was based on the requirement of additional processing steps prior to proteomic analysis when other solvents were used. Sun and coworkers[159] used PBS with the addition of protease inhibitors (a "protease inhibitor cocktail") for the acquisition of liver interstitial fluid. The tissue incubation approach would appear to decrease the amount of protein derived from extravasation and could be accurately considered a secretome, while the direct acquisition of fluid by centrifugation of an excised tissue sample is likely more representative of tissue interstitial fluid.

Ultrasound (sonophoresis) has been used to enhance the permeation of skin for the purpose of drug delivery.[160–163] This technique has also seen application for the acquisition of human skin interstitial fluid.[164] It was possible to obtain 500 μL portions of interstitial fluid with protein concentrations ranging from 0.06 to 4.8 mg/mL and to use these samples for 2-D electrophoresis and Western blot analysis. Two-dimensional electrophoresis showed a greater diversity of protein at longer collection time points (60–90 minutes) than at earlier time points. Western blot analysis demonstrated substantial quantities of albumin and stratifin, with lesser amounts of vascular endothelial growth factor (VEGF). Stratifin is a member of the 14-3-3 protein family, which is important for keratinocyte differentiation.[165]

Skin blister fluid has a long history of use as a source of interstitial fluid as it is relatively easy to obtain and represents the largest portion of total body interstitial fluid (Section 1.8). Worm[54] and others[131] have concluded that skin blister fluid could be considered "average" interstitial fluid.

These studies support the use of interstitial fluid as a source of biomarkers. The issue is how to access interstitial fluid on a routine basis for diagnostic applications. The most promising approaches appear to be spectroscopic techniques, which can be used for noninvasive and continuous monitoring of biomarkers, such as glucose concentration for diabetes. The various applications of Raman spectroscopy for the study of skin[146–150,166] should find value in the study of interstitial fluid. Kiang and coworkers[167] have reviewed some of the issues associated with the use of interstitial fluid for monitoring systemic drug concentration.

1.8   TRANSPORT OF DRUGS AND BIOLOGICALS IN INTERSTITIAL FLUID

The majority of drugs travel to the site of action though the interstitial space. Many biologicals can enter the vascular space via transit in the interstitial space or, as with antibody–drug conjugates, by SC methods directly into the interstitial space. Some biologicals, most notably blood coagulation factors, function primarily in the vascular space.

Transport from the circulation to the interstitial space (*extravasation*) is discussed in Section 1.2. Pharmaceuticals may also enter the interstitial space by transdermal processes.[168,169] Drugs are also absorbed through the gastric and pulmonary epithelia.[170-173] Passage through the interstitium to the target can be challenging and may be complicated by the heterogeneity of the interstitial space (Section 1.6). Binding to components of the ECM, including cell surface proteins, can sequester drugs.[174-177] Interstitial flow[178] is an important factor in the delivery of SC protein drugs by transport to the lymphatic system.[179] Interstitial fluid pressure in tumors can be a problem in the delivery of drugs to tumors from the vasculature.[180,181] Maguire and Juan[182] showed that the use of a hypertonic solution (1 M mannitol) caused tumor cells to shrink, thus increasing the interstitial space within a tumor (sections of a rat fibrosarcoma), improving transport of rhodamine-labeled dextrans; the effect was greatest with smaller (4000 MW) dextran probes but could be observed with 2×10^6 MW probes.

1.8.1 TRANSPORT OF DRUGS IN INTERSTITIAL SPACE

The broad category of pharmaceuticals can be classified into *drugs* and *biologicals* (also referred to as *biopharmaceutics*). Drugs are usually low-molecular-weight chemicals most frequently obtained from organic synthesis, although some may be obtained by the processing of natural products. Drugs can be classified on the basis of their solubility and permeability by use of the biopharmaceutics classification system (BCS).[183] Another system, the biopharmaceutics drug disposition classification system (BDDCS), is based on specific transporter effects into target cells.[184] The BCS is important in considering the uptake from the vascular bed, skin surface, and gastrointestinal epithelium,[185] while the BDDCS is more important for uptake into target cells from the interstitium. Low-molecular-weight drugs can move from the interstitial space into the circulation.

The *lipid solubility* of a drug (LogP) is considered important for the distribution of a drug into the extravascular space.[186,187] There are two mechanisms by which a molecule—either a low-molecular-weight compound, such as a drug, or a high-molecular-weight substance, such as a protein—can pass through a cellular barrier, such as endothelial cells in the vascular system or epithelial cells in the gastric or intestinal wall. Paracellular transport goes "around" the cells through transiently disrupted tight junctions[188-194] and transcellular transport, which involves endocytosis and transport through the cell, followed by exocytosis.[191-196]

We could find few measurements of drug concentration in interstitial fluid. One is the work of Reust and coworkers[127-129] on the distribution of EACA in the interstitial fluid of various tissues (porcine model) after IV administration. Samples of interstitial fluid were collected using a microdialysis apparatus and the concentration of EACA was determined by HPLC. The maximum interstitial concentration of EACA was seen 30 minutes after infusion. The concentration was highest in kidney, with somewhat less in heart; much lower concentrations were observed in liver and quadriceps muscle. The area under the curve (AUC) was also largest for kidney and somewhat less for heart, indicating greater available drug. The approximate ratios of kidney/heart/liver/quadriceps was 1/0.8/0.4/0.2. The reason for the disparity in concentration is not clear. While there is some difference in the capillary permeability (i.e., continuous, fenestrated) between the various tissues, it is not clear that such differences would explain the observed difference in EACA extravasation. Several reports describe the inhibition of capillary permeability by EACA.[62,195–197] Copley and Carrol[195] showed that EACA blocked the extravasation of horseradish peroxidase in a guinea pig skin model, while Don and coworkers[197] showed that EACA inhibited the extravasation of radiolabeled serum albumin (RISA) in a canine posterior paw model. Imatinib (Gleevec®), a monoclonal antibody therapeutic, improves the transport of an albumin–drug conjugate from the interstitium into tumorous and normal tissue.[198]

If one assumes that the substrate used by Reust and coworkers on their studies on the interstitial distribution of EACA[127,128] is specific for plasmin, there would appear to be little correlation between the interstitial concentration of EACA and plasmin inhibition. As discussed by these investigators,[127] the disparity of tissue distribution could be causal for adverse events (off-target reactions). In subsequent work from this group on the interstitial distribution of aprotinin,[129] there was equal distribution to heart, kidney, and liver, but somewhat less to quadriceps (the concentration of aprotinin is inferred from the inhibition of plasmin activity). The presence of aprotinin in the kidney could result in the inhibition of kallikrein activity.

There are some studies on the measurement of drugs in skin blister fluid as compared with the concentration in blood plasma. Tuominen and coworkers[199] measured the concentration of erythromycin base and erythromycin acetate in suction skin blister fluid, saliva, and blood plasma after oral dosage. The concentration in suction skin blister fluid was approximately 50% of that in blood plasma, while the concentration in saliva was approximately 20% of that in blood plasma; approximately 7% was excreted in urine. This group also reported on the concentration of erythromycin in tonsil tissue and found tissue levels comparable with those in skin blister fluid.[200] There is some question as to the validity of the use of skin blister fluid as a surrogate for the interstitial fluid of a specific tissue. Deguchi and coworkers[201] used microdialysis to study the tissue distribution of β-lactam antibiotics in a rodent model. They showed that the concentration of antibiotic in venous flow was only slightly greater than the interstitial concentration of free antibiotic in the interstitial fluid for lung, muscle, and liver. They also observed that the concentration of drug in a tissue homogenate (muscle, lung) was similar to that obtained by microdialysis. These investigators also suggest that the skin blister fluid technique might alter capillary physiology and might just represent the skin interstitium. It is recognized that the skin interstitium is the largest of the various interstitial spaces but may not be representative of interstitial fluid in organs such as the heart, kidney, or liver. Müller and coworkers[202] compared skin blister fluid, saliva, and microdialysis as methods for measurement of interstitial drug concentration. Based on the distribution of theophylline in human subjects, they concluded that microdialysis was the most accurate method. There is significant uptake of erythromycin and other macrolide antibiotics into fibroblasts[203] and epithelial cells.[204] Telithromycin is a ketolide antibiotic that is rapidly internalized by white blood cells. Muller-Serieys and coworkers[205] reported that the concentration of telithromycin in white blood cells greatly exceeded that in plasma after an oral dose of the drug. The concentration of telithromycin in blister fluid was less than that of blood after two hours but was much larger at longer time points. The concentration of the drug in tissue (tonsil), alveolar macrophages, and epithelial lining fluid (bronchoalveolar lavage) was much higher than in blood. The concentration of telithromycin was also higher in saliva than in blood.

Microdialysis is a relatively old method for measuring low-molecular-weight compounds in interstitial fluid,[206] but has recently become popular for measuring interstitial drug concentration. Joukhader and coworkers[206] have reviewed the use of microdialysis for the determination of tissue drug concentration. Traunmüller and coworkers[207] used microdialysis to measure the telithromycin concentration in muscle and SC adipose tissue and found concentrations much lower than that of plasma; approximately one-third of total plasma telithromycin was free (not protein bound). Thus, their results differ from those obtained by Muller-Serieys and coworkers, who used a skin blister fluid technique. Regardless, the results obtained by Traunmüller and coworkers[207] show differences between tissue drug concentration and blood drug concentration. Reust and coworkers,[127,128] who used microdialysis to measure EACA concentration in tissues, also discussed the problem of the difference between blood concentration and tissue concentration.

The concentration of a drug in saliva has been considered to be an approximation of the amount of drug that is not protein bound and thus "available." The disparity between saliva concentration and skin blister fluid, which is considered a surrogate for interstitial fluid, raises a question as to the validity of this assumption. This is supported by the earlier observations of Slevin and coworkers[208] on the saliva concentration of cytosine arabinoside, a drug that binds poorly to plasma proteins. Müller and coworkers[166] observed a higher concentration of theophylline in saliva ($C_{max} = 3.27$ µg/mL) than in microdialysis samples from muscle ($C_{max} = 2.97$ µg/mL) or SC tissue ($C_{max} = 2.22$ µg/mL).

A substantial amount of a drug may be bound to protein in the circulation (and presumably in the interstitial space). Albumin and α_1-acid glycoprotein are two proteins considered to have a major role in the binding of drugs in the intravascular and extravascular space. It is thought that a drug bound to protein is not "available" and the "free" drug is responsible for the pharmacological effect. The majority of total albumin in the interstitial space is derived mostly from extravasation, although there is some synthesis in the extravascular space (Chapter 4). Dancik and coworkers[209] showed that the depth of penetration of a topically applied drug into the dermis was related to the ability of the drug to bind protein. They suggested that the drugs would bind to protein in surface blood capillaries. Although not mentioned by these authors, it is also possible that the drugs bound to protein in the skin interstitium.

1.8.2 TRANSPORT OF BIOLOGICALS IN INTERSTITIAL SPACE

Biologicals are large-molecular-weight drugs, usually proteins, which are given either by IV or intraperitoneal (IP) administration. Alternatives to the IV administration of a drug have considerable technical advantages and also face considerable technical challenges.[210–212] Alternative modes of drug administration may be more cost-effective.[213] While it is true that SC administration is common for drugs such as insulin and other peptide biopharmaceuticals,[214] this approach was seldom used until the rediscovery of the SC administration of immunoglobulin.[215–217]

Biologicals and other large materials such as liposomes cannot move from the interstitial space into the circulation but enter the vascular system though the lymph.[179,218] Low-molecular-weight drugs may be encapsulated in lipid vesicles, yielding a large particle that can be administered via the SC route and then into the lymphatic system.[218] Liposomes are used to deliver chemotherapeutic agents to the lymphatic system after SC administration. It should be noted that dermal administration and oral administration would involve transport across epithelia and the challenge of transport through the interstitial space to the lymphatic system. Takeuchi and coworkers[219] have reported that lactoferrin (bovine) was absorbed from the intestinal lumen after infusion in rats through the duodenal lumen and taken to the vascular system via the lymphatics. Modification of lactoferrin with poly(ethylene) glycol resulted in a 10-fold enhancement of uptake from the intestinal tract.[220] Absorption of antigenic particulates, such as Fc-coated glutaraldehyde-fixed sheep erythrocytes, occur via specific endocytosis by mucosal Fc receptors with direct transfer to hepatic portal blood.[221]

There are several challenges to the successful transport of a protein therapeutic through the interstitial space. The interstitium contains materials, such as collagen and hyaluronan, that complicate the transport of protein drugs.[222] Collagen is discussed in Chapter 2, while hyaluronan is discussed in Chapter 3. Briefly, both collagen and hyaluronan occupy space in the interstitium and can provide a barrier to the diffusion of proteins. In addition, there is the potential of proteins binding to collagen and hyaluronan. Degradation of collagen with collagenase in tumor tissue enhances the transport of IgG, while degradation of hyaluronan with hyaluronidase in tumor tissue enhances the delivery of small drugs, such as doxorubicin.[119] Jiang and coworkers[223] showed that either collagenase or hyaluronidase enhanced the transport of microparticles across the sclera of eye, suggesting that the ECM was a barrier to transport.

There is the possibility that proteolytic activity in the interstitial space could degrade protein biologicals (Chapters 5). The great majority of proteases in the interstitial space are regulatory, not digestive, and not likely expressed except in inflammation and other pathological processes. The inflammasome[224–226] is an example of such activity expressed in pathological situations. While it would appear to be accepted that there is little protease activity in normal SC tissue,[214] there are examples of apparent proteolytic degradation on therapeutic products in the interstitial space. Osikowicz and coworkers[227] showed the inhibition of MMP-2/MMP-9 activity by SC injection of an inhibitor blocked nerve growth factor (NGF) degradation. Shi and coworkers[228] observed that there was an absence of intravascular recovery of factor VIII and vWF factor following SC injection of human therapeutic preparations of these proteins. This interpretation is supported by the work of Fatouros and coworkers,[229] who observed the inactivation of B domain–deleted factor VIII in homogenates of SC tissue. However, there are examples of the cellular expression of factor VIII in SC space resulting in therapeutic levels of the clotting factor in mice.[230,231] While Kashiwakura and coworkers[231] observed weak expression of factor VIII from transduced mesenchymal stem cells with SC implantation, a more robust response was observed with intra-articular injection of transduced mesenchymal stem cells. The SC injection of recombinant human factor VIII in hemophilia A mice elicited a stronger immune response than IV administration.[232] Factor VIII that is injected into the SC space appears to be unstable and immunogenic, while factor VIII expressed *in situ* appears to be stable to the extent of being transported via the lymphatics into the vascular system. There are likely also formulation issues for the SC administration of protein drugs that would have to be addressed, including the use of encapsulation technology.[233] There is more discussion of proteolysis in the interstitial space in Chapter 4.

Regardless of the challenges, there have been successes in the administration, usually SC, of protein therapeutics that would involve transport through the interstitial space. Martinez-Saguer and coworkers[234] compared SC and IV administration of C1-esterase inhibitor (C1-INH) in patients with hereditary angioedema. Maximum IV activity of SC occurred 48 hours after administration with approximately 40% recovery (bioavailability, defined by the AUC compared with IV administration). The functional half-life for the SC material was 120 hours, compared with 64 hours for the IV material. Sang and coworkers[235] compared the IV and SC administration of a His-tagged human recombinant endostatin in a primate model (rhesus monkeys). Pharmacokinetic analysis of an IV-administered product fit a three-compartment model, while SC administration fit a two-component model. Bioavailability of the SC material was approximately 70% of the IV based on AUC at the same dosage level.

The majority of success in the SC administration has been with immunoglobulins.[236] This is, in fact, a "back to the future" story. A crude immunoglobulin therapeutic[237] was developed by Cohn and colleagues during their development of plasma fractionation during World War II.[238] This preparation was successful as an intramuscular injection for the prophylaxis and treatment of measles both in the United States and the United Kingdom.[241] Adverse reactions associated with IV immunoglobulin[240] were a major driver for intramuscular and SC administration. This problem was solved and IV administration became the accepted mode of administration since the dominant (and only approved) use was for primary immune deficiency.[241] The advent of monoclonal antibody–based diagnostics[242–244] and therapeutics[245,246] and other factors[247] have resulted in a return to SC administration of IV immunoglobulin.[248] It is also apparent that SC administration will become the preferred route for monoclonal antibody–based therapeutics.[249–252]

1.9 TUMOR INTERSTITIAL FLUID

Tumor interstitial fluid is physically separate from the bulk interstitium, but flow from the tumor interstitium does enter the bulk interstitial fluid.[253,254] The excessive development of the ECM around the developing tumor encases the tumor interstitial fluid, resulting in the development of tumor interstitial fluid pressure. This makes it difficult for macromolecular drugs to reach the tumor cell mass.[255] Tumor interstitial pressure increases as the tumor develops, with associated increased vascularity.[256] Earlier work by Butler and coworkers[257] noted that the fluid transport in the tumor interstitium is accommodated by lymphatic drainage, resulting in increased tumor interstitial fluid pressure. These investigators also reported an increase in hematocrit on passage from arterial to venous circulation in the tumor. They described this phenomenon as *hemoconcentration*. Butler and coworkers[257] also observed the asymmetry of fluid flow from capillaries. Other investigators[258] have reported areas of fenestration, permitting increased permeability exchange not observed in normal tissue. In addition to the lack of lymphatic drainage, the ECM surrounding the tumor provides a barrier from extravasation into the interstitium.[180,259–260] Børnaes and Rofstad[261] used contrast-enhanced MRI to study the extravasation of a 19 kDa linear molecule [poly-(Gd-DTPA)-co-(1,6-diaminohexane)] in a murine tumor melanoma xenograft model. These investigators used a three-compartment model[262] (a plasma compartment and reversible and irreversible compartments) and concluded that the transport of a protein into tumor cells was limited by interstitial transport, not extravasation into the tumor interstitium.

Tumor interstitial fluid contains proteins secreted by the tumor cells, the tumor secretome.[263,264] Shi and coworkers[265,266] identified 32 proteins secreted from a human colorectal tumor explant. The goal was to identify potential biomarker proteins unique to the tumor and was complicated by the presence of plasma proteins and proteins derived from cell necrosis in the explant. There is also more individual patient variability in tumor samples than normal tissue.[265] As these authors note, there is difficultly in duplicating the tumor microenvironment. There are interactions between tumor cells and surrounding normal tissue that influence tumor secretome content.[267]

REFERENCES

1. Altman, P.L. and Dittmer, D.S., *Blood and Other Body Fluids*, Federation of American Societies for Experimental Biology, Washington, DC, 1961.
2. Abbott, N.J., Evidence for bulk flow of brain interstitial fluid: Significance for physiology and pathology, *Neurochem. Int.* 45, 545–552, 2004.
3. Iliff, J.J., Wang, M., Zeppenfeld, D.M., et al., Cerebral arterial pulsation drives paravascular CSF–interstitial fluid exchange in the murine brain, *J. Neurosci.* 33, 18190–18199, 2013.
4. Thane, A.S., Rangroo, T. V., and Nedergaard, M., Drowning stars: Reassessing the role of astrocytes in brain edema, *Trends Neurosci.* 37, 620–628, 2014.
5. Stukas, S., Robert, J., Lee, J., et al., Intravenously injected human apolipoprotein A-1 rapidly enters the central nervous system via the choroid plexus, *J. Am. Heart Assoc.* 3, e001156, 2014.
6. Weinstein, J.R., Gold, S.J., Cunningham, D.D., and Gall, C.M., Cellular localization of thrombin receptor mRNA in rat brain: Expression by mesencephalic dopaminergic neurons and codistribution with prothrombin mRNA, *J. Neurosci.* 15, 2906–2919, 1995.
7. Almonte, A.G., Qadri, L.H., Sultan, F.A., et al., Protease-activated receptor-1 modulates hippocampal memory formation and synaptic plasticity, *J. Neurochem.* 124, 109–122, 2013.
8. Laurent, T.C., Structure of the extracellular matrix and the biology of hyaluronan, in *Interstitium, Connective Tissue and Lymphatics*, eds. R.K. Reed, N.G. Meltall, J.L. Bert, C.P. Winlove, and G.A. Lane, Chapter 1, pp. 1–12, Portland Press, London, UK, 1995.
9. Holmes, F.L., Claude Bernard, the *milieu intérieur*, and regulatory physiology, *Hist. Phil. Life Sci.* 8, 3–25, 1986.
10. Haslene-Hox H., Tenstad, O., and Wiig, H., Interstitial fluid: A reflection of the tumor microenvironment and secretome, *Biochim. Biophys. Acta* 1834, 2336–2346, 2013.

11. Poulsen, H.L., Jensen, H.A., and Parving, H.-H., Extracellular fluid volume determined by a single injection of inulin in men with untreated essential hypertension, *Scand. J. Clin. Lab. Invest.* 37, 691–697, 1977.
12. Harper, H.A., Water and metabolism, in *Review of Physiological Chemistry*, 15th edn., Chapter 19, p. 422, Lange Medical, Los Altos, CA, 1975.
13. Berson, S.A., Yalow, R.S., Schreiber, S.S., and Post, J., Tracer experiments with I^{131} labeled serum albumin: Distribution and degradation studies, *J. Clin. Invest.* 32, 746–768, 1953.
14. *Oxford English Dictionary*, Oxford University Press, Oxford, UK, 2015.
15. Young, I.M., Mixing of supernatant and interstitial fluids in the Rhum layered intrusion, *Mineral. Mag.* 48, 345–350, 1984.
16. Aquilina, L., Boulegue, J., Sureau, J.-F., Bariac, T., and the GPF Team, Evolution of interstitial waters along the passive margin on the Southeast basin of France: WELCOM (Well Chemical Online Monitoring) applied to Balazuc-1 well (Ardèche), *Appl. Geochem.* 9, 65–675, 1994.
17. Chatziheoldoridis, E., Haigh, S., and Lyon, I., A conspicuous clay ovoid in Nakhla: Evidence for subsurface hydrothermal alteration on Mars with implications for astrobiology, *Astrobiology* 14, 651–693, 2014.
18. Nia, H.T., Han, L., Li, Y., Ortiz, C., and Grodzinsky, A., Poroelasticity of cartilage at the nanoscale, *Biophys. J.* 101, 2304–2313, 2011.
19. Nia, H.T., Han, L., Bozchalooi, S., et al., Aggrecan nanoscale solid-fluid interactions are a primary determinant of cartilage dynamic mechanical properties, *ACS Nano* 9, 2614–2625, 2015.
20. Starling, E.H. and Tubby, A.H., On absorption from and secretion into the serous cavities, *J. Physiol.* 16, 140–158, 1984.
21. Starling, E.H., On the absorption of fluids from the connective tissue spaces, *J. Physiol.* 19, 312–326, 1896.
22. Schäfer, E.A., Notes on the temperature of heat-coagulation of certain of the proteid substances of the blood, *J. Physiol.* 3, 181–187, 1882.
23. Landis, E.M., Microinjection studies of capillary permeability: II. The relation between capillary pressure and the rate at which fluid passes through the walls of single capillaries, *Am. J. Physiol.* 82, 217–238, 1927.
24. Cliff, W.J., *Blood Vessels*, p. 148, Cambridge University Press, Cambridge, UK, 1976.
25. Ruch, T.C. and Fulton, J.F., *Molecular Physiology and Biophysics*, 18th edn., Chapter 34, pp. 752–770, W.B. Saunders, Philadelphia, PA, 1961.
26. Civetta, J.M., A new look at the Starling equation, *Crit. Care Med.* 7, 84–91, 1979.
27. Kongstad, L., Möller, A.D., and Grände, P.O., Reflection coefficient for albumin and capillary fluid permeability in cat calf muscle after traumatic injury, *Acta Physiol. Scand.* 165, 369–377, 1999.
28. White, P., Jr., Brower, R., Sylvester, J.T., et al., Factors influencing measurement of protein reflection coefficient by filtered volume technique, *J. Appl. Physiol.* 74, 1374–1380, 1985.
29. Foster, K.J. and Miklavcic, S.J., On the competitive uptake and transport of ions through differentiated root tissues, *J. Theor. Biol.* 340, 1–10, 2014.
30. Zarkaria, E.R., Mays, C.J., Matheson, P.J., Hurt, R.T., and Garrison, R.N., Plasma appearance rate of intraperitoneal macromolecular tracer underestimates peritoneal lymph flow, *Adv. Perit. Dial.* 24, 16–21, 2008.
31. Zeuthen, T., Alsterfjord, M., Beitz, E., and MacAuley, N., Osmotic water transport in aquaporins: Evidence for a stochastic mechanism, *J. Physiol.* 591, 5017–5029, 2013.
32. Cankova, Z., Huang, J.D., Kruth, H.S., and Johnson, M., Passage of low-density lipoproteins through Burch's membrane and choroid, *Exp. Eye Res.* 93, 947–955, 2011.

33. Lundblad, C., Bentzer, P., and Gränsw, P.O., Inhibition of Rho kinase decreases hydraulic and protein microvascular permeability in cat skeletal muscle, *Microvascul. Res.* 66, 126–133, 2003.

34. Bennett, H.S., Morphological aspects of extracellular polysaccharide, *J. Histochem. Cytochem.* 11, 14–23, 1963.

35. Ito, S., Structure and function of the glycocalyx, *Fed. Proc.* 28, 12–25, 1969.

36. Gipson, I.K., Spurr-Michaud, S., Tisdale, A., and Menon, B.B., Comparison of the transmembrane mucins MUC1 and MUC16 in epithelial barrier function, *PLoS One* 9(6), e100393, 2014.

37. Corfield, A.P., Mucins: A biologically relevant glycan barrier in mucosal protection, *Biochim. Biophys. Acta* 1850, 236–252, 2015.

38. Alphonsus, C.S. and Rodseth, R.N., The endothelial glycocalyx: A review of the vascular barrier, *Anaesthesiology* 69, 777–784, 2014.

39. Curry, F.-R.H. and Noll, T., Spotlight on microvascular permeability, *Cardiovascular Res.* 87, 195–197, 2010.

40. Gao, L. and Lipowsky, H.H., Composition of the endothelial glycocalyx and its relation to its thickness and diffusion of small solutes, *Microvasc. Res.* 80, 394–401, 2010.

41. Jacob, M., Bruegger, D., Rehm, M., et al., The endothelial glycocalyx affords compatibility of Starling's principle and high cardiac interstitial albumin levels, *Cardiovasc. Res.* 73, 575–586, 2007.

42. Mehta, D., Raundarn, K., and Kuebler, W.M., Novel regulators of endothelial barrier function, *Am. J. Physiol. Lung Cell. Mol. Physiol.* 307, L924–L935, 2014.

43. Pries, A.R. and Kuebler, W.M., Normal endothelium, *Handb. Exp. Pharmacol.* 174(Pt 1), 1–40, 2006.

44. Adamson, R.H., Leng, J.F, Zhang, Y., et al., Oncotic pressures opposing filtration across non-fenestrated microvessels, *J. Physiol.* 557, 889–907, 2004.

45. Woodcock, T.E. and Woodcock, T.M., Revised Starling equation and the glycocalyx model of transvascular fluid exchange: An improved paradigm for prescribing intravenous fluid therapy, *Brit. J. Anaesthesia* 108, 384–394, 2012.

46. Levick, J.R., Revision of the Starling principle: New views of tissue fluid balance, *J. Physiol.* 557, 704, 2004.

47. Haraldsson, B., Physiological studies of macromolecular transport across capillary walls: Studies on continuous capillaries in rat skeletal muscle, *Acta Physiol. Scand. Suppl.* 553, 1–40, 1986.

48. Roselli, R.J., Coy, S.R., and Harris, T.R., Models of lung transvascular fluid and protein transport, *Ann. Biomed. Eng.* 15, 127–138, 1987.

49. Katz, M.A., Schaeffer, R.C., Jr., Gratrix, M., et al., The glomerular barrier fits a two-pore-and-fiber-matrix model: Derivation and physiologic test, *Microvasc. Res.* 57, 227–243, 1999.

50. Levick, J.R. and Michel, C.C., Microvascular fluid exchange and the revised Starling principle, *Cardiovasc. Res.* 87, 198–210, 2010.

51. Nakamura, R.M., Spiegelberg, H.L., Lee, S., and Weigle, W.O., Relationship between molecular size and intra- and extravascular distribution of protein antigens, *J. Immunol.* 100, 376–383, 1968.

52. Michel, C.C., Nanjee, M.N., Olszewski, W.L., and Miller, N.E., LDL and HDL transfer rates across peripheral microvascular endothelium agree with those predicted for passive ultrafiltration in humans, *J. Lipid Res.* 56, 122–128, 2015.

53. Brinkhous, K.M. and Walker, S.A., Prothrombin and fibrinogen in lymph, *Am. J. Physiol.* 132, 666–669, 1941.

54. Worm, A.-M., Exchange of macromolecules between plasma and skin interstitium in extensive skin disease, *J. Invest. Dermatol.* 76, 489–492, 1981.

55. Bar, R.S., Boes, M., Clemmons, D.R., et al., Insulin differentially alters transcapillary movement of intravascular IGFBP-1, IGFBP-2 and endothelial cell IGF-binding proteins in the rat heart, *Endocrinology* 127, 497–499, 1990.

56. Areskog, N.-H., Arturson, G., Grotte, G., and Wallenius, G., Studies on heart lymph: II. Capillary permeability of the dog's heart using dextran as a test substance, *Acta Physiol. Scand.* 62, 218–223, 1964.

57. Pollak, M.R., Quaggin, S.E., Hoenig, M.P., and Dworkin, L.D., The glomerulus: The sphere of influence, *Clin. J. Am. Soc. Nephrol.* 9, 1461–1469, 2014.

58. Migliorini, A., Ebid, R., Shcerbaum, C.R., and Anders, H.-J., The danger control concept in kidney disease: Mesangial cells, *J. Nephrol.* 26, 437–449, 2013.

59. Juweld, M., Strauss, H.W., Yaoita, H., et al., Accumulation of immunoglobulin G at focal sites of inflammation, *Eur. J. Nucl. Med.* 19, 159–165, 1992.

60. Reed, R.K. and Rubin, K., Transcapillary exchange: Role and importance of the interstitial fluid pressure the extracellular matrix, *Cardiovasc. Res.* 87, 211–217, 2010.

61. Parving, H.H., Nielsen, S.L., and Lassen, N.A., Increased transcapillary escape rate of albumin, IgG, and IgM during angiotensin-II-induced hypertension in man, *Scand. J. Clin. Lab. Invest.* 34, 111–118, 1974.

62. Eassa, E.-H.M. and Casarett, G.W., Effect of epsilon-amino-n-caproic acid (EACA) on radiation-induced increase in capillary permeability, *Radiology* 106, 679–688, 1973.

63. Vuong, T.T., Prydz, K., and Tveit, H., Differences in the apical and basolateral pathways for glycosaminoglycan biosynthesis in Madin–Darby canine kidney cells, *Glycobiology* 16, 326–332, 2006.

64. Hua, W., Sheff, D., Toomre, D., and Mellman, I., Vectorial insertion of apical and basolateral membrane proteins in polarized epithelial cells revealed by quantitative 3D live cell imaging, *J. Cell Biol.* 172, 1035–1044, 2006.

65. Arin, R.M., Rudea Y., Casis, O., et al., Basolateral expression of GRP94 in parietal cells of gastric mucosa, *Biochemistry* 79, 8–15, 2014.

66. Pillai, D.K., Sankoorikal, B.J., Johnson, E., et al., Directional secretomes reflect polarity-specific functions in an in vitro model of human bronchial epithelium, *Am. J. Respir. Cell Mol. Biol.* 50, 282–300, 2014.

67. Hathout, Y., Approaches to the study of the cell secretome, *Expert Rev. Proteomics* 4, 239–248, 2007.

68. Mukherjee, P. and Mani, S., Methodologies to decipher the cell secretome, *Biochim. Biophys. Acta* 1834, 2226–2232, 2013.

69. Caccia, D., Dugo, M., Callari, M., and Bongarazone, I., Bioinformatics tools for secretome analysis, *Biochim. Biophys. Acta* 1834, 2442–2453, 2013.

70. Wiegert, C., Lehmann, R., Hartwig, S., and Lehr, S., The secretome of the working human skeletal muscle: A promising opportunity to combat the metabolic disaster? *Proteomics Clin. Appl.* 8, 5–18, 2014.

71. Gromov, P., Gromova, I., Olsen, C.J., et al., Tumor interstitial fluid: A treasure trove of cancer biomarkers, *Biochim. Biophys. Acta* 1834, 2259–2270, 2013.

72. Schaaij-Visser, T.B., de Wit, M., Lam, S.W., and Jiménez, C.R., The cancer secretome, current status and opportunities in the lung, breast and colorectal cancer context, *Biochim. Biophys. Acta* 1834, 2242–2258, 2013.

73. Venkatesh, S.G., Tan, J., Gorr, S.-U., and Darling, D.S., Isoproterenol increases sorting of parotid gland cargo proteins to the basolateral pathway, *Am. J. Physiol.* 293, C558–C565, 2007.

74. Eckmann, L., Jung, H.C., Schurer-Maly, C., et al., Differential cytokine expression by human intestinal epithelial cell lines: Regulated expression of interleukin β, *Gastroenterology* 105, 1689–1697, 1993.

75. Fiorentino, M., Ding, H., Blanchard, T.G., et al., *Helicobacter pylori*–induced disruption of monolayer permeability and proinflammatory cytokine secretion in in polarized human gastric epithelial cells, *Infect. Immun.* 81, 876–883, 2013.

76. van Buul-Wortelboer, M.F., Brinkman, H.J., Reinders, J.H., van Aken, W.G., and Mourik, J.A., Polar secretion of von Willebrand factor by endothelial cells, *Biochim. Biophys. Acta* 1011, 129–133, 1989.

77. Sporn, L.A., Marder, V.J., and Wagner, D.D., Differing polarity of the constitutive and regulated secretory pathways for von Willebrand factor in endothelial cells, *J. Cell Biol.* 108, 1283–1289, 1989.

78. Scott, D.M., Kumar, S., and Barnes, M.J., The effect of a native collagen gel substratum on the synthesis of collagen by bovine brain capillary endothelial cells, *Cell. Biochem. Funct.* 6, 209–215, 1988.

79. Levick, J.R., Microvascular architecture and exchange in synovial joints, *Microcirculation* 2, 217–233, 1995.

80. Happonen, K.E., Heinegård, D., Saxne, T., and Blom, A.M., Interactions of the complement system with molecules of extracellular matrix: Relevance for joint diseases, *Immunobiology* 217, 1088–1096, 2012.

81. Hoffman, A., Gath, U., Gross, G., et al., Constitutive secretion of β-trace protein by cultivated porcine choroid plexus epithelial cells: Elucidation of its complete amino acid and cDNA sequences, *J. Cell. Physiol.* 169, 236–241, 1996.

82. Fukuda, H., Hirata, T., Nakamura, N., et al., Identification and properties of a novel variant of NBC4 (Na^+/HCO_3^- co-transporter 4) that is predominately expressed in the choroid plexus, *Biochem. J.* 450, 175–187, 2013.

83. Sakka, L., Coll, G., and Chazal, J., Anatomy and physiology of cerebrospinal fluid, *Eur. Ann. Otorhinolaryngol. Head Neck Dis.* 128, 309–316, 2011.

84. Synmss, N.P. and Oi, S., Theories of cerebrospinal fluid dynamics and hydrocephalus: Historical trend, *J. Neurosurg. Pediatr.* 11, 170–177, 2013.

85. Wilson, E.H., Weninger, W., and Hunter, C.A., Trafficking of immune cells in the central nervous system, *J. Clin. Invest.* 120, 1368–1379, 2010.

86. Engelhardt, B. and Ransohoff, R.M., Capture, crawl, cross: The T cell code to breach the blood–brain barriers, *Trends Immunol.* 33, 579–589, 2012.

87. Apte, R.S. and Niederkorn, J.Y., Isolation and characterization of a unique natural killer cell inhibitory factor present in the anterior chamber of the eye, *J. Immunol.* 156, 2667–2673, 1996.

88. Zhou. R., Horai, R., Mattapallil, M.J., and Caspi, R.R., A new look at immune privilege of the eye: Dual role for the vision-related molecule retinoic acid, *J. Immunol.* 187, 4170–4177, 2011.

89. Strazielle, N. and Ghersi-Egea, J.F., Physiology of blood–brain interfaces in relation to brain disposition of small compounds and macromolecules, *Mol. Pharm.* 10, 1473–1491, 2013.

90. Bressler, J., Clark, K., and O'Driscoll, C., Assessing blood–brain barrier function using *in vitro* assays, *Methods Mol. Biol.* 1066, 67–79, 2013.

91. Ye, D., Raghnaill, M.N., Bramini, M., et al., Nanoparticle accumulation and transcytosis in brain endothelial cell layers, *Nanoscale* 5, 11153–11165, 2013.

92. Johanson, C.E., Stopa, E.G., and McMillan, P.N., The blood–cerebrospinal fluid barrier: Structure and functional significance, *Methods Mol. Biol.* 686, 101–131, 2011.

93. Facchini, L., Bellini, A., and Toro, E.F., A mathematical model for filtration and macromolecule transport across capillary walls, *Microvasc. Res.* 94, 52–69, 2014.

94. Dvorak, H.F., Vascular permeability of plasma, plasma proteins, and cells: An update, *Curr. Opin. Hematol.* 17, 225–229, 2010.

95. Hansen, K., D'Alessandro, A., Clement, C.C., and Santambrogio, L., Lymph formation, composition, and circulation: A proteomic perspective, *Int. Immunol.* 27, 219–227, 2015.
96. Borge, B.Å., Iversen, V.V., and Reed, R.K., Changes in plasma protein extravasation in rat skin during inflammatory challenges by microdialysis, *Am. J. Physiol. Circ. Physiol.* 290, H2108–H2115, 2006.
97. Wiig, H. and Swartz, M.A., Interstitial fluid and lymph formation and transport: Physiological regulation and roles in inflammation and cancer, *Physiol. Rev.* 92, 1005–1060, 2012.
98. Olszewski, W.L., Collection and physiological measurements of peripheral lymph and interstitial fluid in man, *Lymphology* 10, 137–145, 1977.
99. Dzieciatkowska, M., D'Alessandro, A., Moore, E.E., et al., Lymph is not a plasma ultra-filtrate: A proteome analysis of injured patients, *Shock.* 42, 485–498, 2014.
100. Frank, J.S. and Langer, G.A., The myocardial interstitium: Its structure and its role in ionic exchange, *J. Cell Biol.* 60, 586–601, 1974.
101. Borg, T.K., Rubin, K., Carver, W., Samarel, A., and Tarracio, L., The cell biology of the cardiac interstitium, *Trends Cardiovasc. Med.* 6, 65–70, 1976.
102. Scott, J.E., How rational histochemistry produced order out of chaos in the "amorphous ground substance" (with a little help from biochemistry, biophysics, etc.), *Eur. J. Histochem.* 42, 29–34, 1998.
103. Mansek, F.J., Macromolecules in the extracellular compartment of embryonic and mature hearts, *Circ. Res.* 38, 331–335, 1976.
104. Chen, W. and Frangogiannis, N.G., Fibroblasts in post-infarction inflammation and cardiac repair, *Biochim. Biophys. Acta* 1833, 945–953, 2013.
105. Kramann, R., DiRocco, D.P., and Humphreys, B.D., Understanding the origin, activation and regulation of matrix-producing myofibroblasts for treatment of fibrotic disease, *J. Pathol.* 231, 273–289, 2013.
106. Sanders, K.M., Ward, S.M., and Koh, S.D., Interstitial cells: Regulators of smooth muscle function, *Physiol. Rev.* 94, 859–907, 2014.
107. Popescu, L.M. and Faussone-Pellegrine, M.S., Telocytes: A case of serendipity; The winding way from interstitial cells of Cajal (ICC), via interstitial Cajal-like cells (ICLC) to telocytes, *J. Cell. Mol. Med.* 14, 729–740, 2010.
108. Meyer, F.A. and Silberberg, A., Aging and the interstitial content of loose connective tissue: A brief note, *Mech. Aging Dev.* 5, 437–442, 1976.
109. Johansson, B.R., Capillary permeability to interstitial microinjections of macromolecules and influence of capillary hydrostatic pressure on endothelial ultrastructure, *Acta Physiol. Scand. Suppl.* 463, 45–50, 1979.
110. Sage, H., Collagens of basement membranes, *J. Invest. Dermatol.* 79(Suppl. 1), 51s–59s, 1982.
111. Paralkar, V.M., Nandedkar, A.K., Pointer, R.H., et al., Interaction of osteogenin, a heparin binding bone morphogenetic protein, with type IV collagen, *J. Biol. Chem.* 265, 17281–17284, 1990.
112. Saccà, B., Sinner, E.K., Kaiser, J., et al., Binding and docking of synthetic heterotrimeric collagen type IV peptides with $\alpha 1\beta 1$ integrin, *Chembiochem.* 3, 904–907, 2002.
113. Ettelaie, C., Collier, M.E., Mei, M.P., et al., Enhanced binding of tissue factor–microparticles to collagen-IV and fibronectin leads to increased tissue factor activity *in vitro*, *Thromb. Haemost.* 109, 61–71, 2013.
114. Paavola, K.J., Sidik, H., Zuchero, J.B., et al., Type IV collagen is an activating ligand for the adhesion G protein–coupled receptor GPR125, *Sci. Signal.* 7(338), ra76, 2014.
115. Fitzgerald, J., Holden, P., and Hansen, U., The expanded collagen VI family: New chains and new questions, *Connect Tissue Res.* 54, 345–350, 2013.

116. Henthorn, T.K., Avram, M.J., Frederiksen, M.C., and Atkinson, A.J., Jr., Heterogeneity of interstitial fluid space demonstrated by simultaneous kinetic analysis of the distribution and elimination on inulin and gallamine, *J. Pharmacol. Expt. Therapeut.* 222, 389–394, 1982.

117. Wiig, H., Gyenge, C., Iverson, P.O., Gullberg, D., and Tenstad, O., The role of the extracellular matrix in tissue distribution of macromolecules in normal and pathological tissues: Potential therapeutic consequences, *Microcirculation* 15, 283–296, 2008.

118. Haslene-Hox, H., Overland, E., Woie, K., et al., Distribution volumes of macromolecules in human ovarian and endometrial cancers: Effects of extracellular matrix structure, *Am. J. Physiol. Heart Circ. Physiol.* 308, H18–H28, 2015.

119. Erikson, A., Tufto, I., Bjønnum, A.B., Bruland, Ø., and Davies, Cde. L., The impact of enzymatic degradation on the uptake of differently sized therapeutic molecules, *Anticancer Res.* 28, 3557–3566, 2008.

120. Choi, J., Credit, K., Henderson, K., et al., Intraperitoneal immunotherapy for metastatic ovarian carcinoma: Resistance of intratumoral collagen to antibody penetration, *Clin. Cancer Res.* 12, 1906–1912, 2006.

121. Magzoub, M., Jin, S., and Verkman, A.S., Enhanced macromolecule diffusion deep in tumors after enzymatic digestion of extracellular matrix collagen and its associated proteoglycan decorin, *FASEB J.* 22, 276–284, 2008.

122. Hynes, W.L. and Ferretti, J.J., Assays for hyaluronidase activity, *Methods Enzymol.* 235, 606–616, 1994.

123. Wells, A.F., Larsson, E., Tengblad, A., et al., The localization of hyaluronan in normal and rejected human kidneys, *Transplantation* 50, 240–243, 1990.

124. Stridh, S., Palm, F., and Hansell, P., Renal interstitial hyaluronan: Functional aspects during normal and pathological conditions, *Am. J. Physiol. Regul. Integr. Comp. Physiol.* 302, R1235–R11249, 2012.

125. Hansell, P., Maric, C., Alcorn, D., et al., Renomedullary interstitial cells regulate hyaluronan turnover depending on growth media osmolality suggesting a role in renal water handling, *Acta Physiol. Scand.* 165, 115–116, 1999.

126. Plante, G.E., Impact of aging on the body's vascular system, *Metabolism* 52(Suppl. 2), 31–35, 2003.

127. Reust, D.L., Reeves, S.T., Abernathy, J.H., III, et al., Interstitial plasmin activity with epsilon aminocaproic acid: Temporal and regional heterogeneity, *Ann. Thorac. Surg.* 89, 1538–1545, 2010.

128. Reust, D.L., Reeves, S.T., Abernathy, J.H, III, et al. Temporally and regionally disparate differences in plasmin activity by tranexamic acid, *Anesth. Analg.* 110, 694–701, 2010.

129. Reust, D.L., Dixon, J.A., McKinney, R.A., et al., Continuous localized monitoring of plasmin activity identifies differential and regional effects of the serine protease inhibitor aprotinin: Relevance to antifibrinolytic therapy, *J. Cardiovasc. Pharmacol.* 57, 400–406, 2011.

130. Haaverstad, R., Romslo, I., and Myhre, H.O., The concentration of high molecular weight compounds in interstitial tissue fluid: A study in patients with post-reconstructive leg oedema, *Eur. J. Vasc. Endovasc. Surg.* 13, 355–360, 1997.

131. Haaverstad, R., Romslo, I., Larsen, S., and Myhre, H.O., Protein concentration of subcutaneous interstitial fluid in the human leg, *Int. J. Microcirc.* 16, 111–116, 1996.

132. Anvar, M.D., Khiabani, H.Z., Lande, K., et al., The concentration of protein-compounds in interstitial tissue of patients with chronic critical limb ischaemia and oedema, *Vasa* 30, 14–20, 2001.

133. Butler, H.J., Ashton, L., Bird, B., et al., Using Raman spectroscopy to characterize biological materials, *Nat. Protoc.* 11, 664–687, 2016.

134. Russell, S., Nguyen, T.A., Torres, C.R., et al., Spatial frequency analysis of high-density lipoprotein and iron-oxide nanoparticle transmission electron microscope image structure for pattern recognition in heterogeneous fields, *J. Biomed. Opt.* 19, 15004, 2014.

135. Oveland, E., Karlsen, T.V., Haslene-Hox, H., et al., Proteomic evaluation of inflammatory proteins in rat spleen interstitial fluid and lymph during LPS-induced systemic inflammation reveals increased levels of ADAMTS1, *J. Proteome Res.* 11, 5338–5349, 2012.

136. Haslene-Hox, H., Overland, E., Woie, K., et al., Increased WD-repeat containing protein 1 in interstitial fluid from ovarian carcinomas shown by comparative proteomic analysis of malignant and healthy gynecological tissue, *Biochim. Biophys. Acta* 1834, 2347–2359, 2013.

137. Baronzio, G., Parmar, G., Baronzio, M., and Kiselevsky, M., Tumor interstitial fluid: Proteomic determination as a possible source of biomarkers, *Cancer Genomics Proteomics* 11, 225–237, 2014.

138. Haslene-Hox, H., Overland, E., Woie, K., et al., Distribution volumes of macromolecules in human ovarian and endometrial cancers: Effects of extracellular matrix structure, *Am. J. Physiol. Heart Circ. Physiol.* 308, H18–H28, 2015.

139. Pleitez, M., von Lilienfeld-Toal, H., and Mäntele, W., Infrared spectroscopic analysis of human interstitial fluid *in vitro* and *in vivo* using FT-IR spectroscopy and pulsed quantum cascade lasers (QCL): Establishing a new approach to non invasive glucose measurements, *Spectrochim. Acta A Mol. Biomol. Spectrosc.* 85, 61–65, 2012.

140. Vrancic, C., Kroger, N., Gretz, N., et al., A quantitative look inside the body: Minimally invasive infrared analysis *in vivo*, *Anal. Chem.* 86, 10511–10514, 2014.

141. Liakat, S., Michel, A.P.M., Bors, K.A., and Gmachl, C.F., Mid-infrared ($\lambda = 8.4$–9.9 μm) light scattering from porcine tissue, *Appl. Phys. Lett.* 101(9), 093705, 2012.

142. Rebrin, K. and Steil, G.M., Can interstitial glucose measurement replace blood glucose measurement? *Diabetes Technol. Ther.* 2, 461–472, 2000.

143. Keenan, D.B., Mastrototara, J.J., Wienzimer, S.A., and Steil, G.M., Interstitial fluid glucose time-lag correction for real-time continuous glucose monitoring, *Biomed. Signal. Process. Control* 8, 81–89, 2013.

144. Barman, I., Kong, C.R., Singh, C.P., Dasari, R.R., and Feld, M.S., Accurate spectroscopic calibration for noninvasive glucose monitoring by modeling the physiological glucose dynamics, *Anal. Chem.* 82, 6104–6114, 2010.

145. Ma, K., Yuen, J.M., Shah, N.C., et al., *In vivo*, transcutaneous glucose sensing using surface-enhanced spatially offset Raman spectroscopy: Multiple rats, improved hypoglycemic accuracy, low incident power, and continuous monitoring for greater than 17 days, *Anal. Chem.* 83, 9146–9152, 2011.

146. Ermakov, I.V. and Gellermann, W., Optical detection methods for carotenoids in human skin, *Arch. Biochem. Biophys.* 572, 101–111, 2015.

147. Holt, E.W., Wei, E.K., Bennett, N., and Zhang, L.M., Low skin carotenoid concentration measured by resonance Raman spectroscopy is associated with metabolic syndrome in adults, *Nutr. Res.* 34, 821–826, 2014.

148. Mateus, R., Moore, D.J., Hadgraft, J., and Lane, M.E., Percutaneous absorption of salicylic acid: *In vitro* and *in vivo* studies, *Int. J. Pharm.* 475, 471–474, 2014.

149. Chen, X., Grégoire, S., Formanek, F., Galey, J.B., Quantitative 3D molecular cutaneous absorption in human skin using label free nonlinear microscopy, *J. Control. Release* 200, 78–86, 2015.

150. Silveira, F.L., Pacheco, M.T., Bodanese, B., et al., Discrimination of non-melanoma skin lesions from non-tumor skin tissues *in vivo* using Raman spectroscopy and multivariate statistics, *Lasers Surg. Med.* 47, 6–16, 2015.

151. Azagury, A., Khoury, L., Enden, G., and Kost, J., Ultrasound mediated transdermal drug delivery, *Adv. Drug Deliv. Rev.* 72, 127–143, 2014.

152. Benitez, A., Edens, H., Fishman, J., Moran, K., and Asgharnejad, M., Rotigotine transdermal system developing continuous dopaminergic delivery to treat Parkinson's disease and restless legs syndrome, *Ann. N.Y. Acad. Sci.* 1329, 45–66, 2014.

153. Magistroni, R., Canto, M., Ligabue, G., et al., Interstitial fluid obtained from kidney biopsy as new source of renal biomarkers, *J. Nephrol.* 24, 329–337, 2012.

154. Semaeva, E., Tenstad, O., Bletsa, A., Gjerde, E.-A.B., and Wiig, H., Isolation of rat trachea interstitial fluid and demonstration of local cytokine production in lipopolysaccharide-induced systemic inflammation, *J. Appl. Physiol.* 104, 809–820, 2008.

155. Olausson, P., Gerdle, B., Ghafouri, N., Larsson, B., and Ghafouri, B., Identification of proteins from interstitium of trapezius muscle in women with chronic myalgia using microdialysis in combination with proteomics, *PLoS One* 7(12), e53560, 2012.

156. Celis, J.E., Gromov, P., Cabezón, T., et al., Proteomic characterization of the interstitial fluid perfusing the breast tumor microenvironment: A novel resource for biomarker and therapeutic target discovery, *Mol. Cell. Proteomics* 3, 327–344, 2004.

157. Celis, J.E., Moreira, J.M.A., Cabezón, T., et al., Identification of extracellular and intracellular signaling components of the mammary adipose tissue and its interstitial fluid in high risk breast cancer patients, *Mol. Cell. Proteomics* 4, 493–522, 2005.

158. Teng, P.-N., Rungruang, B.J., Hood, B.L., et al., Assessment of buffer systems for harvesting proteins from tissue interstitial fluid for proteomic analysis, *J. Proteome Res.* 9, 4161–4169, 2010.

159. Sun, W., Ma, J., Wu, S., et al., Characterization of the liver tissue interstitial fluid (TIF) proteome indicates potential for application in liver disease biomarker discovery, *J. Proteome Res.* 9, 1020–1031, 2010.

160. Smith, M.B., Applications of ultrasonic skin permeation in transdermal drug delivery, *Expert Opin. Drug Deliv.* 5, 1107–1120, 2008.

161. Polat, B.E., Seto, J.E, Blankschtein, D., and Langer, R., Application of the aqueous porous pathway model to quantify the effect of sodium lauryl sulfate on ultrasound-induced skin structural perturbation, *J. Pharm. Sci.* 100, 1387–1397, 2011.

162. Krishnan, G., Grice, J.E., Roberts, M.C., Benson, H.A., and Plow, T.W., Enhanced sonophoretic delivery of 5-aminolevulinic acid: Preliminary human *ex vivo* permeation data, *Skin. Res. Technol.* 19, e283–289, 2013.

163. Has, T. and Das, D.B., Permeability enhancement for transdermal delivery of large molecule using low-frequency sonophoresis combined with microneedles, *J. Pharm. Sci.* 102, 3614–3622, 2013.

164. Lecomte, M.M., Atkinson, K.R, Kay, D.P., Simons, J.L., and Ingram, J.R., A modified method using the SonoPrep ultrasonic skin permeation system for sampling human interstitial fluid is compatible with proteomic techniques, *Skin Res. Technol.* 19, 27–34, 2013.

165. Medina, A., Ghaffari, A., Kilani, R.T., and Chahary, A., The role of stratifin in fibroblast–keratinocyte interaction, *Mol. Cell. Biochem.* 305, 255–264, 2007.

166. Schleusener, J., Gluszczynska, P., Reble, C., et al., Perturbation factors in the clinical handling of a fiber-coupled Raman probe for cutaneous *in vivo* diagnostic Raman spectroscopy, *Appl. Spectrosc.* 69, 243–256, 2015.

167. Kiang, T.K., Schmidt, V., Ensom, M.H.H., Chua, B., and Häfei, U.O., Therapeutic drug monitoring in interstitial fluid: A feasibility study using a comprehensive panel of drugs, *J. Pharm. Sci.* 101, 4642–4652, 2012.

168. Quinn, H.L., Kearney, M.C., Courtenay, A.J., McCrudden, M.T., and Donnelly, R.F, The role of microneedles for drug and vaccine delivery, *Expert Opin. Drug Deliv.* 11, 1769–1780, 2014.

169. Han, T. and Das, D.B., Potential of combined ultrasound and microneedles for enhanced transdermal drug permeation: A review, *Eur. J. Pharm. Biopharm.* 89, 312–328, 2015.

170. Tronded, A., Nordén, B., Jeppsson, A.B., et al., Drug absorption from the isolated perfused rat lung: Correlations with drug physicochemical properties and epithelial permeability, *J. Drug Target.* 11, 61–74, 2003.

171. Hamman, J.H., Schultz, C.M., and Kotzé, A.F., N-Trimethyl chitosan chloride: Optimum degree of quaterization for drug absorption enhancement across epithelial cells, *Drug Dev. Ind. Pharm.* 29, 1161–1172, 2003.

172. Zhu, W., Liu, Z., Li, P., and Cheng, Z., Drug interaction studies reveal that simotinib upregulates intestinal absorption by increasing the paracellular permeability of intestinal epithelial cells, *Drug Metab. Pharmacokinet.* 29, 317–324, 2014.

173. Tanaka, T., Harada, N., and Kuze, J., Human small intestinal epithelial cells differentiated from adult intestinal stem cells as a novel system for predicting oral drug absorption in humans, *Drug. Metab. Dispos.* 42, 1947–1954, 2014.

174. Zhang, Y., Lukacova, V., Bartus, V., and Balaz, S., Structural determinants of binding of aromates to extracellular matrix: A multi-species multi-mode CoMFA study, *Chem. Res. Toxicol.* 20, 11–19, 2007.

175. Di Paolo, A. and Bocci, G., Drug distribution in tumors: Mechanisms, role in drug resistance, and methods for modification, *Curr. Oncol. Rep.* 9, 109–114, 2007.

176. Zhang, Y., Lukacova, V., Bartus, V., et al., Binding of matrix metalloproteinase inhibitors to extracellular matrix: 3D-QSAR analysis, *Chem. Biol. Drug Design* 72, 237–248, 2008.

177. Levina, A., Mitra, A., and Lay, P.A., Recent developments in ruthenium anticancer drugs, *Metallomics* 1, 458–470, 2009.

178. Swartz, M.A. and Fleury, M.E., Interstitial flow and its effects in soft tissues, *Annu. Rev. Biomed. Eng.* 9, 229–256, 2007.

179. Porter, C.J., Edwards, G.A., and Charman, S.A., Lymphatic transport of proteins after s.c. injection: Implications of animal model selection, *Adv. Drug Deliv. Rev.* 50, 157–171, 2001.

180. Heldin, C.H., Rubin, K., Pietras, K., and Ostman, A., High interstitial fluid pressure: An obstacle in cancer therapy, *Nat. Rev. Cancer* 4, 806–813, 2004.

181. Katz, F. and Warnecke, A., Finding the optimal balance: Challenges of improving conventional cancer chemotherapy using suitable combinations with nano-sized drug delivery systems, *J. Control. Release* 164, 221–235, 2012.

182. McGuire, S. and Yuan, F., Improving interstitial transport of macromolecules through reduction in cell volume fraction in tumor tissues, *Nanomedicine* 8, 1088–1095, 2012.

183. Amidon, G.L., Lennernäs, H., Shah, V.P., and Crison, J.E., A theoretical basis for a biopharmaceutic drug classification: The correlation of *in vitro* drug product dissolution and *in vivo* bioavailability, *Pharm. Res.* 12, 413–420, 1995.

184. Benet, L.Z., The role of BCS (Biopharmaceutics Classification System) and BDDCS (Biopharmaceutics Drug Disposition Classification System) in drug disposition, *J. Pharm. Sci.* 102, 34–42, 2013.

185. Fagerholm, U., Evaluation and suggested improvements of the Biopharmaceutics Classification System (BCS), *J. Pharm. Pharmacol.* 59, 751–757, 2007.

186. Tuominen, R.K., Männistö, P.T., Solkinen, A., et al., Antibiotic concentration in suction skin blister fluid and saliva after repeated dosage of erythromycin acetate and erythromycin base, *J. Antimicrob. Chemother.* 21(Suppl. D), 57–65, 1988.

187. Waters, N.J. and Lombardo, F., Use of the Øie–Tozer model in understanding mechanisms and determinants of drug distribution, *Drug. Metab. Dispos.* 38, 1159–1165, 2010.

188. Lemmer, H.J. and Hamman, J.H., Paracellular drug absorption enhancement through tight junction modulation, *Expert Opin. Drug Deliv.* 10, 103–114, 2013.

189. Kirschner, N., Rosenthal, R., Furuse, M., et al., Contribution of tight junction proteins to ion, macromolecule, and water barrier in keratinocytes, *J. Invest. Dermatol.* 133, 1161–1169, 2013.

190. Ghaffiarian, R. and Muro, S., Models and methods to evaluate transport of drug delivery systems across cellular barriers, *J. Vis. Exp.* 80, e50638, 2013.

191. Kolosov, D. and Kelly, S.P., A role for tricellulin in the regulation of gill epithelium permeability, *Am. J. Physiol. Regul. Integr. Comp. Physiol.* 304, R1139–1148, 2013.

192. Cavarelli, M., Foglieni, C., Rescigno, M., and Scarlatti, G., R5 HIV-1 envelope attracts dendritic cells to cross the human intestinal epithelium and sample luminal virions via engagement of the CCR5, *EMBO Mol. Med.* 5, 776–794, 2013.

193. Tordesillas, L., Gómez-Casado, C., Garrido-Arandia, M., et al., Transport of Pru p 3 across gastrointestinal epithelium: An essential step towards the induction of food allergy? *Clin. Exp. Allergy* 43, 1374–1383, 2013.

194. Girgagossian, C., Clark, T., Piché-Nicholas, N., and Bowman, C.J., Neonatal Fc receptor and its role in the absorption, distribution, metabolism and excretion of immunoglobulin G–based biotherapeutics, *Curr. Drug Metab.* 14, 764–790, 2013.

195. Copley, A.L. and Carol, B., Inhibiting action of epsilon aminocaproic acid on capillary permeability in guinea pigs tested with new quantitative method based on Straus peroxidase procedure: Variance and covariance analyses, *Life Sci.* 3, 65–76, 1964.

196. Katz, F. and Feher, P.J., Vascular permeability of human skin, *Dermatologica* 134, 173–176, 1967.

197. Don, F., Grosu, L., Pavel, T., et al., Influence of some inhibitors and activators on fibrinolysis on transcapillary transport of macromolecules, *Physiologie* 24, 153–160, 1987.

198. Fiume, L., Baglioni, M., Busi, C., Manerb, M., and Di Stefano, G., The enhancement of interstitial transport of a doxorubicin–lactosaminated albumin conjugate by imatinib: In rat hepatocellular carcinoma it is not preferentially higher than in liver and bone marrow, *Eur. J. Pharmaceut. Biopharmaceut.* 72, 630–631, 2009.

199. Tuokinen, R.K., Männistö, P.T., Solkinen, A., et al., Antibiotic concentration in suction skin blister fluid and saliva after repeated dosage of erythromycin acistrate and erythromycin base, *J. Antimicrob. Chemother.* 21(Suppl. D), 57–65, 1988.

200. Savolalnen, S., Männistö, P.T., Gordin, A., et al., Tonsillar penetration of erythromycin and its 2'acetyl ester in patients with chronic tonsillitis, *J. Antimicrob. Chemother.* 21(Suppl. D), 73–84, 1988.

201. Deguchi, Y., Terasaki, T., Yamada, H., and Tsuji, A., An application of microdialysis to drug tissue distribution study: *In vivo* evidence for free-ligand hypothesis and tissue binding of β-lactam antibiotics in interstitial fluid, *J. Pharmacobio-Dynamics* 15, 79–89, 1992.

202. Müller, M., Brunner, M., Schmid, R., et al., Comparison of three different experimental methods for the assessment of peripheral compartment pharmacokinetics in humans, *Life Sci.* 62, 227–234, 1996.

203. Gladue, R.P. and Snider, M.E., Intracellular accumulation of azithromycin by cultured human fibroblasts, *Antimicrob. Agents Chemother.* 34, 1056–1060, 1990.

204. Hariharan, S., Gunda, S., Mishra, G.P., Pal, D., and Mitra, A.K., Enhanced corneal absorption of erythromycin by modulating P-glycoprotein and MRP mediated efflux with corticosteroids, *Pharm. Res.* 26, 1270–1282, 2009.

205. Muller-Serieys, C., Andrews, J., Vacheron, F., and Cantalloube, C., Tissue kinetics of telithromycin, the first ketolide antibacterial, *J. Antimicrob. Chemother.* 53, 149–157, 2004.

206. Joukhadar, C., Derendorf, H., and Müller, M., Microdialysis. A novel tool for clinical studies of anti-infective agents, *Eur. J. Clin. Pharmacol.* 57, 211–219, 2001.

207. Traunmüller, F., Fille, M., Thallinger, C., and Joukhadar, C., Multiple-dose pharmacokinetics of telithromycin in peripheral soft tissues, *Int. J. Antimicrob. Agents* 34, 72–75, 2009.

208. Slevin, M.L., Wollard, R.D., Lister, T.A., et al., Relationship between protein binding and extravascular drug concentrations of a water-soluble drug, cytosine arabinoside, *J. R. Soc. Med.* 76, 365–368, 1983.

209. Dancik, Y., Anissimov, Y.G., Jepps, O.G., and Roberts, M.S., Convective transport of highly plasma protein bound drugs facilitates direct penetration into deep tissues after topical application, *Br. J. Clin. Pharmacol.* 73, 564–578, 2012.
210. Oussoren, C. and Storm, G., Liposomes to target the lymphatics by subcutaneous administration, *Adv. Drug Deliv. Rev.* 50, 143–156, 2001.
211. Brown, L.R., Commercial challenge of protein drug delivery, *Expert Opin. Drug Deliv.* 2, 29–42, 2005.
212. Vaishya, R., Khurana, B., Patel, S., and Mitra, A.K., Long-term delivery of protein therapeutics, *Expert Opin. Drug Deliv.* 12, 415–440, 2015.
213. Lin, J., Kelsberg, G., and Safranek, S., Clinical inquiry: Is high-dose oral B_{12} a safe and effective alternative to a B_{12} injection? *J. Fam. Pract.* 61, 162–163, 2012.
214. Kinnunen, H.M. and Mrsny, R.J., Improving the outcomes of biopharmaceutical delivery via the subcutaneous route by understanding the chemical, physical and physiological properties of the subcutaneous injection site, *J. Control. Release* 182, 22–32, 2014.
215. Abolhassani, H., Sadaghiani, M.S., Aghamohammadi, A., Och, H.D., and Rezaei, N., Home-based subcutaneous immunoglobulin versus hospital-based intravenous immunoglobulin in treatment of primary antibody deficiencies: Systematic review and meta analysis, *J. Clin. Immunol.* 32, 1180–1192, 2012.
216. Chapel, H. and Gardulf, A., Subcutaneous immunoglobulin replacement therapy: The European experience, *Curr. Opin. Allergy Clin. Immunol.* 13, 623–629, 2013.
217. Ali Khan, A., Mudassir, J., Montar, N., and Darwin, Y., Advanced drug delivery to the lymphatic system: Lipid-based nanoformulations, *Int. J. Nanomedicine* 8, 2733–2744, 2013.
218. Jolles, S., Orange, J.S., Gardulf, A., et al., Current treatment options with immunoglobulin G for the individualization of care in patients with primary immunodeficiency disease, *Clin. Exp. Immunol.* 179, 146–160, 2015.
219. Takeuchi, T., Kitagawa, H., and Harada, E., Evidence of lactoferrin transportation into blood circulation from intestine via lymphatic pathway in adult rats, *Exp. Physiol.* 89, 263–270, 2004.
220. Nojima, Y., Suzuki, Y., Iguchi, K., et al., Development of poly(ethylene glycol)-conjugated lactoferrin for oral administration, *Bioconjug. Chem.* 19, 2253–2259, 2008.
221. Yugi, M., Fujimoto, M., Zi, W.-M., et al., Persorption of IgG-Fc-coated particulates from intestinal lumen into portal blood via villous columnar epithelial cells in rat small intestine, *J. Vet. Med. Sci.* 74, 1447–1452, 2012.
222. Aukland, K. and Reed, R.K., Interstitial-lymphatic mechanisms in the control of extracellular fluid volume, *Physiol. Rev.* 73, 1–78, 1993.
223. Jiang, J., Moore, J.S., Edelhauser, H.F., and Prausnitz, M.R., Intrascleral drug delivery in the eye using hollow microneedles, *Pharm. Res.* 26, 395–403, 2009.
224. Stienstra, R., Joosten, L.A., Koenen, T., et al., The inflammasome-mediated caspace-1 activation controls adipocyte differentiation and insulin sensitivity, *Cell Metab.* 12, 593–605, 2010.
225. Lupfer, C., Malik, A., and Kaneganti, T.D., Inflammasome control of viral infection, *Curr. Opin. Virol.* 12, 38–46, 2015.
226. Vanaja, S.K., Rathinam, V.A., and Fitzgerald, K.A., Mechanism of inflammasome activation: Recent advances and novel insights, *Trends Cell Biol.* 25, 308–315, 2015.
227. Osikowicz, M., Longo, G., Allard, S., Cuello, A.C., and Rebeiro-da-Silva, A., Inhibition of endogenous NGF degradation induces mechanical allodynia and thermal hyperalgesia in rats, *Mol. Pain* 9, 37, 2013.
228. Shi, Q., Kuether, E.L., Schroeder, J.A., Fahs, S.A., and Montgomery, R.R., Intravascular recovery of VWF and FVIII following intraperitoneal injection and differences from intravenous and subcutaneous injection in mice, *Haemophilia* 18, 639–646, 2012.

229. Fatouros, A., Liden, Y., and Sjöström, B., Recombinant factor VIII SQ: Stability of VIII: C in homogenates from porcine, monkey, and human subcutaneous tissue, *J. Pharm. Pharmacol.* 52, 797–805, 2000.

230. Tatsumi, K., Sugimoto, M., Lillicrap, D., et al., A novel cell-sheet technology that achieves durable factor VIII delivery in a mouse model of hemophilia A, *PLoS One* 8(12), e83280, 2013.

231. Kashiwara, Y., Ohmori, T., Mimuro, J., et al., Intra-articular injection of mesenchymal stem cells expressing coagulation ameliorates hemophilic arthropathy in factor VIII–deficient mice, *J. Thromb. Haemost.* 10, 1802–1813, 2012.

232. Peng, A., Gaitonde, P., Kosloski, M.P., et al., Effect of route of administration of human recombinant factor VIII on its immunogenicity in hemophilia A mice, *J. Pharm. Sci.* 98, 4480–4484, 2009.

233. Schwendeman, S.P., Shah, R.B., Bailey, B.A., and Schwendeman, A.S., Injectable controlled release depots for large molecules, *J. Control Release* 190, 240–253, 2014.

234. Martinez-Saguer, I., Cicardi, M., Suffritti, C., et al., Pharmacokinetics of plasma-derived C1-esterase inhibitor after subcutaneous versus intravenous administration in subjects with mild or moderate hereditary angioedema: The PASSION study, *Transfusion* 54, 1552–1561, 2014.

235. Song, H.-F., Liu, X.-W., Zhang, H.-N., et al., Pharmacokinetics of His-tag recombinant human endostatin in Rhesus monkeys, *Acta Pharmacol. Sin.* 26, 124–128, 2005.

236. Berger, M., Subcutaneous IgG in neurologic diseases, *Immunotherapy* 6, 71–83, 2014.

237. Enders, J.F., Chemical, clinical and immunological studies on the products of human plasma fractionation: X. The concentrations of certain antibodies in globulin fractions derived from human blood plasma, *J. Clin. Invest.* 23, 510–530, 1944.

238. Cohn, E.J., Oncley, J.L., Strong, L.E., Hughes, W.L., and Armstrong, S.H., Chemical, clinical, and immunological studies on the products of human plasma fractionation: I. Characterization of the protein fractions of human plasma, *J. Clin. Invest.* 23, 417–432, 1944.

239. Stokes, J., Jr., Maris, E.P., and Gellis, S.S., Chemical, clinical and immunological studies on the products of human plasma fractionation: XI. The use of concentrated normal human serum gamma globulin (human immune serum globulin) in the prophylaxis and treatment of measles, *J. Clin. Invest.* 23, 531–549, 1944.

240. Ellis, E.F. and Henney, C.S., Adverse reactions following administration of human gamma globulin, *J. Allergy* 43, 45–54, 1969.

241. Lundblad, R.L., Plasma immunoglobulins, in *Biotechnology of Plasma Proteins*, Chapter 4, pp. 183–232, CRC Press/Taylor and Francis, Boca Raton, FL, 2013.

242. Paganelli, G., Riva, P., Moscatelli, G., et al., Improved immunoscintigraphy by subcutaneous injection of ^{99m}Tc or ^{111}In labelled F(ab')$_2$ fragments of an anti-melanoma monoclonal antibody, *Int. J. Rad. Appl. Instrum.* B 13, 423–428, 1986.

243. Keenan, A.M., Weinstein, J.N., Mulshine, J.L., et al., Immunolymphoscintigraphy in patients with lymphoma after subcutaneous injection of indium-111-labeled T101 monoclonal antibody, *J. Nucl. Med.* 28, 42–46, 1987.

244. Walh, R.L., Laino, L., Schteingart, M., and Beierwaltes, W.H., Improved radioimmunolocalization of human tumor xenografts following subcutaneous delivery on monoclonal antibodies, *Eur. J. Nucl. Med.* 13, 530–536, 1988.

245. Schnitzer, T.J., Yocum, D.E., Michalska, M., et al., Subcutaneous administration of CAMPATH-1H: Clinical and biological outcomes, *J. Rheumatol.* 24, 1031–1036, 1997.

246. Yang, M.X., Shenoy, B., Disttler, M., et al., Crystalline monoclonal antibodies for subcutaneous delivery, *Proc. Natl. Acad. Sci. USA* 100, 6934–6939, 2003.

247. Chinen, J. and Shearer, W.T., Subcutaneous immunoglobulins: Alternative for the hypogammaglobulinemic patient? *J. Allergy Clin. Immunol.* 114, 934–935, 2004.
248. Saeedian, M. and Randhawa, I., Immunoglobulin replacement therapy: A twenty-year review and current update, *Int. Arch. Allergy Immunol.* 164, 151–166, 2014.
249. Pinto, A.C., Ades, F., de Azambuja, E., and Piccart-Gebhart, M., Trastuzumab for patients with HER2 positive breast cancer: Delivery, duration and combination therapies, *Breast* 22(Suppl. 2), S152–S155, 2013.
250. Normansell, R., Walker, S., Milan, S.J., Walters, E.H., and Nair, P., Omalizumab for asthma in adults and children, *Cochrane Database Syst. Rev.* 1, CD003559, 2013.
251. Leveque, D., Subcutaneous administration of anticancer agents, *Anticancer Res.* 34, 1579–1586, 2014.
252. Cicero, A.F., Tartagni, E., and Ertek, S., Efficacy and safety profile of evolocumab (AMG145), an injectable inhibitor of the proprotein convertase subtilisin/kexin type 9: The available clinical evidence, *Expert Opin. Biol. Ther.* 14, 863–868, 2014.
253. Pathak, A.P., Artemov, D., Ward, B.D., et al., Characterizing extravascular fluid transport of macromolecules in the tumor interstitium by magnetic resonance imaging, *Cancer Res.* 65, 1425–1432, 2005.
254. Matsuo, M., Matsumoto, S., Mitchell, J.B., et al., Magnetic resonance imaging of the tumor microenvironment in radiotherapy: Perfusion, hypoxia, and metabolism, *Semin. Radiat. Oncol.* 24, 210–217, 2014.
255. Persson, A.I., Ikhanizadeh, S., Miroshnikova, Y.A., et al., High interstitial fluid pressure regulates tumor growth and drug uptake in human glioblastoma, *Neuro. Oncol.* 16(Suppl. 3), iii32, 2014.
256. Boucher, Y., Leunig, M., and Jain, R.K., Tumor angiogenesis and interstitial hypertension, *Cancer Res.* 56, 4264–4266, 1996.
257. Butler, T.P., Grantham, F.H., and Gullino, P.M., Bulk transport of fluid in the interstitial compartment of mammary tumors, *Cancer Res.* 35, 3084–3088, 1975.
258. Roy, S. and Sarkar, C., Ultrastructural study of micro-blood vessels in human brain tumors and peritumoral tissue, *J. Neurooncol.* 7, 283–292, 1989.
259. Brekken, C., Bruland, Ø.S., and de Lange Davies, C., Interstitial fluid pressure in human osteosarcoma xenografts: Significance of implantation site and the response to intratumoral injection of hyaluronidase, *Anticancer Res.* 20, 3503–3512, 2000.
260. Jacobsen, A., Salnikov, A., Lammerts, E., et al., Hyaluronan content in experimental carcinoma is not correlated to interstitial fluid pressure, *Biochem. Biophys. Res. Commun.* 305, 1017–1023, 2003.
261. Bjørnes, I. and Rofstad, E.K., Transvascular and interstitial transport of a 19 kDa linear molecule in human melanoma xenografts measured by contrast-enhanced magnetic resonance imaging, *J. Magn. Reson. Imaging* 14, 606–616, 2001.
262. Pathak, C.S., Blasberg, R.G., and Fenstermacher, J.D., Graphical evaluation of blood-to-brain transfer constants from multiple-time uptake data, *J. Cereb. Blood Flow Metab.* 3, 1–7, 1983.
263. Huang, C.M., Ananathaswamy, H.N., Barnes, S., et al., Mass spectrometric proteomics profiles of *in vivo* tumor secretomes: Capillary ultrafiltration sampling of regressive tumor masses, *Proteomics* 6, 6107–6116, 2006.
264. Wang, H., Tang, H.Y., Tan, G.C., and Speicher, D.W., Data analysis strategy for maximizing high-confidence protein identifications in complex proteomes such as human tumor secretomes and human serum, *J. Proteome Res.* 10, 4993–5005, 2011.
265. Shi, H.J., Stubbs, R., and Hood, K., Characterization of *de novo* synthesized proteins released from human colorectal tumor explants, *Electrophoresis* 30, 2442–2453, 2009.

266. Shi, H., Hood, K.A. Hayes, M.T., and Stubbs, R.J., Proteomic analysis of advanced colorectal cancer by laser capture microdissection and two-dimensional electrophoresis, *J. Proteomics* 75, 339–351, 2011.

267. Zeng, X., Yang, P., Chen, B., et al., Quantitative secretome analysis reveals the interactions between epithelia and tumor cells by an *in vitro* modulating colon cancer microenvironment, *J. Proteomics* 89, 51–70, 2013.

2 The Extracellular Matrix, Basement Membrane, and Glycocalyx

2.1 MATRICES THAT MODULATE INTERSTITIAL FLUID COMPOSITION

Unlike blood or the digestive tract, proteolytic enzymes in the interstitial space function within a matrix consisting of collagen, other proteins such as vitronectin and fibronectin, and sulfated proteoglycans such as syndecan and chondroitin sulfate. The macromolecules have the potential to modulate the activity of various proteases, as described in subsequent chapters on various groups of proteases. For example, vitronectin accelerates the inactivation of thrombin by plasminogen activator inhibitor-1 (PAI-1) by several orders of magnitude.[1] The activation of plasminogen to plasmin by urokinase-type plasminogen activator (uPA) is slightly enhanced by the extracellular matrix (ECM).[2] Subsequent work from this group[3] showed that collagen I was most effective in stimulating plasminogen activation by uPA, while collagen IV and vitronectin were less effective; inhibition of uPA activation of plasminogen was observed with fibronectin and laminin. Collagen IV is a unique component of basement membrane (BM), while laminin is a major component (Section 2.3). Moser and coworkers[3] did report that uPA bound to vitronectin with higher affinity than that observed for the other ECM components. There is a paucity of studies on the effect of the ECM or ECM components on proteolytic activity in the interstitial space and there are few studies other than that of Moser and coworkers that have solid kinetic data. Such studies are needed to determine the effect of such interactions on interstitial physiology.

There are two so-called membranes—or, more accurately, matrices—that are important to the composition of the interstitial fluid: the glycocalyx and the BM. The glycocalyx and the BM are referred to as membranes on the basis that they restrict passage. The ECM is not as much a membrane as it is a matrix or zone that surrounds cells,[4–7] and can also be referred to as the mesenchyme or stroma. The interstitial fluid is contained within the ECM.[7] Wiig and coworkers[7] suggest that the interstitium consists of two phases: the interstitial fluid and the ECM. The glycocalyx can act as a filter for the process of extravasation. The BM and ECM bind components of the interstitial fluid such as growth factors and proteolytic enzymes, serving both as a storage site and a microenvironment separate from bulk interstitial solution. An examination of several histology texts suggests that the ECM should be considered a connective tissue but with characteristics quite different from bone and cartilage, the connective tissues responsible for the support of skeletal elements. The

BM (Section 2.3) is considered to be distinct from the ECM but similar in composition in that both contain collagen, protein, proteoglycans, and mucopolysaccharides. Farquhar[8] defines the BM as a "continuous sheet of ECM material composed of collagens and non-collagenous glycoproteins." Elsewhere, Farquhar[9] observes that the definition of structures such as the ECM and BM resulted from developments in electron microscopy. The BM can be distinguished from the ECM by its content of collagen type IV;[10,11] collagen type IV is absent from the ECM. Laminin, a large, complex glycoprotein with isoforms, is also mostly found in the BM.[11,12] The glycocalyx (Section 2.3) is a polysaccharide-rich lining that can be found on intestinal epithelium and on the vascular luminal endothelium;[13] a glycocalyx also surrounds most cells, including bacteria. The glycocalyx is thought to have a role in capillary permeability, influencing the composition of the interstitial fluid, while components of the interstitial fluid can interact with the ECM and BM.

2.2   EXTRACELLULAR MATRIX

The ECM is produced by the cells for which it will provide support[14–16] in multicellular organisms (metazoa).[17–19] The composition of the ECM is complex, consisting of structural components (Table 2.1) such as collagen, proteoglycans, elastin, fibronectin, von Willebrand factor, and heparan sulfate proteoglycans.[20,21] Several proteins, such as collagens and fibronectin, would be considered intrinsic to the ECM and, as noted by Timpl and Martin,[22] are multidomain proteins capable of interaction with other proteins and cells. It is also apparent that glycosaminoglycans (mucopolysaccharides) such as chondroitin sulfate and keratin sulfate are also important structural components; heparan may also be a structural component, while hyaluronan, another proteoglycan, is considered a component of the interstitial fluid (Chapter 3). The ECM is not a static, homogeneous structure but rather varies within a tissue and from one tissue to another.[7,23]

While the term *extracellular matrix* did not appear until the latter half of the twentieth century, it was recognized by earlier investigators as "loose connective tissue," the first citation of which appeared in 1919.[24] Early work described the function of loose connective tissue composed of collagen fibers with an interstitium occupied by a mucopolysaccharide such as hyaluronan.[25] From this observation and other studies, it would appear that the loose connective tissue described in these early studies may be closely related to the ECM.[26–28] Ragan[28] mentioned support, transport, storage, and wound healing as functions of loose connective tissue (loose areolar tissue). However, the first citation that we could find to the actual term extracellular matrix was in the title of a conference sponsored by the Columbia University School of Medicine in 1964.[29] During the next decade, there were sporadic reports on the formation and function of the ECM. In early studies, Cooper and Prockop[30] demonstrated the extrusion of collagen by connective tissues and the transfer of collagen from "ground cytoplasm" to the ECM. Elsedale and Foley[31] showed that the lung fibroblasts in culture secreted layers of collagen, which in turn served as a surface for colonization; a matrix is only secreted by immobilized cells. Other early work[32,33] had suggested that nucleic acids were an important component of the ECM. Subsequent work suggested that it was likely that the presence of nucleic acids was

TABLE 2.1
Some Macromolecular Constituents of Extracellular Matrix and Basement Membrane[1-5]

Constituent	Comment
Aggrecan	A large chondroitin sulfate containing proteoglycan (2.5×10^6), which is a major constituent of cartilage ECM. Aggrecan is an asymmetric proteoglycan where the N-terminal G1 domain interacts with hyaluronan, forming a ternary complex with the link protein, thus retaining aggrecan in cartilage.[6] The C-terminal G3 domain contains two EGF-like repeats, a C-type lectin domain and a complement regulatory protein (CRP). The function of the terminal G3 domain is not defined, but defects have phenotypic consequences. Aggrecan is degraded by ADAMTS-4 (aggrecanase-1) and ADAMTS-5 (aggrecanase-2)[7] by cleavage of the Glu^{373}-Ala^{374} peptide bond, which is considered important in cartilage destruction.[8] ADAMTS-4 is bound to chondroitin sulfate and heparan sulfate on syndecan-1 following activation by MMP-17.[9] As with other components of cartilage and similar tissue, aggrecan has a longer half-life than, for example, plasma proteins, which are measured in hours and, with albumin and immune globulin, days. The half-life of aggrecan as determined by aspartic acid racemization is, dependent on region, 5–23 years.[10]
Chondroitin sulfate	Chondroitin sulfate is a viscous anionic polysaccharide with a molecular weight of approximately 50 kDa, composed of N-acetylchondrosine, a repeating sulfated disaccharide. Chondroitin sulfate, dermatan sulfate, and heparan sulfate are components of conjugate proteoglycans such as versican, considered important for interaction with cell surface integrins,[3] and ECM components such as fibulin-1 and collagen.[11] Chondroitin sulfate has been shown to promote the autoactivation of cathepsin K and subsequent collagen degradation.[12] Chondroitin sulfate likely binds thrombin at one of the anion-binding sites and may influence its activity in zymogen activation.[13,14] As an anionic moiety in a proteoglycan, chondroitin sulfate does not bind proteins as tightly as heparan sulfate proteoglycans.[15,16] There are regional differences in the degree of sulfation of chondroitin sulfate proteoglycans.[17] Chondroitin sulfate has been reported to occur as a complex hybrid glycosaminoglycan with keratin and heparan sulfate in perlecan found in the BM in epithelial cells.[18]
COMP	COMP (cartilage oligomeric matrix protein; thrombospondin-5) is a large (524 kDa) protein consisting of five identical subunits linked by disulfide bonds.[2,19] Electron microscopy has established the structure as having a central "assembly domain" with five arms, giving a "star-like" appearance with peripheral globular domains.[20] These domains interact with a variety of ECM proteins including collagen I, collagen III, and fibronectin.[2] Data have been presented suggesting that COMP is an inhibitor of thrombin.[21] This inhibition may be similar to the interaction of heparan sulfate proteoglycan with thrombin, which is important for the regulation of MMP-2 activity.[22] ADAMTS-7 and ADAMTS-12 degrade COMP.[23,24]

(Continued)

TABLE 2.1 (CONTINUED)
Some Macromolecular Constituents of Extracellular Matrix and Basement Membrane[1-5]

Constituent	Comment
Collagen I	Collagen I forms fibrils in the interstitial space, giving rise to the early description of the ECM as "loose connective tissue." Collagen I is the predominant collagen in the interstitial space and provides binding sites for other structural proteins such as fibronectin.[25] Collagen I, together with hyaluronan, provides the major barrier to drug transport in the interstitial space.[26] MMP-9 has been demonstrated to bind to collagen I, and the binding may serve to regulate enzyme activity.[27] There have been mixed reports on the ability of MMP-9 to digest collagen, with recent work showing that MMP-9 can digest soluble triple-helix collagens.[28] The interaction of matrix metalloproteinases with collagen is complex; MMP-9 can move along a collagen fragment to a susceptible site and "unwind" the soluble fibril with "helicase" activity.[29] Collagen type I has also been reported to bind osteopontin[30] and has been shown to enhance the binding of MMP-2 and MMP-9 to fibrin.[31-] Collagen I (and collagens II and III) are known for a close association with fibronectin in the ECM.[32] It is suggested that fibronectin is required for the *in vivo* formation of fibrils.[33] Fibrin(ogen) also binds to collagen I, providing a link to integrins on cells such as fibroblasts.[34] The binding of fibrin(ogen) to collagen I occurs at a site known to bind MMP-1. As with MMP-9, the interaction of MMP-1 with collagen is complex, with the unwinding of the triple helix only taking place after the first peptide bond cleavage.[35]
Collagen III	Together with collagen I, collagen III is a structural component of the ECM in the interstitial space.[36,37] Collagen III can form heterotypic fibrils with collagen I.[36,38] Collagen II also contributes to fibrillar structure together with fibril-associated collagen with interrupted triplet (FACIT).[39]
Collagen IV	Collagen IV is a nonfibrillar collagen unique to the BM that interacts with other BM components such as nidogen, perlecan, and laminin.[40-42] Matrikines can be derived from the fragmentation of collagen IV, which can inhibit angiogenesis and limit tumor growth.[43] Collagen IV binds other proteins including blood coagulation factor IX,[44] osteogenin,[45] integrins,[46] IGFBP-5,[47] osteopontin,[30] tissue factor microparticles,[48] and pro-MMP-9 (latent MMP-9).[49] The specific binding of pro-MMP-9 may have a role in the degradation of collagen IV or in targeting cell–matrix interactions. Collagen IV has also been reported to enhance the binding of MMP-2 and MMP-9 to fibrin.[31]
Collagen VII	Collagen VII is a major component of anchoring fibrils, which connect the BM to the underlying matrix (stroma)[50,51] via terminal nonhelical globular NC-1 domains.[52] Anchoring fibrils are responsible for connecting the epidermis and dermis layers in skin and a defect in the function of collagen VII has devastating consequences.[53,54] The IV administration of recombinant collagen VII has shown promise in reversing phenotypes in a murine model of recessive dystrophic epidermolysis bullosa.[55]

TABLE 2.1 (CONTINUED)
Some Macromolecular Constituents of Extracellular Matrix and Basement Membrane[1-5]

Constituent	Comment
Dermatan sulfate	Dermatan sulfate (chondroitin sulfate B) is similar to chondroitin sulfate in being an anionic polysaccharide composed of a repeating sulfated disaccharide, which differs from chondroitin sulfate in that dermatan sulfate contains iduronic acid, whereas chondroitin sulfate contains glucuronic acid. Dermatan sulfate proteoglycans are associated with the BM collagen IV matrix[56-58] and with fibrillar collagen in the ECM.[59,60] Biglycan and decorin are two proteoglycans containing dermatan sulfate that bind to ECM collagen and accelerate the inactivation of thrombin by heparin cofactor II.[61] Dermatan sulfate and chondroitin sulfate are found as a hybrid glycosaminoglycan in some large proteoglycans.[62-64]
Elastin	Elastin is the primary component (90%) of elastic fibers in the ECM in tissues such as skin, lungs, and ligaments where shape change (deformability) is required.[65] Elastin (tropoelastin) is composed of large hydrophobic domains, containing proline, glycine, and valine, interspersed with lysine-rich regions, which can participate in cross-linking reactions.[3,65] Elastin is formed from a precursor, tropoelastin, which is deposited on a glycoprotein, fibrillin. The splicing of tropoelastin mRNA is tissue specific and developmentally specific.[66] Elastin has an extremely long half-life estimated at 70 years,[67] resulting in significant glycation as part of the aging process.[68] Lysozyme has been reported to bind to elastin and protects degradation by several elastases.[69,70] The binding appears to be specific in that BSA does not compete for binding; the bound lysozyme is inactive.
Fibrillins	Fibrillins are large glycoproteins (M_r 350 kDa) found in the ECM.[3] It is interesting in that fibrillin contains 14% total cysteine/cystine, of which one-third is present as cysteine.[71] The average content of cysteine in proteins is usually 0.3%–1.7%.[72] Fibrillin is associated with the framework for the formation of elastin fibers.[73,74] Fibrillin 1 has been suggested to provide extracellular control of growth factor signaling[75] with the involvement of ADAMTS proteins.[75,76]
Fibrinogen	Fibrinogen is deposited into the ECM.[77,78] There is no evidence for the deposition of fibrin into an *in vivo* ECM. However, earlier work has shown that the binding of fibrin to a plastic surface[79] or to platelet receptor[80] also induced conformational changes that, on the basis of immunological reactivity, are similar to those observed on the conversion of fibrinogen to fibrin. It is therefore likely that fibrinogen bound in the ECM acts like fibrin in binding other constituents in the interstitial space. MMP-2 and MMP-9 have been shown to bind to fibrin[31] and it has been suggested that this binding protects the enzymes from inactivation by inhibitors such as TIMPs. Thrombin binds to fibrin with retention of activity.[81] Thrombin and fibrin can also form a ternary complex with heparin.[62] It is not unreasonable to suggest that a ternary complex could be formed between thrombin, fibrinogen, and heparan sulfate proteoglycan in the ECM. Basic FGF,[82] factor Xa,[83] and plasminogen[84] have also been shown to bind to fibrin(ogen).

(Continued)

TABLE 2.1 (CONTINUED)
Some Macromolecular Constituents of Extracellular Matrix and Basement Membrane[1-5]

Constituent	Comment
Fibromodulin	Fibromodulin is a keratin sulfate proteoglycan, which is one of several leucine-rich proteoglycans that are constituents in the ECM.[2] Fibromodulin, together with other leucine-rich proteoglycans, is suggested to be involved in the inflammatory response by interacting with toll-like receptors.[85] Fibromodulin and other leucine-rich proteoglycans are associated with collagen and important for fibrillogenesis.[86,87] Fibromodulin has been shown to interact with complement component C1q, resulting in a limited complement activation response, as fibromodulin also binds complement inhibitor factor H and C4b-binding protein.[88] There is a suggestion that the binding of TGFβ-1/latent TGFβ-1 by fibromodulin is a regulatory mechanism for the expression of this growth factor in the ECM.[89] Trappin-2 (pre-elafin), a small serine protease inhibitor secreted by epithelial cells and some immune cells,[90] is bound to fibromodulin in cartilage by the action of tissue transglutaminase.[91]
Fibronectin	Fibronectin is a plasma protein as well as a structural component of the ECM associated with collagen in the ECM and the BM.[92,93] Fibronectin is a monomer of 220 kDa composed of three domains—FN1, FN2, and FN3—forming a disulfide-linked dimer,[3,4,94] which, as result of variable splicing of mRNA, provides a multiplicity of variants.[95,96]
	Partially as a result of the production of variants, fibronectin is truly a pleiotropic protein with a multiplicity of functions,[3,4,97] including the organization of matrix proteins[3,98] and cell adhesion.[99] A variety of cells including fibroblasts, endothelial cells, and macrophages synthesize and secrete fibronectin.[94] Endothelial cells secrete fibronectin at the basolateral (subendothelial) surface, contributing to the formation of the BM.[100] Tissue transglutaminase binds to a specific site in fibronectin[101,102] with high affinity.[103] The binding of transglutaminase to fibronectin is noncovalent and enzymatic activity is retained.[104] Transglutaminase bound to fibronectin has been shown to cross-link plasminogen activator inhibitor-2 (PAI-2) to fibronectin[105] as well as elafin/trappin-2, with retention of inhibitory activity.[106,107]
Fibulin	Fibulins are a group of structural glycoproteins associated with ligands in the BM and the ECM (loose connective tissue).[108–110] Fibulins are divided into two classes based on length and domain structure. Fibulin-1 and fibulin-2 are structurally associated with other BM components such as nidogen, elastin, and laminin.[2,109,110] The function of short fibulins is enhanced by calcium ions, but calcium ions do not appear to be an obligate requirement.[2,111] Fibulin-1 has been shown to enhance ADAMTS-1 degradation of aggrecan.[112] Fibulin-5 has been shown to bind uPA, promoting its cleavage by plasmin, resulting in the dissociation of fibulin-5 from cell surface β1 integrin and facilitating cell migration.[113]
Laminin	Laminins are a family of large (500–800 kDa) glycoproteins that are closely associated with the basolateral surface of cells, forming a network with other BM components, supporting the subsequent development of a collagen IV network that associates with perlecan and nidogen.[114] As with other matrix components, laminins are suggested to have functions other than structural, such as signaling via the binding to integrins.[3,115] Thrombin and plasmin cleave laminin and the fragments maintain the ability to bind epithelial cells to collagen IV.[116]

TABLE 2.1 (CONTINUED)
Some Macromolecular Constituents of Extracellular Matrix and Basement Membrane[1-5]

Constituent	Comment
Nidogen (entactin)	Nidogen-1 (150 kDa) is a protein containing approximately 5% carbohydrate and 1–2 sulfated tyrosine residues.[2,117] Nidogen-1 is considered to have an important role in connecting laminins and collagen IV in the BM. Nidogen-2 (approximately 200 kDa) is a protein with homology to nidogen-1 but a higher degree of glycosylation.[118] Nidogen-2 has similar binding characteristics as nidogen-1 in that it binds to collagen IV and laminins. Nidogen-2 is also capable of binding to a transmembrane, collagen XIII, which can be found in the BM.[119]
Perlecan	Perlecan is a large (approximately 450 kDa) heparan sulfate proteoglycan in the BM.[2,120] While usually described as a heparan sulfate proteoglycan, perlecan is a hybrid proteoglycan containing chondroitin sulfate and heparan sulfate.[121] Perlecan binds to the cell surface and to other BM components. As with other proteoglycans found in both the ECM and the BM, perlecan binds peptide growth factors such as VEGF and FGF,[122,123] which can be released via degradation by proteolytic enzymes and heparanase.[124] The binding of TIMP-3 to perlecan (heparan sulfate and/or chondroitin sulfate) increases affinity for ADAMTS-5.[125] Thrombin has been shown to bind to the subendothelial matrix,[126,127] but receptor site(s) have not been identified; it is possible that perlecan could be responsible for the binding of thrombin as well as lipoprotein lipase.[128]
Tenascins	Tenascins are a group of glycoproteins composed of repeated domains ranging in weight from 150 to 380 kDa and associating in multimers.[2,3] Tenascins are considered matricellular proteins, which bind to matrix components, cell surfaces, and other components such as proteases.[129]
Thrombospondins	Thrombospondins (thrombin sensitive proteins) are a group of five multimeric matricellular proteins with a monomer weight of approximately 140 kDa.[130] Thrombospondin-1 forms a complex with MMP-2, which is recognized by the low-density lipoprotein-related protein receptor.[131] Thrombospondin has also been reported to inhibit plasmin[132,133] and neutrophil elastase,[134] as well as forming a complex with urokinase-type plasminogen activator (uPA), with retention of activity and protection from inactivation by PAI-1.[135] The binding of uPA to thrombospondin provides a mechanism for concentrating uPA within the ECM. Thrombospondin-1 has been reported to enhance the formation of the prothrombinase complex initiated by tissue factor on a fibroblast surface.[136]
Vitronectin	Vitronectin (serum spreading factor) is a plasma protein that is also a component of the ECM. While there are some minor extravascular sites of vitronectin synthesis,[137] the bulk of vitronectin is transported through endothelial cells via a facilitated pathway and deposited in the ECM.[138] Vitronectin has been described as a "master controller" or "micromanager" of the ECM environment.[137] Vitronectin binds to components of the ECM such as collagen and glycosaminoglycans.[137,139] Vitronectin is best known for binding components of the interstitial space including plasminogen activator inhibitor-1 (PAI-1).[140,141] Vitronectin binds a number of peptide growth factors and integrins.[137]

Note: It is acknowledged that this table is incomplete so as to emphasize the influence of ECM and BM components on the expression of proteolytic activity in the interstitial space.

REFERENCES FOR TABLE 2.1

1. Ayad, S., Boot-Handford, R. P., Humphries, M. J., Kadler, K.E., and Schuttleworth, C.A., *The Extracellular Matrix Facts Book*, Academic Press, San Diego, CA, 1998.
2. Kreis, T. and Vale, R., eds., *Guidebook to the Extracellular Matrix, Anchor, and Adhesion Proteins*, Oxford University Press, Oxford, UK, 1999.
3. Halper, J. and Kjaer, M., Basic components of connective tissues and extracellular matrix: Elastin, fibrillin, fibrinogen, fibronectin, laminin, tenascins and thrombospondins, *Adv. Exp. Med. Biol.* 802, 31–47, 2014.
4. Huxley-Jones, J., Foord, S.M., and Barnes, M.R., Drug discovery in the extracellular matrix, *Drug Discov. Today* 13, 685–694, 2008.
5. Coats, W.D., Jr. and Faxon, D.P., The role of the extracellular matrix in arterial remodeling, *Semin. Intervent. Cardiol.* 2, 167–176, 1997.
6. Aspberg, A., The different roles of aggrecan interaction domains, *J. Histochem. Cytochem.* 60, 987–996, 2012.
7. Verma, P. and Dalal, K., AMAMTS-4 and ADAMTS-5: Key enzymes in osteoarthritis, *J. Cell. Biochem.* 112, 3507–3514, 2011.
8. Fushimi, K., Troeberg, L., Nakamura, H., Lim, N.H., Nagase, H., Functional differences of the catalytic and non-catalytic domains in human ADAMTS-4 and ADAMTS-5 in aggrecanolytic activity, *J. Biol. Chem.* 283, 6706–6716, 2008.
9. Gao, G., Plaas, A., Thompson, V.P., et al., ADAMTS-4 (aggrecanase-1) activation on the cell surface involves C-terminal cleavage by glycosylphosphatidyl inositol–anchored membrane type 4-matrix metalloproteinase and binding of the activated proteinase to chondroitin sulfate and heparan sulfate on syndecan-1, *J. Biol. Chem.* 279, 10042–10051, 2004.
10. Sivan, S.S., Tsitron, E. Wachtel, E., et al., Aggrecan turnover in human intervertebral disc as determined by the racemization of aspartic acid, *J. Biol. Chem.* 281, 13009–13014, 2006.
11. Wu, Y.J., La Pierre, D.P., Wu, J., Yee, A.J., and Yang, B.B., The interaction of versican with its binding partners, *Cell Res.* 15, 483–494, 2005.
12. Lemaire, P.A., Huang, L., Zhuo, Y., et al., Chondroitin sulfate promotes activation of cathepsin K, *J. Biol. Chem.* 289, 21562–21572, 2014.
13. Galiani, D. and Broze, G.J., Jr., Effect of glycosaminoglycans on factor XI activation by thrombin, *Blood Coag. Fibrinol.* 4, 15–20, 1993.
14. Liu, L.W., Rezazie, A.R., Carson, C.W., Esmon, N.L., and Esmon, C.T., Occupancy of anion binding exosite 2 on thrombin determines Ca^{2+} dependence of protein C activation, *J. Biol. Chem.* 269, 11807–11812, 1994.
15. Chajek-Shaul, T., Friedman, G., Bengtsson-Olivecrona, G., Vlodavsky, T., and Bar-Shavit, R., Interaction of lipoprotein lipase with subendothelial extracellular matrix, *Biochim. Biophys. Acta* 1042, 168–174, 1990.
16. Billings, P.C. and Pacifici, M., Interaction of signaling proteins, growth factors and other proteins with heparan sulfate: Mechanisms and mysteries, *Connect. Tissue Res.* 56, 272–280, 2015.
17. Hoffman-Kim, D., Lander, A.D., and Jhaveri, S., Patterns of chondroitin sulfate immunoreactivity in the developing tectum reflect regional differences in glycosaminoglycan biosynthesis, *J. Neurosci.* 18, 5881–5890, 1998.
18. Knox, S., Fosang, A.J., Last, K., Melrose, J., and Whitelock, J., Perlecan from human epithelial cells is a hybrid heparan/chondroitin/keratan sulfate proteoglycan, *FEBS Lett.* 579, 5019–5023, 2005.
19. Hedbom, E., Antonsson, P., Hjerpe, A., et al., Cartilage matrix proteins: An acidic oligomeric protein (COMP) detected only in cartilage, *J. Biol. Chem.* 267, 6132–6136, 1992.

20. Mörgelin, M., Heinegård. D., Engel, J., and Paulsson, M., Electron microscopy of native cartilage oligomeric matrix protein purified from the Swarm rat chondrosarcoma reveals a five-armed structure, *J. Biol. Chem.* 267, 6137–6141, 1992.
21. Liang, Y., Fu, Y., Qi, R., et al., Cartilage oligomeric matrix protein is a natural inhibitor of thrombin, *Blood* 1226, 905–914, 2015.
22. Koo, B.H., Han, J.H., Yeom, Y.I., and Kim, D.S., Thrombin-dependent MMP-2 activity is regulated by heparan sulfate, *J. Biol. Chem.* 285, 41270–41279, 2010.
23. Kelwick, R., Desanlis, I., Wheeler, G.N., and Edwards, D.R., The ADAMTS (a distintegrin and metalloproteinase with thrombospondin motifs) family, *Genome Biol.* 16, 113, 2015.
24. Liu, C.J., Kong, W., Ilalov, K., et al., ADAMTS-7: A metalloproteinase that directly binds to and degrades cartilage oligomeric matrix protein, *FASEB J.* 20, 988–990, 2006.
25. Kubow, K.E., Vukmirovic, R., Zhe, L., et al., Mechanical forces regulate the interactions of fibronectin and collagen I in extracellular matrix, *Nat. Commun.* 6, 8026, 2015.
26. Eikenes, L., Tufto, I., Schnell, E.A., Bjørkøy, A., and de Lange Davies, C.., Effect of collagenase and hyaluronidase on free and anomalous diffusion in multicellular spheroids and xenografts, *Anticancer Res.* 30, 359–368, 2010.
27. Makela, M., Salo, T., and Larjava, H., MMP-9 from TNF α-stimulated keratinocytes binds to cell membranes and type I collagen: A cause for extended degradation in inflammation? *Biochem. Biophys. Res. Commun.* 253, 325–335, 1998.
28. Bigg, H.F., Rowan, A.D., Barker, M.D., and Cawston, T.E., Activity of matrix metalloproteinase-9 against native collagen types I and III, *FEBS J.* 274, 1246–1255, 2007.
29. Van Doren, S.R., Matrix metalloproteinase interactions with collagen and elastin, *Matrix Biol.* 44–46, 224–231, 2015.
30. Kaartinen, M.T., Pirhonen, A., Linnala-Kankkunen, A., and Mäenpää, P.H., Crosslinking of osteopontin by tissue transglutaminase increases its collagen binding properties, *J. Biol. Chem.* 274, 1729–1735, 1999.
31. Makowski, G.S. and Ramsby, M.L., Differential effect of calcium phosphate and calcium pyrophosphate on binding of matrix metalloproteinases to fibrin: Comparison to a fibrin-binding protease from inflammatory joint fluids, *Clin. Exp. Immunol.* 136, 176–187, 2004.
32. Engvall, E., Ruoslahti, E., and Miller, E.J., Affinity of fibronectin to collagens of different genetic types and to fibrinogen, *J. Exp. Med.* 147, 1584–1595, 1978.
33. Kadler, K.E., Hill, A., and Canty-Laird, E.G., Collagen fibrillogenesis: Fibronectin, integrins, and minor collagens as organizers and nucleators, *Curr. Opin. Cell Biol.* 20, 495–501, 2008.
34. Reyhani, V., Seddigh, P., Guss, B., et al., Fibrin binds to collagen and provides a bridge for αVβ3 integrin-dependent contraction of collagen gels, *Biochem. J.* 462, 113–123, 2014.
35. Fasciglione, G.F., Gioia, M., Tsukada, H., et al., The collagenolytic action of MMP-1 is regulated by the interaction between the catalytic domain and the hinge region, *J. Biol. Inorg. Chem.* 17, 663–672, 2012.
36. Fleischmajer, R., Perlish, J.S., Burgeson, R.E., Shaikh-Bahai, E., and Timpl, R., Type I and type III collagen interact during fibrillogenesis, *Ann. N.Y. Acad. Sci.* 580, 161–175, 1990.
37. Voss, B. and Rauterberg, J., Localization of collagen types I, III, IV, V, fibronectin and laminin in human arteries by the indirect immunofluorescence method, *Pathol. Res. Pract.* 181, 562–575, 1986.
38. Hulmes, D.J.S., Collagen diversity, synthesis and assembly, in *Collagen Structure and Mechanics*, ed. P. Fratzl, Chaper 2, pp. 15–47, Springer Science, New York, 2008.

39. Shaw, L.M. and Olsen, B.R., FACIT collagens: Diverse molecular bridges in extracellular matrices, *Trends Biochem. Sci.* 16, 191–194, 1991.

40. Timpl, R., Fujiwara, S., Dziadek, M., et al., Laminin, proteoglycan, nidogen and collagen IV: Structural models and molecular interactions, *Ciba Found. Symp.* 108, 25–43, 1984.

41. Pőschl, E., Schlőtzer-Schredhardt, U., Brachvogel, B., et al., Collagen IV is essential for basement membrane stability but dispensable for initiation of its assembly during early development, *Development* 131, 1619–1628, 2004.

42. Mayer, U., Zimmerman, K., Mann, K., et al., Binding properties and protease stability of recombinant nidogen, *Eur. J. Biochem.* 227, 681–686, 1995.

43. Monboisse, J.C., Oudart, J.B., Ramont, L., Brassart-Pasco, S., and Maquart, F.X., Matrikines from basement membrane collagens: A new anti-cancer strategy, *Biochim. Biophys. Acta* 1840, 2589–2598, 2014.

44. Cheung, W.F., van den Born, J., Kühn, K., et al., Identification of the endothelial cell binding site for factor IX, *Proc. Natl. Acad. Sci. USA* 93, 11068–11073, 1996.

45. Paralkar, V.M., Nandedkar, A.K., Pointer, R.H., Kleinman, H.K., and Reddi, A.H., Interaction of osteogenin, a heparin binding bone morphogenetic protein, with type IV collagen, *J. Biol. Chem.* 265, 17281–17284, 1990.

46. Aggeli, A.S., Kitsiou, P.V., Tzinia, A.K., et al., Selective binding of integrins from different renal cell types to the NC1 domain of $\alpha 3$ and $\alpha 1$ chains of type IV collagen, *J. Nephrology* 22, 130–136, 2009.

47. Clemmons, D.R., Busby, W.H., Arai, T., et al., Role of insulin-like growth factor binding proteins in control of IGF actions, *Prog. Growth Factor Res.* 6, 357–366, 1995.

48. Ettalaie, C., Collier, M.E.W., Mei, M.P., Xiao, Y.P., and Maraveyas, A., Enhanced binding of tissue factor–microparticles to collagen-IV and fibronectin leads to increased tissue factor activity *in vitro*, *Thromb. Haemost.* 109, 61–71, 2013.

49. Olson, M.W., Toth, M., Gervasi, D.C., et al., High affinity binding of latent matrix metalloproteinase-9 to the $\alpha 2$ (IV) chain of collagen IV, *J. Biol. Chem.* 273, 10672–10681, 1998.

50. Keene, D.R., Sakai, L.Y., Lunstrum, G.P., Morris, N.P., and Burgeson, R.E., Type VII collagen forms an extended network of anchoring fibrils, *J. Exp. Med.* 104, 611–621, 1987.

51. Bachinger, H.P., Morris, N.P., Lunstrum, G.P., et al., The reiationship of the biophysical characteristics of type VII collagen to the function of the anchoring fibrils, *J. Biol. Chem.* 265, 10095–10101, 1990.

52. Brittingham, R., Uitto, J., and Fertala, A., High-affinity binding of the NC1 domain of collagen VII to laminin 5 and collagen IV, *Biochem. Biophys. Res. Commun.* 34, 692–699, 2006.

53. Chung, H.J. and Uitto, J., Type VII collagen: The anchoring fibril protein at fault in dystrophic epidermolysis bullosa, *Dermatol. Clin.* 28, 93–105, 2010.

54. Skinkuma, S., Dystrophic epidermolysis bullosa: A review, *Clin. Cosmet. Invest. Dermatol.* 8, 275–284, 2015.

55. Hou, Y., Guey, L.T., Wu, T., et al., Intravenously administered recombinant human type VII collagen derived from Chinese hamster ovary cells reverses the disease phenotype in recessive dystrophic epidermolysis bullosa mice, *J. Invest. Dermatol.*, in press, 2015.

56. Vőlker, W., Schmidt, A., and Buddecke, E., Mapping of proteoglycans in human arterial tissue, *Eur. J. Biochem.* 45, 72–79, 1987

57. Faber, V., Quentin-Hoffman, E., Breuer, B., et al., Colocalization of a large heterodimeric proteoglycan with basement membrane proteins in cultured cells, *Eur. J. Cell Biol.* 59, 37–46, 1992.

58. Couchman, J.R., Kapoor, R., Sthanam, M., and Wu, R.R., Perlecan and basement membrane chondroitin sulfate proteoglycan (bamacan) are two basement membrane chondroitin sulfate/dermatan sulfate proteoglycans in the Engelbreth-Holm-Swarm tumor matrix, *J. Biol. Chem.* 271, 9595–9602, 1996.

59. Schönherr, E., Hausser, H., Beavan, L., and Kresse, H., Decorin-type I collagen interaction: Presence of separate core protein–binding domains, *J. Biol. Chem.* 270, 8877–8883, 1995.

60. Tenni, R., Viola, M., Welser, F., et al., Interaction of decorin with CNBr peptides from collagens I and II: Evidence for multiple binding sites and essential lysine residues in collagen, *Eur. J. Biochem.* 269, 1428–1437, 2002.

61. Whinna, H.C., Choi, H.U., Rosenberg, L.C., and Church, F.C., Interaction of heparin cofactor II with biglycan and decorin, *J. Biol. Chem.* 268, 3920–3924, 1993.

62. Sugahara, K. and Mikami, T., Chondroitin/dermatan sulfate in the central nervous system, *Curr. Opin. Struct. Biol.* 17, 536–545, 2007.

63. Du, W.W., Yang, W., and Yee, A.J., Roles of versican in cancer biology: Tumorogenesis, progress and metastasis, *Histol. Histopathol.* 28, 701–713, 2013.

64. Robu, A.C., Poescu, L., Muneanu, C.V., Seidler, D.G., and Zamfir, A.D., Orbitrap mass spectrometry characterization of hybrid chondroitin/dermatan sulfate hexasaccharide domains expressed in brain, *Anal. Biochem.* 485, 122–131, 2015.

65. Kielty, C.M., Elastic fibres in health and disease, *Exp. Rev. Mol. Med.* 8, 1–23, 2006.

66. Heim, R.A., Pierce, R.A., Deak, S.B., et al., Alternative splicing of rat tropoelastin mRNA is tissue-specific and developmentally regulated, *Matrix* 11, 359–366, 1991.

67. Urry, D.W., Pattanaik, A., Xu, J., et al., Elastic protein-based polymers in soft tissue augmentation and generation, *J. Biomater. Sci. Polym. Ed.* 9, 1015–1048, 1998.

68. Konova, E., Baydanoff, S., Atanasova, M., and Velkova, A., Age-related changes in the glycation of human aortic elastin, *Exp. Gerontol.* 39, 249–254, 2004.

69. Park, P.W., Biedermann, K., Mecham, L., Bissett, D.L., and Mecham, R.P., Lysozyme binds to elastin and protects elastin from elastase-mediated degradation, *J. Invest. Dermatol.* 106. 1075–1080, 1996.

70. Seite, S., Zucchi, H., Septier, D., et al., Elastin changes during chronological and photoaging: The important of lysozyme, *J. Eur. Acad. Dermatol. Venerol.* 20, 980–987, 2006.

71. Sakai, L.Y., Keene, D.R., Glanville, R.W., and Bachinger, H.P., Purification and partial characterization of fibrillin, a cysteine-rich structural component of connective tissue microfibrils, *J. Biol. Chem.* 266, 14763–14770, 1991.

72. Belitz, H.-D., Grosch, W., and Schieberle, P., *Food Chemistry*, 4th edn., Springer-Verlag, Heidelberg, Germany.

73. Rosenbloom, J., Abrams, W.R., and Mecham, R., Extracellular matrix 4: The elastic fiber, *FASEB J.* 7, 1208–1218, 1993.

74. Ramirez, F. and Sakai, L.Y., Biogenesis and function of fibrillin assemblies, *Cell Tissue Res.* 339, 71–82, 2010.

75. Sengle, G., Tsutsui, K., Keene, D.R., et al., Microenvironmental regulation by fibrillin-1, *PLoS Genet.* 8(1), e1002425, 2012.

76. Hubmacher, D. and Apte, S.S., ADAMTS proteins as modulators of microfibril formation and function, *Matrix Biol.* 47, 34–43, 2015.

77. Guadiz, G., Sporn, L.A., and Simpson-Haidaris, P.J., Thrombin cleavage–independent deposition of fibrinogen in extracellular matrix, *Blood* 90, 2644–2653, 1997.

78. Simpson-Haidaris, P.J. and Rybarczyk, B., Tumors and fibrinogen: The role of fibrinogen as an extracellular matrix protein, *Ann. N.Y. Acad. Sci.* 936, 406–425, 2001.

79. Zamarron, C., Ginsberg, M.H., and Plow, E.F., Monoclonal antibodies specific for a conformationally altered state of fibrinogen, *Thromb. Haemost.* 64, 41–46, 1990.

80. Zamarron, C., Ginsberg, M.H., and Plow, E.F., A receptor-induced binding site in fibrinogen elicited by its interaction with platelet membrane glycoprotein IIb-IIIa, *J. Biol. Chem.* 266, 16193–16199, 1991.

81. Hogg, P.J. and Jackson, C.M., Formation of a ternary complex between thrombin, fibrin monomer, and heparin influences the action of thrombin on its substrates, *J. Biol. Chem.* 265, 248–255, 1990.

82. Sahni, A., Odrljin, T., and Francis, C.W., Building of basic fibroblast growth factor to fibrinogen and fibrin, *J. Biol. Chem.* 273, 7554–7559, 1998.

83. Iino, M., Takeya H., Takemitsu, T., et al., Characterization of the binding of factor Xa to fibrinogen/fibrin derivatives and localization of the factor Xa binding site on fibrinogen, *Eur. J. Biochem.* 232, 90–97, 1995.

84. Adelman, B. and Quynn, P., Plasminogen interactions with immobilized fibrinogen, *Thromb. Haemost.* 62, 1078–1082, 1989.

85. Frey, H., Schroeder, N., Manon-Jensen, T., Iozzo, R.V., and Schaefer, L., Biological interplay between proteoglycans and their innate immune receptors in inflammation, *FEBS J.* 280, 2165–2179, 2013.

86. Yoon, J.H. and Halper, J., Tendon proteoglycans: Biochemistry and function, *J. Musculoskelet. Neuronal Interact.* 5, 22–34, 2005.

87. Halper, J., Proteoglycans and diseases of soft tissues, *Adv. Exp. Med. Biol.* 802, 49–58, 2014.

88. Happanen, K.E., Sjöberg, A.P., Mőrgelin, M., Heinegård, D., and Blom, A.M., Complement inhibitor C4b-binding protein interacts directly with small glycoproteins of the extracellular matrix, *J. Immunol.* 182, 1518–1525, 2009.

89. Hildebrand, A., Romaris, M., Rasmussen, L.M., et al., Interaction of the small interstitial proteoglycans biglycan, decorin and fibronectin with transforming growth factor β, *Biochem. J.* 302, 527–534, 1994.

90. Verrier, T., Solhonne, B., Sallenave, J.M., and Garcia-Verdugo, I., The WAP protein trappin-2/elafin: A handyman in the regulation of inflammatory and immune responses, *Int. J. Biochem. Cell Biol.* 44, 1377–1380, 2012.

91. Jaovisidha, K., Etim, A., Yamakawa, K., et al., The serine protease inhibitor trappin-2 is present in cartilage and synovial fluid in osteoarthritis, *J. Rheumatol.* 33, 318–325, 2006.

92. Engvall, E. and Ruoslahti, E., Binding of soluble form of fibroblast surface protein, fibronectin, to collagen, *Int. J. Cancer* 20, 1–5, 1977.

93. Jaffe, E.A. and Mosher, D.F., Synthesis of fibronectin by cultured human endothelial cells, *J. Exp. Med.* 147, 1779–1791, 1978.

94. Pankov, R. and Yamada, K.M., Fibronectin at a glance, *J. Cell. Sci.* 115, 3861–3863, 2002.

95. Schwarzbauer, J.E., Alternative splicing of fibronectin: Three variants, three functions, *BioEssays* 13, 527–553, 1991.

96. White, E.S., Baralle, F.E., and Muro, A.F., New insights into form and function of fibronectin splice variants, *J. Pathol.* 216, 1–14, 2008.

97. Hynes, R.O. and Yamada, K.M., Fibronectins: Multifunctional modular glycoproteins, *J. Cell Biol.* 95, 369–377, 1982.

98. Sabatier, L., Chen, D., Fagotto-Kaufmann, C., et al., Fibrillin assembly requires fibronectin, *Mol. Biol. Cell* 20, 846–858, 2009.

99. Lark, M.W., Laterra, J., and Culp, L.A., Close and focal contact adhesions of fibroblasts to a fibronectin-containing matrix, *Fed. Proc.* 44, 394–405, 1985.

100. Kowalczyk, A.P., Tulloh, R.H., and McKeown-Longo, P.J., Polarized fibronectin secretion and localized matrix assembly sites correlated with subendothelial matrix formation, *Blood* 75, 2335–2342, 1990.

101. Hang, J., Zemskov, E.A., Lorand, L., and Belkin, A.M., Identification of a novel recognition sequence for fibronectin within the NH$_2$-terminal β-sandwich domain of tissue transglutaminase, *J. Biol. Chem.* 280, 23675–23683, 2005.
102. Turner, P.M. and Lorand, L., Complexation of fibronectin with tissue transglutaminase, *Biochemistry* 28, 628–635, 1989.
103. Radek, J.T., Jeong, J.-M., Murthy, S.N.P., Ingham, K.C., and Lorand, L., Affinity of human erythrocyte transglutaminase for a 42-kDa gelatin-binding fragment of human plasma fibronectin, *Proc. Natl. Acad. Sci. USA* 90, 3152–3156, 1993.
104. Upchurch, H.F., Conway, E., Patterson, M.K., Jr., and Maxwell, M.D., Localization of cellular transglutaminase on the extracellular matrix after wounding: Characteristics of the matrix bound enzyme, *J. Cell. Physiol.* 149, 375–382, 1991.
105. Jensen, P.H., Lorand, L., Ebbesen, P., and Gliemann, J., Type-2 plasminogen activator inhibitor is a substrates for trophoblast transglutaminase and factor XIIIa: Transglutaminase-catalyzed cross-linking to cellular and extracellular structures, *Eur. J. Biochem.* 214, 141–146, 1993.
106. Guyot, N., Zani, M.-L., Manuel, M.C., Dallet-Choisy, S. and Moreau, T., Elafin and its precursor trappin-2 still inhibit neutrophil serine proteases when they are covalently bound to extracellular matrix proteins by tissue transglutaminase, *Biochemistry* 44, 15610–15618, 2005.
107. Baranger, K., Zani, M.-L., Labas, V., Dallet-Choisy, S., and Moreau, T., Secretory leukocyte protease inhibitor (SLPI) is, like its homologue trappin-2 (pre-elafin), a transglutaminase substrate, *PLoS One* 6(6), e20976, 2011.
108. Segade, F., Molecular evolution of the fibulins: Implications on the functionality of the elastic fibulins, *Gene* 464, 17–31, 2010.
109. Cooley, M.A. and Argraves, W.S., The fibulins, in *The Extracellular Matrix: An Overview*, ed. R.P. Mecham, Chapter 10, pp. 337–367, Springer-Verlag, Berlin, Germany, 2011.
110. Timpl, R., and Brown, J.C., The laminins, *Matrix Biol.* 14, 275–281, 1994.
111. Yanagisawa, H. and Davis, E.C., Unraveling the mechanism of elastic fiber assembly: The roles of short fibulins, *Int. J. Biochem. Cell Biol.* 42, 1084–1093, 2010.
112. Lee, N.V., Rodriguez-Manzaneque, J.C., Thai, S.N., et al., Fibulin-1 acts as a cofactor for the matrix metalloprotease ADAMTS-1, *J. Biol. Chem.* 280, 34706–37804, 2005.
113. Kapustin, A., Stepanova, V., Aniol, N., et al., Fibulin-5 binds urokinase-type plasminogen activator and mediates urokinase-stimulated β1-integrin-dependent cell migration, *Biochem. J.* 443, 491–503, 2012.
114. Hohenester, E. and Yurchenco, P.D., Laminins in basement membrane assembly, *Cell Adh. Migr.* 7, 56–63, 2013.
115. Domogatskaya, A., Rodin, S., and Ryggvason, K., Functional diversity of laminins, *Annu. Rev. Cell Dev. Biol.* 28, 523–553, 2012.
116. Liotta, L.A., Goldfarb, R.H., and Terranova, V.P., Cleavage of laminin by thrombin and plasmin: Alpha thrombin selectively cleaves the beta chain of laminin, *Thromb. Res.* 21, 663–673, 1981
117. Yurchenco, P.D., and Schittny, J.C., Molecular architecture of basement membranes, *FASEB J.* 4, 1577–1590, 1990.
118. Kohfeldt, E., Sasdaki, T., Göhring, W., and Timpl, R., Nidogen-2: A new basement membrane protein with diverse binding properties, *J. Mol. Biol.* 282, 99–109, 1998.
119. Tu, H., Sasaki, T., Snellman, A., et al., The type XIII collagen ectodomain is a 150-nm rod and capable of binding to fibronectin, nidogen-2, perlecan, and heparin, *J. Biol. Chem.* 277, 23092–23099, 2002.
120. Farach-Carson, M.C., Warrne, C.R., Harrington, D.A., and Carson, D.D., Border patrol: Insights into the unique role of perlecan/heparan sulfate proteoglycan 2 at cell and tissue borders, *Matrix Biol.* 34, 64–79, 2014.

121. Knox, S., Fosang, A.J., Last, K., Melrose, J., and Whitelock, J., Perlecan from human epithelial cells is a hybrid heparan/chondroitin/keratin sulfate proteoglycan, *FEBS Lett.* 579, 5019–5023, 2005.

122. Vincent, T.L., McLean, C.J., Full, L.E., Peston, D., and Saklatvala, J., FGF-2 is bound to perlecan in the pericellular matrix of articular cartilage, where it acts as a chondrocyte mechanotransducer, *Osterarthr. Cartil.* 15, 752–763, 2007.

123. Ishijima, M., Suzuki, N., Hozumi, K., et al., Perlecan modulates VEGF signaling and is essential for vascularization in endochondral bone formation, *Matrix Biol.* 31, 234–245, 2012.

124. Whitelock, J.M., Murdoch, A.D., Iozzo, R.V., and Underwood, P.A., The degradation of human endothelial cell-derived perlecan and release of bound basic fibroblast growth factor by stromelysin, collagenase, plasmin, and heparanases, *J. Biol. Chem.* 271, 10079–10086, 1996.

125. Troeberg, L., Lazenbatt, C., Anower-E-Khuda, M.F., et al., Sulfated glycosaminoglycans control the extracellular trafficking and the activity of the metalloprotease inhibitor TIMP-3, *Chem. Biol.* 21, 1300–1309, 2014.

126. Hatton, M.W. and Moar, S.L., A role for pericellular proteoglycan in the binding of thrombin or antithrombin III by the blood vessel endothelium? The effects of proteoglycan-degrading enzymes and the glycosaminoglycan-binding proteins on ^{125}I thrombin by the rabbit aorta *in vitro*, *Thromb. Haemost.* 53, 228–234, 1985.

127. Bar-Shavit, R., Eldor, A., and Vlodavsky, I., Binding of thrombin to subendothelial extracellular matrix: Protection and expression of functional properties, *J. Clin. Invest.* 84, 1096–1104, 1989.

128. Chajek-Shaul, T., Friedman, G., Bengtsson-Olivecrona, G., Vlodavsky, I., and Bar-Shavit, R., Interaction of lipoprotein lipase with subendothelial extracellular matrix, *Biochim. Biophys. Acta* 1042, 168–175, 1990.

129. Bornstein, P., Diversity of function is inherent in matricellular proteins: An appraisal of thrombospondin 1, *J. Cell. Biol.* 130, 503–506, 1995.

130. Lawler, J., The structural and functional properties of thrombospondin, *Blood* 67, 1197–1209, 1986.

131. Hornebeck, W., Emonard, H., Monboisse, J.C., and Bellon, G., Matrix-directed regulation of pericellular proteolysis and tumor progression, *Semin. Cancer Biol.* 12, 231–241, 2002.

132. Hogg, P.J., Stenflo, J., and Mosher, D.F., Thrombospondin is a slow tight-binding inhibitor of plasmin, *Biochemistry* 31, 265–269, 1992.

133. Mosher, D.F., Misenheimer, T.M., Stenflo, J., and Hogg, P.J., Modulation of the fibrinolysis by thrombospondin, *Ann. N.Y. Acad. Sci.* 667, 64–69, 1992.

134. Hogg, P.J., Owensby, D.A., Mosher, D.F., Misenheimer, T.M., and Chesterman, C.N., Thrombospondin is a tight-binding competitive inhibitor of neutrophil elastase, *J. Biol. Chem.* 268, 7139–7145, 1993.

135. Silverstein, R.L., Nachman, R.L., Pannell, R., Gurewich, V., and Harpel, P.C., Thrombospondin forms complexes with single-chain and two-chain forms of urokinase, *J. Biol. Chem.* 265, 11289–11294, 1990.

136. Rico, M.C., Rough, J.J., Manns, J.M., et al., Assembly of the prothrombinase complex on the surface of human foreskin fibroblasts: Implications for connective tissue growth factor, *Thromb. Res.* 129, 801–806, 2012.

137. Leavesley, D.I., Kashyap, A.S., Croll, T., et al., Vitronectin: Master controller or micromanager? *IUBMB Life* 65, 807–818, 2013.

138. Preissner, K.T. and Pötzsh, B., Vessel wall–dependent metabolic pathways of the adhesive proteins, von-Willebrand factor and vitronectin, *Histol. Histopathol.* 10, 239–251, 1995.

139. Schvartz, I., Seger, D., and Shaltiel, S., Vitronectin, *Int. J. Biochem. Cell Biol.* 31, 539–544, 1999.
140. Seiffert, D., Mimuro, J., Schleef, R.R., and Loskutoff, D.J., Interactions between type 1 plasminogen activator inhibitor, extracellular matrix and vitronectin, *Cell Differ. Dev.* 32, 287–292, 1990.
141. Hertig, A. and Rondeau, E., Plasminogen activator inhibitor type 1: The two faces of the same coin, *Curr. Opin. Nephrol. Hypertens.* 13, 39–44, 2004.

due to contaminating cells.[34] The removal of nucleic acid is considered important for the use of isolated ECMs in regenerative medicine.[35,36] Early works also referred to the ECM as a ground substance composed of collagen, polysaccharides, and tissue glycoproteins.[37,38] It became apparent that the ground substance was composed of polysaccharide, glycoproteins, proteoglycans, and protein, and was an integral component of the ECM.[39,40]

In what might be considered a more expansive definition, the ECM could also be defined as all secreted molecules in the interstitial space that are subsequently immobilized outside the cell.[41] The term *secretome*[42–45] has been used to describe the proteins secreted by a specific tissue, such as the liver secretome,[46] or more frequently by a specific cell, such as an adipocyte.[47] There has been particular interest in the secretome of tumor cells as a source of biomarkers.[48–50] The interstitial fluid is a product of several secretomes of various cells, such as epithelial cells, smooth muscle cells, and fibroblasts, which are intrinsic to the interstitial space; leukocytes, which enter the interstitial space by diapedesis (transmigration);[51,52] and substances derived from the vascular space by extravasation. Other "omics" terms used to describe the ECM are the matridome,[16] the degradome,[16] and N-terminomics.[16]

The ECM also serves as a substructure for cell movement,[53] a repository for growth factors,[54–59] provides signaling for cell differentiation and communication,[41,60–63] and absorbs stress and compression. This latter characteristic, the ability to act as a shock absorber, is of particular importance in cartilage ECM.[64,65] There is considerable work on the mechanical function of the ECM.[66–69]

The role of the ECM in the control of growth factor activity involves the reversible binding of growth factors. As an example, consider the role of ECM proteins fibronectin and fibrillin in the regulation of TGFβ activity.[54] TGFβ is synthesized as pro-TGFβ bound to the latent TGFβ-binding protein by disulfide linkages; this is referred to as the large latent complex, which is secreted and then bound to fibrillin and fibronectin in the ECM. Activation of TGFβ, which involves cleavage to the active dimer form and release from the latent TGFβ-binding protein, can be achieved by a number of substances, including MMP2, MMP9, MMP14, plasmin, kallikrein, α integrin, or β integrin.

Several fibroblast growth factors (FGFs) can bind to a heparan sulfate proteoglycan both in the ECM and in solution, as well as to other sulfated oligosaccharides and sulfated polysaccharides such as heparin.[59,70] Such interaction in solution is important for the productive binding of FGFs to FGF receptors (FGFRs)[70,71] as well as for the stabilization of FGFs in solution.[72,73] Antiangiogenic antithrombin (Chapter 9) is a conformation isomer (conformer) of the metastable protease inhibitor antithrombin and blocks the formation of a productive complex of heparin or heparin analogue, FGF, and FGFR.[74] Adenosine triphosphate also binds to the FGF–heparin binding site and stabilizes FGF in solution.[75,76] The effect is not unique to ATP but is also observed with other nucleotide triphosphates such as GTP.[75]

FGFs can be released from the ECM by heparanase,[77] heparitinase,[78] elastase,[79,80] matrix metalloproteinases,[81] and thrombin.[82] Sanderson and coworkers[83] discuss the role of heparanase in the fragmentation of the heparan sulfate moiety as one of several mechanisms of heparan sulfate proteoglycans that would result in the release of FGFs and increased angiogenesis. The expression of heparanase in tumors is associated with tumor growth and metastasis.[84] Plasmin and thrombin cleave the heparan sulfate–rich ectodomain from heparin sulfate proteoglycans such as syndican-1 and syndican-4,[85] with the release of FGF–heparan sulfate complex into the interstitial space; the FGF–heparan sulfate complex then forms a ternary complex with the FGF receptor tyrosine kinase.[66,82] Earlier work by Benezra[82] has demonstrated the thrombin-catalyzed release of heparan sulfate proteoglycan–FGF2 complex from subendothelial ECM, as shown by immunoprecipitation with anti-FGF2 antibodies. Elastase degrades several proteins in the ECM,[87,88] resulting in the release of heparan sulfate and heparan sulfate proteoglycan, which would contain bound growth factors such as FGF2. The presence of the myeloperoxidase/peroxide/chloride system greatly increases the extent of degradation and the release of heparan sulfate/heparan sulfate proteoglycan as measured by ^{35}S release.[89]

Material is deposited into the ECM during development. An example is provided by the cross-linking of fibronectin in the development of the ECM, catalyzed by factor XIIIa.[90] Factor XIIIa also catalyzes the cross-linking of fibronectin and fibrinogen,[91] resulting in a matrix for cell adhesion,[92] and catalyzes the cross-linking of fibronectin to collagens.[93] The possible roles of factor XIII in the ECM have been discussed by Greenberg and coworkers[94] as well as others.[95–97] The incorporation of fibrinogen into the ECM is independent of thrombin activity[98] but is dependent on the presence fibronectin.[99,100] While fibrin is extensively used for *in vitro* 3D matrices for the study of cell migration, there are few data to support the presence of fibrin in the interstitial space except in disease situations.[101–105]

2.3 BASEMENT MEMBRANE

The BM is located on the basal (basolateral) surfaces of cells and is also known as the basal lamina; histological analysis shows the presence of three layers or zones: lamina lucida, lamina densa, and lamina reticularis. One authority[106] argues that the term *basement membrane* is inappropriate as it contains no lipid, which is characteristic of cell membranes. There is a tendency to refer to the BM as an extracellular membrane.[107,108] The BM contains collagen type IV and laminin, which together with proteoglycans are the primary structural components. Both collagen IV and laminin have the property of self-association, which forms the BM matrix.[109–111] The presence of collagen IV is unique to the BM and laminin is also characteristic. Collagen IV is considered to be an unconventional collagen[112] in that it does not have the canonical tripeptide repeat Gly-Xaa-Yaa and does not form a classical fibril, such as that seen with collagens I, II, and III. It would appear that laminin deposition and network formation are necessary for the subsequent formation of the collagen IV network.

The collagen IV is cross-linked via oxidation of lysine residues to form an aldehyde derivative, which can react with an unmodified lysine residue or other nucleophile to form a covalent cross-link.[113] Monomeric type IV collagen is cross-linked by disulfide exchange through the NC1 domain to yield dimers and further cross-linked at the N-terminal region, also by disulfide exchange, to yield higher-order polymers.[114,115] Laminin associates with collagen IV via interaction with nidogen (entactin).[116] Heparin sulfate proteoglycan is also a structural component of the BM.[117,118] It has been shown that heparan sulfate gradients exist in the endothelial lining of blood vessels with much greater amounts of heparan sulfate on the basolateral aspect.[119] Perlecan (heparan sulfate proteoglycan 2) is a heparan sulfate proteoglycan unique to the BM and has been suggested to be more important than nidogen in interacting with type IV collagen and laminin.[120] Farach-Carson and coworkers[118] have catalogued proteins that bind to perlecan and are thus considered structural components of the BM. The list includes collagen IV, collagen V, elastin, laminin, fibronectin, and fibulin.

The BM can be considered to be contiguous with the extracellular matrix. This relationship is based on interactions such as that involving collagen VII.[121,122] Brittingham and coworkers[123] reported that the NC1 domain of collagen VII bound to laminin 5 and collagen VI with a nanomolar dissociation constant, providing attachment of the BM to the ECM. Collagen IV has been reported to specifically bind a number of proteins, including blood coagulation factor IX,[123] von Willebrand factor,[124] certain chemokines,[125] oncostatin M,[126] transforming growth factor β type 1,[127] and tissue factor microparticles.[128] Collagen type IV is less effective than other collagen species in binding oncostatin M; collagen type III is the most effective collagen species tested in the binding of oncostatin M with collagen type I; and collagen type II is less effective than type III but more effective than type IV.[126] Transforming growth factor β type 1 was effective in stimulating cell growth while bound to collagen type IV.[127] Perlecan can also bind transforming growth factor β.[129] The binding of tissue factor to collagen type IV is suggested as a mechanism for enhancing tissue factor activity.[128]

2.4   GLYCOCALYX

The glycocalyx is a layer of glycoproteins[13,130] on the apical surface of epithelial and endothelial cells. The mucin of the gastrointestinal epithelia is a glycocalyx composed largely of mucin glycoproteins.[131] The glycocalyx on the luminal surface of endothelial cells is composed of membrane-bound proteoglycans and glycoproteins.[132] The glycocalyx has a major role in maintaining vascular integrity and membrane transport,[132,133] and in controlling protein transport from the vascular bed to the interstitial space.[134–136] The elucidation of its structure was seminal in the revision of the Starling principle for vascular transport (Chapter 1).

REFERENCES

1. Rezaie, A.R., Roles of exosites 1 and 2 in thrombin reaction with plasminogen activator inhibitor-1 in the absence and presence of cofactors, *Biochemistry* 38, 14592–14599, 1999.

2. Stack, M.S., Rinehart, A.R., and Pizzo, S.V., Comparison of plasminogen binding and activation on extracellular matrices produced by vascular smooth muscle and endothelial cells, *Eur. J. Biochem.* 226, 937–943, 1994.
3. Moser, T.L., Enghild, J.J., Pizzo, S.V., and Stack, M.S., Specific binding of urinary-type plasminogen activator (uPA) to vitronectin and its role in mediating u-PA-dependent adhesion of U937 cells, *Biochem. J.* 307, 867–873, 1995.
4. Hay, E.D., Introductory remarks, in *Cell Biology of Extracellular Matrix*, ed. E.D. Hay, pp. 1–5, Plenum Press, New York, 1981.
5. Coats, W.D., Jr. and Faxon, D.P., The role of the extracellular matrix in arterial remodeling, *Semin. Interv. Cardiol.* 2, 167–176, 1997.
6. Franz, C., Stewart. K.M., and Weaver, V.M., The extracellular matrix at a glance, *J. Cell. Sci.* 123, 4195–4200, 2010.
7. Wiig, H., Gyenge, C., Iversen, P.O., Gullberg, D., and Tenstad, O., The role of the extracellular matrix in tissue distribution of macromolecules in normal and pathological tissues: Potential therapeutic consequences, *Microcirculation* 15, 283–296, 2008.
8. Farquhar, M.G., The glomerular BM: A selective macromolecular filter, in *Cell Biology of Extracellular Matrix*, ed. E.D. Hay, Chapter 11, pp. 335–378, Plenum Press, New York, 1981.
9. Farquhar, M.G., Structure and function of glomerular capillaries: Role of the BM in glomerular filtration, in *Biology and Chemistry of BMs*, ed. N.A. Kefalides, pp. 43–80, Academic Press, New York, 1978.
10. Khoshnoodi, J., Pedchenko, V., and Hudon, B.G., Mammalian collagen IV, *Microsc. Res. Tech.* 71, 357–370, 2008.
11. Timpl, R., Fujiwara, S., Dziadek, M., et al., Laminin, proteoglycan, nidogen and collagen IV: Structural models and molecular interactions, *Ciba Found. Symp.* 108, 25–43, 1984.
12. Hohenester, E. and Yurchenco, P.D., Laminins in BM assembly, *Cell Adh. Migr.* 7, 56–63, 2013.
13. Alphonsus, C.S. and Rodseth, R.N., The endothelial glycocalyx: A review of the vascular barrier, *Anaesthesia* 69, 777–784, 2014.
14. Engel, J. and Chiquet, M., An overview of extracellular matrix structure and function, in *The Extracellular Matrix: An Overview*, ed. R.P. Mecham, Chapter 1, pp. 1–39, Springer, Berlin, Germany, 2011.
15. Kleinman, H.K., Malinda, K.M., and Ponce, M.L., ECM, in *Inflammatory Diseases of Blood Vessels*, ed. G.S. Hoffman and C.M. Weyand, Chapter 3, pp. 29–36, Marcel Dekker, New York, 2002.
16. Patterson, N.L., Iyer, R.P., de Castro Brás, L.E., et al., Using proteomics to uncover extracellular matrix interactions during cardiac remodeling, *Proteomics Clin. Appl.* 7, 516–527, 2013.
17. Adams, J.C., Extracellular matrix evolution: An overview, in *Evolution of the ECM*, ed. R.W. Keely and R.P. Mecham, Chapter 1, pp. 1–25, Springer, Berlin, Germany, 2013.
18. Nichols, S.A., Dirks, W., Pearse, J.S., and King, N., Early evolution of animal cell signaling and adhesion genes, *Proc. Natl. Acad. Sci. USA* 103, 12451–12456, 2006.
19. Huxley-Jones, J., Foord, S.M., and Barnes, M.R., Drug discovery in the extracellular matrix, *Drug Discov. Today* 13, 685–694, 2008.
20. Haralson, M.A. and Hassell, J.R., The extracellular matrix: An overview, in *Extracellular Matrix: A Practical Approach*, Chapter 1, pp. 1–30, IRL Press, Oxford, UK, 1995.
21. Halper, J. and Kjaer, M., Basic components of connective tissues and extracellular matrix: Elastin, fibrillin, fibulins, fibrinogen, fibronectin, laminin, tenascins, and thrombospondins, *Adv. Exp. Med. Biol.* 802, 31–47, 2014.

22. Timpl, R. and Martin, G.R., Components of BM, in *Immunochemistry of the Extracellular Matrix*, Vol. II, ed. H. Furthmayer, Chapter 5, pp. 119–150, CRC Press, Boca Raton, FL, 1981.
23. Byron, A., Humphries, J.D., and Humphries, M.J., Defining the extracellular matrix using proteomics, *Int. J. Exp. Pathol.* 94, 75–92, 2013.
24. Foot, N.C., Studies on endothelial reactions (First paper): The macrophage of the loose connective tissue, *J. Med. Res.* 40, 353–370, 1919.
25. Meyer, F.A. and Silberberg, A., *In vitro* study of the influence of some factors important for any physicochemical characterization of loose connective tissue in the microcirculation, *Microvasc. Res.* 8, 263–273, 1974.
26. Hedman, K., Kurkinen, M., Alitalo, K., et al., Isolation of the pericellular matrix of human fibroblast cultures, *J. Cell Biol.* 81, 83–91, 1979.
27. Waugh, D.F., Physical properties of protoplasm, *Annu. Rev. Physiol.* 14, 13–30, 1952.
28. Ragan, C., The physiology of connective tissue (loose areolar), *Annu. Rev. Physiol.* 14, 51–76, 1952.
29. Conference on biology and chemistry of the extracellular matrix, Department of Medicine, Columbia University, New York, November 2–4, 1964.
30. Cooper, G.W. and Prockop, D.J., Intracellular accumulation of protocollagen and extrusion of collagen by embryonic cartilage cells, *J. Cell Biol.* 38, 523–537, 1968.
31. Elsdale, T. and Foley, R., Morphogenetic aspects of multilayering in petri dish cultures of human fetal lung fibroblasts, *J. Cell Biol.* 41, 298–311, 1969.
32. Dempsey, M. and Haines, B.M., Nature of the ground substance in interstitial connective tissue, *Nature* 164, 368, 1949.
33. Steinberg, M.S., "ECM": Its nature, origin and function in cell aggregation, *Exp. Cell Res.* 30, 257–279, 1963.
34. Moscona, A.A., Cell aggregation: Properties of specific cell-ligands and their role in the formation of multicellular systems, *Dev. Biol.* 18, 250–277, 1968.
35. Choi, Y.C., Choi, J.S., Kim, B.S., et al., Decellularized extracellular matrix derived from porcine adipose tissue as a xenogenic biomaterial for tissue engineering, *Tissue Eng. Part C Methods* 18, 866–876, 2012.
36. Filippo, N., Paola, A., Laura, I., Michele, S., and Gino, G., Biocompatibility evaluation criteria for novel xenograft materials: Distribution and quantification of remnant nucleic acid and alpha-gal epitope, *Stem Cell Res. Ther.* S6(009), 2013.
37. Goldsmith, E.D., Ground substance of the mesenchyme and hyaluronidase, *Nature* 163, 184, 1949.
38. Schubert, M. and Pras, M., Ground substance protein polysaccharides and the precipitation of calcium phosphate, *Clin. Orthop. Relat. Res.* 60, 235–255, 1968.
39. Schliwa, M. and van Blerkom, J., Structural interaction of cytoskeletal components, *J. Cell Biol.* 90, 222–235, 1981.
40. Coats, W.D., Jr. and Faxon, D.P., The role of the extracellular matrix in arterial remodeling, *Semin. Interv. Cardiol.* 2, 167–176, 1997.
41. Reichardt, L.F., Extracellular matrix and their receptors, in *Guidebook to the Extracellular Matrix and Adhesive Proteins*, ed. T. Kreis and R. Vale, Oxford University Press, Oxford, UK, 1995.
42. Dupont, A., Tokarski, C., Dekeyzer, O., et al., Two-dimensional maps and databases of the human macrophage proteome and secretome, *Proteomics* 4, 1761–1778, 2004.
43. Dupont, A., Corseaux, D., Dekeyzer, O., et al., The proteome and secretome of human arterial smooth muscle cells, *Proteomics* 5, 585–596, 2005.
44. Zwicki, H., Traxler, E., Staettner, S., et al., A novel technique to specifically analyze the secretome of cells and tissues, *Electrophoresis* 26, 2779–2785, 2005.
45. Mukherjee, P. and Mani, S., Methodologies to decipher the cell secretome, *Biochim. Biophys. Acta* 1834, 2220–2232, 2013.

46. Zhang, Y., Wang, Y., Sun, W., et al., Strategy for studying the liver secretome on the organ level, *J. Proteome Res.* 9, 1894–1901, 2010.

47. Renes, J., Rosenow, A., Roumans, N., et al., Calorie restriction–induced changes in the secretome of human adipocytes, comparison with resveratrol-induced secretome effects, *Biochim. Biophys. Acta* 1844, 1511–1522, 2014.

48. Gromov, P., Gromova, I., Olsen, C.I., et al., Tumor interstitial fluid: A treasure trove of cancer biomarkers, *Biochim. Biophys. Acta* 1834, 2259–2270, 2013.

49. Shaaij-Visser, T.B., de Wit, M., Lam, S.Q.W., and Jiménez, C.R., The cancer secretome, current status and opportunities in the lung, breast, and colorectal cancer context, *Biochim. Biophys. Acta* 1834, 2242–2258, 2013.

50. Haslene-Hox, H., Tenstad, O., and Wiig, H., Interstitial fluid: A reflection of the tumor cell microenvironment and secretome, *Biochim. Biophys. Acta* 1834, 2336–2346, 2013.

51. Nourshargh, S. and Marelli-Berg, F.M., Transmigration through venular walls: A key regulator of leukocyte phenotype and function, *Trends Immunol.* 26, 157–165, 2005.

52. Olsson, J., Paulsson, J., Dadfar, E., et al., Monocyte and neutrophil chemotactic activity at the site of interstitial inflammation in patients on high-flux hemodialysis or hemofiltration, *Blood Purif.* 28, 47–52, 2009.

53. Humphries, M.J., Mould, A.P., and Yamada, K.M., Matrix receptors in cell migration, in *Receptors for ECM*, ed. J.A. McDonald and R.P. Mecham, pp. 195–253, Academic Press, San Diego, CA, 1991.

54. Zhu, J. and Clark, R.A., Fibronectin at select sites binds multiple growth factors and enhances their activity: Expansion of the collaborative ECM-GF paradigm, *J. Invest. Dermatol.* 134, 895–901, 2014.

55. Robertson, I.B. and Rifkin, D.B., Unchaining the beast: Insights from structural and evolutionary studies on TGFβ secretion, sequestration, and activation, *Cytokine Growth Factor Rev.* 24, 355–372, 2013.

56. Vlodavsky, I., Bar-Shavit, R., Ishai-Michaeli, R., et al., Extracellular sequestration and release of fibroblast growth factor: A regulatory mechanism? *Trends Biochem. Sci.* 16, 268–271, 1991.

57. Vlodavsky, I., Miao, H.Q., Medalion, B., et al., Involvement of heparan sulfate and related molecules in sequestration and growth promoting activity of fibroblast growth factor, *Cancer Metastasis Rev.* 15, 177–186, 1996.

58. Casu, B., Naggi, A., and Torri, G., Heparin-derived heparan sulfate mimics to modulate heparan sulfate–protein interaction in inflammation and cancer, *Matrix Biol.* 29, 442–452, 2010.

59. Guerrini, M., Hricovini, M., and Torri, G., Interaction of heparins with fibroblast growth factors: Conformation aspects, *Curr. Pharm. Des.* 13, 2045–2056, 2007.

60. Fan, D., Creemers, E.E., and Kassin, Z., Matrix as an interstitial transport system, *Circ. Res.* 114, 889–902, 2014.

61. Øien, A.H., Justad, S.R., Tenstad, O., and Wiig, H., Effect of hydration on steric and electric charge–induced interstitial volume exclusion: A model, *Biophys. J.* 105, 1276–1284, 2013.

62. Brizzi, M.F., Tarone, G., and Defilippi, P., Extracellular matrix, integrins, and growth factors as tailors of the stem cell niches, *Curr. Opin. Cell Biol.* 24, 645–651, 2012.

63. Olsen, J.G. and Kragelund, B.B., Who climbs the tryptophan ladder? On the structure and function of the WSXWS motif in cytokine receptors and thrombospondin repeats, *Cytokine Growth Factor Rev.* 25, 337–341, 2014.

64. Jimenez, S.A., Alal-Kokko, L., Prockop, D.J., et al., Characterization of human type II procollagen and collagen-specific antibodies and their application to the study of human type II collagen processing and ultrastructure, *Matrix Biol* 16, 29–39, 1997.

65. Gruber, H.E., Hoelscher, G.L., Ingram, J.A., et al., Variations in aggrecan localization and gene expression patterns characterize increasing stages of human intervertebral disk degeneration, *Exp. Mol. Pathol.* 91, 534–539, 2011.
66. Silver, F.H., *Mechanosensing and Mechanochemical Transduction in ECM*, Springer, New York, 2006.
67. Huang, C., Dai, J., and Zhang, X.A., Environmental physical cues determine the linage specification of mesenchymal stem cells, *Biochim. Biophys. Acta* 1850, 1261–1266, 2015.
68. Freedman, B.R., Bade, N.D., Riggin, C.N., et al., The (dys)functional extracellular matrix, *Biochim. Biophys. Acta* 1853, 3153–3164, 2015.
69. Manninen, A., Epithelial polarity: Generating and integrating signals from the ECM with integrins, *Exp. Cell Res.* 334, 337–349, 2015.
70. Zhang, F., Zhang, Z., Lin, X., et al., Compositional analysis of heparin/heparan sulfate interacting with fibroblast growth factor: Fibroblast growth factor receptor complexes, *Biochemistry* 48, 8379–8386, 2009.
71. Robinson, C.J, Harmer, N.J., Goodger, S.J., et al., Cooperative dimerization of fibroblast growth factor 1 (FGF1) upon a single heparin saccharide may drive the formation of 2:2:1 FGF.FGFR2c.heparin ternary complexes, *J. Biol. Chem.* 280, 42274–42282, 2005.
72. Uniewicz, K.A., Ori, A., Xu, R., et al., Differential scanning fluorimetry measurement of protein stability changes upon binding to glycosaminoglycans: A screening test for binding specificity, *Anal. Chem.* 82, 3796–3802, 2010.
73. Nguyen, T.H., Kim, S.-H., Decker, C.G., et al., A heparin-mimicking polymer conjugate stabilizes basic fibroblast growth factor, *Nature Chem.* 5, 221–227, 2013.
74. Zhang, W., Swanson, R., Xiong, Y., et al., Antiangiogenic antithrombin blocks the heparan sulfate-dependent binding of proangiogenic growth factors to their endothelial cell receptors: Evidence for differential binding of antiangiogenic and anticoagulant forms of antithrombin to proangiogenic heparan sulfate domains, *J. Biol. Chem.* 281, 37302–37310, 2006.
75. Chavan, A.J., Haley, B.E., Volkin, D.B., et al., Interaction of nucleotides with acidic fibroblast growth factor (FGF-1), *Biochemistry* 33, 7193–7202, 1994.
76. Rose, K., Interaction of ATP with fibroblast growth factor 2: Biochemical characterization and consequence of growth factor stability, *BMB Biochem.* 12(14), 2011.
77. Elkin, M., Llan, N., Ishai-Michaeli, R., et al., Heparanase as mediator of angiogenesis: Mode of action, *FASEB J.* 15, 1661–1663, 2001.
78. Bashkin, P., Doctrow, S., Klagsbrun, M., et al., Basic fibroblast growth factor binds to subendothelial ECM and is released by heparitinase and heparin-like molecules, *Biochemistry* 28, 1737–1743, 1989.
79. Thompson, K. and Rabinovitch, M., Exogenous leukocyte and endogenous elastase can mediate mitogenic activity in pulmonary artery smooth muscle cells by release of extracellular matrix-bound basic fibroblast growth factor, *J. Cell. Physiol.* 166, 495–505, 1996.
80. Buczek-Thomas, J.A. and Nugent, M.A., Elastase-mediated release of heparan sulfate proteoglycan from pulmonary fibroblast cultures: A mechanism of basic fibroblast growth factor (bFGF) release and attenuation of bFGF binding following elastase-induced injury, *J. Biol. Chem.* 24, 25167–25172, 1999.
81. Tamura, T., Nakanishi, T., Kimura, Y., et al., Nitric oxide mediates interleukin-1-induced matrix degradation and basic fibroblast growth factor release in cultured rabbit articular chondrocytes: A possible mechanism of pathological neovascularization in arthritis, *Endocrinology* 137, 3729–3737, 1990.
82. Benezra, M., Vlodavsky, I., Ishai-Micheali, R., et al., Thrombin-induced release of active basic fibroblast growth factor–heparan sulfate complexes from subendothelial extracellular matrix, *Blood* 81, 3324–3331, 1993.

83. Sanderson, R.D., Yang, Y., Kelly, T., et al., Enzymatic remodeling of heparan sulfate proteoglycans within the tumor microenvironment: Growth regulation and the prospect of new cancer therapies, *J. Cell. Biochem.* 96, 897–905, 2005.

84. Pisano, C., Vlodavsky, I., Ilan, N., and Zunino, F., The potential of heparanase as a therapeutic target in cancer, *Biochem. Pharmacol.* 89, 12–19, 2014.

85. Schmidt, A., Echtermeyer, F., Alozie, A., et al., Plasmin- and thrombin-accelerated shedding of syndecan-4 ectodomain generates cleavage sites at Lys^{114}–Arg^{115} and Lys^{129}–Val^{130} bonds, *J. Biol. Chem.* 280, 34441–34446, 2005.

86. Guimond, S.E., Rudd, T.F., Skidmore, M.A., et al., Cations modulate polysaccharide structure to determine FGF-FGFR signaling: A comparison of signaling and inhibitory polysaccharide interactions with FGF-1 in solution, *Biochemistry* 48, 4772–4779, 2009.

87. Buczek-Thomas., J.A. and Nugent, M.A., Elastase-mediated release of heparan sulfate proteoglycans from pulmonary fibroblast cultures: A mechanism for basic fibroblast growth factor (bFGF) release and attenuation of bFGF binding following elastase-induced injury, *J. Biol. Chem.* 274, 25167–25172, 1999.

88. Liu, J., Rich, C.B., Buczek-Thomas, J.A., et al., Heparin-binding EGF-like growth factor regulates elastin and FGF-2 expression in pulmonary fibroblasts, *Am. J. Physiol. Lung Cell. Mol. Physiol.* 285, L1106–L1115, 2003.

89. Klebanoff, S.J., Kinsella, M.G., and Wright, T.N., Degradation of endothelial cell matrix heparan sulfate proteoglycan by elastase and the myeloperoxidase-H_2O_2-chloride system, *Am. J. Pathol.* 143, 907–917, 1993.

90. Mosher, D.F., Fogerty, F.J., Chernousov, M.A., and Barry, E.L., Assembly of fibronectin into ECM, *Ann. N.Y. Acad. Sci.* 614, 167–180, 1991.

91. Procyk, R. and Blomback, B., Factor XIII-induced crosslinking in solutions of fibrinogen and fibronectin, *Biochim. Biophys. Acta* 967, 304–313, 1988.

92. Corbett, S.A., Lee, L., Wilson, C.L., and Schwarzbauer, J.E., Covalent cross-linking of fibronectin to fibrin is required for maximal cell adhesion to a fibronectin–fibrin matrix, *J. Biol. Chem.* 272, 24999–25005, 1997.

93. Mosher, D.F., Cross-linking of fibronectin to collagenous proteins, *Mol. Cell. Biochem.* 58, 63–68, 1984.

94. Greenberg. C.S., Sone, D.C., and Lai, T.-S., Factor XIII and fibrin stabilization, in *Thrombosis and Haemostasis*, eds. R.W. Colman, V.J. Marder, A.W. Clowes, J.N. George, and S.Z. Goldhaber, Chapter 17, pp. 312–334, Lippincott Williams & Wilkins, Philadelphia, PA, 2006.

95. Bonvin, C., Overney, J., Shieh, A.C., Dixon, J.B., and Schwartz, M.A., A multichamber fluidic device for 3D cultures under interstitial flow with live imaging: Development, characterization, and applications, *Biotechnol. Bioeng.* 105, 982–991, 2010.

96. Malara, A., Gruppi, C., Rebuzzini, P., et al., Megakaryocyte-matrix interaction within bone marrow: New roles for fibronectin and factor XIII-A, *Blood* 117, 2476–2783, 2014.

97. Cui, C., Wang, S., Myneni, V.C., Hitomi, K., and Kaartinen, M.T., Transglutaminase activity arising from factor XIIIA is required for stabilization and conversion of plasma fibronectin into matrix is osteoblast cultures, *Bone* 59, 127–138, 2014.

98. Guadiz, G., Sporn, L.A., and Simpson-Haidaris, P.J., Thrombin cleavage–independent deposition of fibrinogen in extracellular matrixes, *Blood* 90, 2644–2653, 1997.

99. Pereira, M., Rybarczyk, B.J., Odrijin, T.M., et al., The incorporation of fibrinogen into ECM is dependent on active assembly of a fibronectin matrix, *J. Cell Sci.* 115, 609–617, 2002.

100. Tzoneva, R., Groth, T., Altankov, G., and Paul, D., Remodeling of fibrinogen by endothelial cells in dependence on fibronectin matrix assembly: Effect of substratum, *J. Mater. Sci. Mater. Med.* 13, 1235–1244, 2002.

101. Fujita, T., Yamabe, H., Shimada, M., et al., Thrombin enhances the production of monocyte chemoattractant protein-1 in cultured rat glomerular epithelial cells, *Nephrol. Dial. Transplant.* 23, 3412–3417, 2008.
102. Chapman, J., Allen, C.L., and Stone, O.L., Abnormalities in pathways of alveolar fibrin turnover among patients with interstitial lung disease, *Am. Rev. Respir. Dis.* 133, 437–443, 1986.
103. Idell, S., James, K.K., Gillies, C., Fair, D.S., and Thrall, R.S., Abnormalities of pathways of fibrin turnover in lung lavage of rats with oleic acid and bleomycin-induced lung injury support alveolar fibrin deposition, *Am. J. Pathol.* 135, 387–399, 1989.
104. Schnitt, S.J., Stillman, I.E., Ownings, D.V., et al., Myocardial fibrin deposition in experimental viral myocarditis that progresses to dilated cardiomyopathy, *Circ. Res.* 72, 914–920, 1993.
105. Claudy, A.L., Mirshahi, M., Soria, C., and Soria, J., Detection of undegraded fibrin and tumor necrosis factor-α in venous leg ulcers, *J. Am. Acad. Dermatol.* 25, 623–627, 1991.
106. Fawcett, D.W., *A Textbook of Histology* (Bloom and Fawcett), 12th edn., Chapman & Hall, New York, 1994.
107. Kefalides, N.A., Chemistry of antigenic components isolated from glomerular BM, *Connective Tissue Res.* 1, 3–13, 1972.
108. Korpos, E., Vu, C., Song, J., Hallmann, R., and Sorokin, L., Role of the extracellular matrix in lymphocyte migration, *Cell Tissue Res.* 339, 47–57, 2010.
109. Yurchenco, P.D. and Schittny, J.C., Molecular architecture of BMs, *FASEB J.* 4, 1577–1590, 1990.
110. Smyth, N., Vatansever, H.S., Murray, P., et al., Absence of a BM after targeting the *LACM1* gene results in embryonic lethality due to failure of endoderm differentiation, *J. Cell. Biol.* 144, 151–160, 1999.
111. Kar, K., Wang, Y.H., and Brodsky, B., Sequence dependent of kinetics and morphology of collagen model peptide self-assembly into higher order structures, *Protein Sci.* 17, 1086–1095, 2008.
112. Richard-Blum, S., Dublet, G., and van der Rest, M., *Unconventional Collagens Types VI, VII, VIII, IX, X, XII, XIII, XV, XIX*, Oxford University Press, Oxford, UK, 2000.
113. Levene, C.I., Heale, G., and Robins, S.P., Collagen cross-link synthesis in cultured vascular endothelium, *Br. J. Exp. Pathol.* 70, 621–626, 1989.
114. Ries, A., Engle, J., Lustig, A., and Kühn, K., The function of the NC1 domains in type IV collagen, *J. Biol. Chem.* 270, 23790–23794, 1995.
115. Sielbold, B., Deutzmann, R., and Kühn, K., The arrangement of intra- and intermolecular disulfide bonds in the carboxyterminal, non-collagenous aggregation and cross-linking domain of basement-membrane type IV collagen, *Eur. J. Biochem.* 176, 617–624, 1988.
116. Aumailley, M., Wiedermann, H., Mann, K., and Timpl, R., Binding of nidogen and the laminin–nidogen complex to the BM collagen type IV, *Eur. J. Biochem.* 184, 241–248, 1989.
117. Danielson, K.G., Martinez-Hernandez, A., Hassell, J.R., and Iozzo, R.V., Establishment of a cell line from the EHS tumor: Biosynthesis of basement membrane constituents and characterization of a hybrid proteoglycan containing heparan and chondroitin sulfate chains, *Matrix* 12, 22–35, 1992.
118. Farach-Carson, M.C., Warren. C.R., Harrington, D.A., and Carson, D.D., Border patrol: Insights into the unique role of perlecan/heparan sulfate proteoglycan 2 at cell and tissue borders, *Matrix Biol.* 34, 64–79, 2014.
119. Stoler-Barak, L., Mousslon, C., Shezen, E., et al., Blood vessels pattern heparan sulfate gradients between their apical and basolateral aspects, *PLoS One* 9(11), 85699, 2014.

120. Behrens, D.T., Villone, D., Koch, M., et al., The epidermal basement membrane in a composite of separate laminin or collagen IV–containing networks connected by aggregated perlecan, but not by nidogens, *J. Biol. Chem.* 287, 18700–18709. 2012.

121. van der Rest, M. and Garrone, R., Collagen family of proteins, *FASEB J.* 5, 2814–2823, 1991.

122. Brittingham, R., Uitoo, J., and Fertala, A., High-affinity binding of the NC1 domain of collagen VII to laminin 5 and collagen IV, *Biochem. Biophys. Res. Commun.* 343, 692–699, 2006.

123. Wolberg, A.S., Stafford, D.W., and Erie, D.A., Human factor IX binds to specific sites on the collagenous domain of collagen IV, *J. Biol. Chem.* 272, 16717–16720, 1997.

124. Flood, V.H., Schlauderaff, A.C., Haberichter, S.L., et al., Crucial role the VWF A1 domain in binding to type IV collagen, *Blood* 125, 2297–2304, 2015.

125. Yang, B.-G., Tanaka, T., Jang, M.H., et al., Binding of lymphoid chemokines to collagen IV that accumulates in the basal lamina of high endothelial venules: Its implications in lymphocyte trafficking, *J. Immunol.* 179, 4376–4382, 2007.

126. Somasundaram, R., Ruehl, M., Schaefer, B., et al., Interstitial collagens I, II, and VI sequester and modulate the multifunctional cytokine oncostatin M, *J. Biol. Chem.* 277, 3242–3246, 2002.

127. Paralkar, V.M., Vukicevic, S., and Reddi, A.H., Transforming growth factor β type 1 binds to collagen IV of basement membrane matrix: Implications for development, *Develop. Biol.* 143, 303–308, 1991.

128. Ettalaie, C., Collier, M.E.W., Mei, M.P., Xiao, Y.P., and Maraveyas, A., Enhanced binding of tissue factor–microparticles to collagen-IV and fibronectin leads to increased tissue factor activity *in vitro, Thromb. Haemost.* 109, 61–71, 2013.

129. Harrison, C.A., Al-Musawi, S.L., and Walton, K.L., Prodomains regulate the synthesis, extracellular localisation and activity of TGF-β superfamily ligands, *Growth Factors* 29, 174–186, 2011.

130. Nieuwdorp, M., Meuwese, M.C., Vink, H., et al., The endothelial glycocalyx: A potential barrier between health and vascular disease, *Curr. Opin. Lipidol.* 16, 507–511, 2005.

131. Linden, S.K., Sutton, P., Karlsson, N.B., Korolik, V., and McGuckin, M.A., Mucins in the mucosal barrier to infection, *Mucosal Immunol.* 1, 183–197, 2008.

132. Reitsma, S., Slaaf, D.W., Vink, H., Zandvoort, M.A., oude Egbrink, M.G., The endothelial glycocalyx: Composition, functions, and visualization, *Pflugers Arch.* 454, 345–359, 2007.

133. Weinbaum, S., Tarbell, J.M., and Damiano, E.R., The structure and function of the endothelial glycocalyx layer, *Annu. Rev. Biomed. Eng.* 9, 121–167, 2007.

134. Salmon, A.H., Neal, C.R., Sage, L.M., et al., Angiopoietin-1 alters microvascular permeability coefficients *in vivo* via modification of endothelial glycocalyx, *Cardiovasc. Res.* 83, 24–33, 2009.

135. Perrin, R.M., Harper, S.J., and Bates, D.O., A role for the endothelial glycocalyx in regulating microvascular permeability in diabetes mellitus, *Cell Biochem. Biophys.* 49, 65–72, 2007.

136. Becker, B.F., Chappell, D., and Jacob, M., Endothelial glycocalyx and coronary vascular permeability: The fringe benefit, *Basic. Res. Cardiol.* 105, 687–701, 2010.

3 The Biochemistry of Hyaluronan in the Interstitial Space

3.1 HYALURONAN

Hyaluronan is a very large carbohydrate heteropolymer that is a major constituent of the interstitial space and is of great importance in synovial fluid. In addition to its physical functions as a lubricant and a cushioning agent, it is vital to cellular function. It is also a key component of hydrogels used for drug delivery[1–3] and tissue augmentation.[4–6] The hyaluronan is generally internally cross-linked or cross-linked with a protein, such as fibrin. The focus of the current chapter is on the effect of hyaluronan on proteolytic activity in the interstitial space. The reader is directed to the recent book by Garg and Hales[7] for more information on hyaluronan.

3.1.1 Introduction to Hyaluronan

First, from a protein chemist's perspective, hyaluronan—a very large polysaccharide composed of a repeating disaccharide—is a dull molecule, and this view is shared by others.[8,9] It is remarkable, then, that hyaluronan binds to specific cell surface receptors and other proteins described as hyaladherins, which have great diversity.[9] The interaction of hyaluronan with proteins can be complex, considering its homogeneous nature. Hyaluronan may influence the activity of enzymes, including proteases, within the interstitial space as well as protease substrates such as fibrinogen. The response of some cells via the CD44 receptor or other hyaluronan receptors can depend on the size of the hyaluronan ligand; the response to low-molecular-weight hyaluronan fragments can differ from that observed for high-molecular-weight hyaluronan. The degradation of hyaluronan frequently occurs as a result of inflammation and includes the action of reactive oxygen species (ROS). High-molecular-weight hyaluronan may be anti-inflammatory, while low-molecular-weight hyaluronan fragments can be proinflammatory. Hyaluronan in the interstitial space has multiple functions including lubrication, water homeostasis, partition of plasma proteins, and regulation of macromolecular transport.[10] Hyaluronan is the primary material in the pericellular coat seen in various cells including fibroblasts and mesothelial cells.[10]

3.1.2 Physical Characteristics of Hyaluronan

Hyaluronan is a large polydisperse glycosaminoglycan with an average molecular weight of $2–4 \times 10^6$ Da.[11] Hyaluronan is composed of a repeating disaccharide, glucuronic acid–N-acetylglucosamine, and thus has a negative charge; however, it is not as anionic as sulfated glycosaminoglycans such as heparin. Despite its relatively simple structure, hyaluronan has considerable secondary structure in solution, driven by the formation of a water bridge between the uronate carboxyl group of glucuronic acid and the amide group in N-acetylglucosamine.[12–16] There are also hydrogen bonds involving hydroxyl groups and the ring oxygen. This leads to the formation of long, rigid, coiled structures that are sensitive to ionic strength.[13] There is some evidence for the existence of secondary and tertiary structures in hyaluronan.[15] It is possible that hyaluronan can develop higher-order structures upon interaction with proteins.

3.1.2.1   Effect of Protein on Hyaluronan Conformation

The interaction of hyaluronan with specific proteins is discussed in Section 3.4.4. Day and Prestwich[9] reviewed the structural organization of hyaladherins, which differ in tissue and cellular location and expression, specificity, primary structure, and binding affinity. A large number of hyaladherins contain a Link domain of approximately one hundred amino acids. This Link domain is found in hyaladherins such as aggrecan, versican, and the cell surface receptors CD44 and LYVE-1. Another receptor for hyaluronan, RHAMM, does not contain a Link domain. Day and Prestwich[9] also catalog the Link domains by size, including a single Link module of 90 amino acids, a Link domain with C- and N-terminal extensions (160 amino acids), and a Link pair (approximately 200 residues). As noted by Day and Prestwich,[9] it is assumed that basic amino acids are critical for binding hyaluronan, although the importance of other amino acid residues such as tyrosine and phenylalanine has been demonstrated. Finally, Day and Prestwich[9] mention the possibility of hyaladherins stabilizing a given conformation of hyaluronan. The smallest hyaluronan fragment is a decasaccharide (five disaccharide units) that binds to several hyaladherins including hyaluronectin,[17] aggrecan,[18] and keratinocyte CD44 receptor.[19] Courel and coworkers[17] used an enzyme-linked sorbent assay (ELSA) to measure the binding of hyaluronan to hyaluronectin as the basis for the quantitative assay of hyaluronan. The hyaluronan sample was absorbed to a plastic microplate, which was then measured by binding to a hyaluronectin–alkaline phosphatase conjugate (p-nitrophenyl acetate substrate). When native hyaluronan (human umbilical cord) was digested with hyaluronidase, the amount of hyaluronan increased as a function of digestion time and then markedly decreased. These data support the hypothesis that some hyaluronectin-binding sites are masked in the native hyaluronan but exposed during fragmentation of native hyaluronan, eventually reaching a point where only fragments less the five decasaccharides were present in the digestion mixture. Cowman and coworkers[20] used atomic force microscopy to study the conformational changes of hyaluronan on binding to surfaces and in cartilage. These investigators describe a number of possible conformations for hyaluronan and speculate that interaction with a protein, including receptors, could induce a conformational change in hyaluronan. While there are limited studies on the conformation of hyaluronan bound to proteins, Banerji and coworkers[21] report a conformational change in the hyaluronan-binding domain (HABD) of murine CD44 receptor (residues 25–174) on binding hyaluronan; attempts to use the human CD44 receptor HABD were frustrated by the inability to crystallize the protein. These investigators suggest that there is a conformational change in the sequence of hyaluronan that binds to the HABD and that there are also conformational changes in the HABD involving the orientation of a specific arginine residue, resulting in two conformers. Banerji and coworkers further suggest that hydrogen bonding is the dominant interaction between hyaluronic acid and HABD. Higman and coworkers[22] show conformational changes in hyaluronan octomer bound to tumor necrosis factor–stimulated gene-6 protein. There are other studies on the importance of a conformational transition in the CD44 receptor[23,24] but no further work on hyaluronan conformation. There is a suggestion that binding hyaluronan to a receptor could stabilize mobile hydrogen bonds.

The work on the conformational change of hyaluronan on binding to CD44 and other hyaladherins has been done with very small hyaluronan fragments at the lower end of measurable binding to such proteins.[17–19] Thus, in considering the binding of high- or low-molecular-weight hyaluronan, any conformational change would likely involve only a small portion of hyaluronan molecules.

3.1.3 SOLVENT AND HYALURONAN

Water plays a significant role in several of the functions of hyaluronan. Hyaluronan occupies a large volume in solution; estimates show that 1 g occupies between 1–5 L of volume in water.[25,26] The solution behavior of hyaluronan is remarkably sensitive to ionic strength, with a marked decrease in solution volume (a decrease in hydrodynamic radius from 99 nm to 33 nm), measured by the diffusion coefficient in the transition from H_2O to 100 mM NaCl.[27] This represents a greater than 90% reduction in volume.[28] While this effect of ionic strength is of interest from a physical chemistry perspective, it is of little consequence in the majority of the interstitial space (skin), where the concentration of sodium chloride is likely in excess of 100 mM; the concentration of sodium in human thoracic lymph is 127 meq/L, which is equal to that in blood serum or plasma.[29] Bretag[30] has developed an artificial interstitial fluid for the storage of tissues with a sodium concentration in excess of 100 mM. The hydration properties of hyaluronan are suggested to be of considerable consequence to the kidney for the maintenance of water homeostasis[31] and to the function of the skin,[32–34] as well as to the cosmetic industry, where the goal is to maintain hyaluronan, particularly during the aging process.[35] A recent study[36] has shown that the oral delivery of medium-sized hyaluronan (800 and 300 kDa) improves skin condition by increasing moisture content.

Studies on the effect of ionic strength on hyaluronan[26,27] were performed with relatively small hyaluronan molecules of 500 and 830 kDa; both species showed a 2.8-fold increase in the diffusion coefficient in the transition to 100 mM NaCl. It is suggested that this represents contraction of a coil structure caused by the electrostatic shielding of carboxyl groups. It is likely that the very large hyaluronan molecules present in the interstitial space undergo a similar change with an increase in ionic strength. Vincent[26] discusses the role of hyaluronan in organizing water for load bearing and application in the interstitial space. As a large molecule, hyaluronan occupies a large volume in space. A single molecule of hyaluronan occupies the volume of a sphere of 1 μm (10,000 Å) in diameter. To put this into perspective, the hydrodynamic radius of fibrinogen monomer is 9.7 nm (97 Å),[37] while lysozyme has a hydrodynamic radius of 20.5 Å.[38] Thus, hyaluronan is much larger than most of the hyaladherins. The size of hyaluronan also means there will be an overlap at relatively low polymer concentration (80% overlap at 0.1% hyaluronan).[26] Exceeding the overlap concentration for a polymer such as hyaluronan results in the interaction of chains, resulting in entanglement (transition from dilute to semidilute solutions)[39,40] and a sharp increase in viscosity.[40,41] Values for the critical overlap concentration for "native" high-molecular-weight hyaluronan vary between 0.5[42] and 4 g/L.[43] The latter figure is for high-molecular-weight hyaluronan (4×10^6 M) obtained from *Streptococcus zooepidemicus*. Maintenance of hyaluronan concentration above the critical overlap concentration is important for load bearing and other mechanical functions.

3.2   HYALURONAN IN INTERSTITIAL SPACE

There is regional variability in hyaluronan distribution, with skin containing approximately 50% of the total body hyaluronan.[11] The concentration in blood is low (0.01–0.1 mg/L in human serum), higher in thoracic lymph (8–18 mg/L) and dermis (200 mg/L), and the highest in synovial fluid (1420–3600 mg/L) and umbilical cord (Wharton's Jelly). Hyaluronan can be degraded at the local level by a receptor-mediated process[8] or quickly from the circulation after passage through the lymph by the liver.[11] The distribution of hyaluronan is asymmetric within the interstitial space,[31,41,44] resulting in regions rich in hyaluronan and others with less. For example, hyaluronan concentration is high in the interstitium of the renal medulla[45–49] and low in the renal cortex.[50,51] Schweinfurth and Thibeault[52] have suggested that the distribution of hyaluronan in the larynx is responsible for the relative intensity of infant vocalization when compared to adults. The use of a microgels containing hyaluronan has been proposed for therapeutic use in vocal cord scarring.[53]

Hyaluronan (hyaluronic acid) is the most abundant polysaccharide in the interstitial space and associates with hyaladherins, proteins such as CD44 (a cell surface receptor), and aggrecan (a component of the extracellular matrix [ECM]), which specifically bind to hyaluronan.[54–56] Some workers consider hyaluronan to be a component of the ECM. For the purpose of the current work, hyaluronan is a component of the interstitial fluid, which permeates the ECM but is separate from it. This is consistent with the early work on ground substance,[57] the proteoglycan-rich interstitial fluid.

The amount of fluid in the interstitial space is greater than the amount of fluid in the vascular system[49] but is compromised by the presence of hyaluronan and collagen,[44,45] which restrict the access of macromolecules to the total interstitial space.[58–60] Excessive deposition of collagen in the interstitial space contributes to the pathology of fibrotic lesions.[61] Collagen I and hyaluronan can be thought of as occupying a large amount of interstitial space and blocking large molecules from the total interstitial space in a manner similar to that seen in gel filtration (size-exclusion chromatography), where separation is based on exclusion from a polysaccharide network.[62] A second concept is derived from the heterogeneity of hyaluronan distribution within the interstitium, where there would be areas/channels of unrestricted passage. It is likely the net effect on large molecules will be the same; large molecules, such as proteins, are distributed more slowly than small molecules. Watson and coworkers[63] proposed a model involving a gel composed of hyaluronan and/or collagen and which had a low permeability to large molecules such as fibrinogen, the analogy being that a protein passes through a G-25 Sephadex® column more rapidly than a buffer salt.[64] The observation of Watson and coworkers[63] is that while the lymph/plasma ratio of fibrinogen (0.04) is less than albumin (0.24), a smaller protein, fibrinogen reaches its equilibrium concentration more rapidly than albumin. This is consistent with the physical process of extravasation determining the size of plasma proteins passing into the interstitial space (Chapter 1). The data of Watson and coworkers[63] are also consistent with the regional differences in hyaluronan distribution. The concentration of a protein such as albumin in the interstitial fluid phase will increase with excluded volume fraction (decreased access to the gel network); such a situation could occur with increased water concentration.[65] Laurent[66] used equilibrium dialysis to show that the exclusion of albumin from hyaluronan gels is dependent on hyaluronan concentration; these experiments used a 0.45 µ membrane that was permeable to all proteins used in the study but impervious to the hyaluronan gel (0.1%). Laurent[66] also used chromatography on a hyaluronan gel column (1.4%) to show that the molecule size was the determining factor in exclusion from the gel. This work contributed to the development of a theory of gel filtration, as discussed in a retrospective by Laurent in 1993.[67] Collagen also contributes to the exclusion of proteins in the interstitial space. Shaw and Schy[68] measured the diffusion of various materials in a 5% collagen gel. They observed a value of 0.24 for the ratio of the diffusion constant in the gel to that in tritiated water, while a value of 0.13 was obtained for ovalbumin and 0.17 for glucose. Sharon[25] also stated that a hyaluronan gel excludes macromolecules.

As a charged polymer, hyaluronan can also partition on the basis of electrostatic attraction or repulsion.[58,69] Positively charged proteins partition into the hyaluronan mesh more rapidly than anionic proteins. Gandhi and Bell[70] prepared aminoethyl amido derivatives of carboxyl groups in albumin by reaction with diethylamine in the presence of carbodiimide, with the effect of raising the isoelectric point (making the protein more basic). They then compared the transvascular transport of these derivatives with native albumin. The most basic derivative ($I_p = 8.1$) was cleared 80% more rapidly than native albumin ($I_p = 5.0$). Similar results were obtained subsequently by Wiig and coworkers[71] using a in vitro dermis model. Sagestad and coworkers[69] demonstrated a positive correlation between protein size (Stokes–Einstein radius) and the fraction of protein excluded from the interstitial space, but showed a negative correlation between the isoelectric point and the fraction of protein excluded from the interstitial space. Early work on gel filtration with an agarose matrix (Sephadex) showed interaction between basic proteins, and Sephadex showed adsorption of basic proteins in H_2O; elution from the column was accomplished with 100 mM NaCl.[72] It was earlier suggested that the adsorption properties of Sephadex reflected the presence of carboxyl groups in the matrix resulting from oxidation of the polysaccharide matrix.[73]

Hyaluronan could also be considered as one phase of a two-phase system, such as that described by Albertsson.[74] In the case of the interstitium, the two-phase system is composed of hyaluronan and plasma protein, primarily albumin.[75] This presents the possibility of phase separation of low-molecular-weight compounds in the interstitial space; however, there is no work to support such a process.

3.3 EFFECT OF HYALURONAN ON ENZYME ACTIVITY

Considering the presence of hyaluronan in the interstitium and other extravascular spaces such as the synovium, we are surprised that there are so few studies on the effect of this biopolymer on enzyme activity. Sage and coworkers[76] reported a modest stimulation by hyaluronan of the degradation of collagen IV by cathepsin S; a similar stimulation of cathepsin S was observed with dextran sulfate and heparin, while inhibition of cathepsin S degradation of collagen IV was observed with chondroitin 4-sulfate. A modest stimulation of cathepsin S hydrolysis of benzyloxycarbonyl-phenylalanyl-arginine-4-methylcoumarin was also observed with hyaluronan, while inhibition was observed with chondroitin 4-sulfate. Iwanicki and coworkers[77] observed that hyaluronan inhibited the action of phospholipase A_2 in the hydrolysis of dipalmitoyl phosphatidylcholine-N-(4-nitrobenzo-2-oxa-1,3-diazole).

Hyaluronan shows a modest stabilizing effect on cathepsin K as a well a small effect on the activity toward a synthetic substrate, Z-Leu-Arg-MCA (carbobenzoxy-leucine-arginine-4-methyl-7-coumarylamide); however, there was no stimulation of activity toward a collagen substrate.[78] Cathepsin K is an important enzyme for osteoclast-mediated bone remodeling. Cathepsin K is also involved in the metabolism of interstitial collagen.[79,80] While the effects of hyaluronan are slight, Li and coworkers[81] did observe a large effect of chondroitin sulfate on cathepsin K activity. These investigators used *cumulative activity* (CA), a combination of the effect on enzyme activity and the effect on enzyme stability, to express the effects of modulating substances on cathepsin K activity. Chondroitin sulfate provided a 200-fold increase in CA,ʹ while hyaluronan had a 10-fold effect. Subsequent work from this group[81] showed that a complex of chondroitin sulfate with cathepsin K is the active catalytic species in bone resorption.

Hyaluronan binds to tissue kallikrein (KLK-1); digestion of hyaluronan releases KLK-1 with an increase in enzyme activity,[82] suggesting that the bound KLK-1 is less active than KLK-1 in solution. Since KLK-1 and hyaluronan are both secreted by bronchial epithelial cells, binding to hyaluronan is a potential mechanism for regulating postsecretion KLK-1 activity in the lung. Further work from this group[83] suggested that oxidative stress degrades hyaluronan, increasing bronchial KLK-1, which could process pro-EGF to EGF (epidermal growth factor), which in turn binds to EGF receptor activation. EGF receptor activation causes submucosal gland hypertrophy and hyperplasia and mucus hypersecretion with airway obstruction. Yu and coworkers[84] extended the observations of the role of ROS in hyaluronan degradation, leading to the release of KLK-1 and the conversion of pro-EGF to EGF. They propose that hyaluronan fragments induce epidermal growth factor receptor (EGFR) to interact with CD44, leading to MUC5AC expression and mucus formation. Other investigators[85] have suggested that TGF-β1 stimulation of fibroblasts involves hyaluronan synthesis; the hyaluronan then stimulates CD44, coupled with EGFR stimulation by EGF. The binding of hyaluronan by CD44 and EGF by EGF4 results in cell proliferation driven by MAP kinase (ERK1/2). These investigators do not describe a mechanism for EGF formation, but it is possible that it could involve KLK-1. The physical state of the hyaluronan is not described, but it does seem that native hyaluronan would be effective.[86] Since this work on the interaction of hyaluronan with KLK-1, a number of KLK-1-related peptidases (Chapter 7) have been described,[87] but there is no information on the possible effect of hyaluronan on their activities.

Molecular crowding in the interstitial space is a consequence of the ability of hyaluronan and other components of the ECM to exclude molecules from bulk solution. Molecular crowding is most often considered from the perspective of intracellular events.[88] Laurent[89] discusses the early work on the function of hyaluronan as a molecular crowder.[74] Other than Laurent's comments on the potential role of hyaluronan, we could find no studies on hyaluronan as a molecular crowder. Molecular crowding would likely affect enzyme activity[90,91] and protein–protein interactions.[92,93]

3.4 SPECIFIC INTERACTION OF HYALURONAN WITH RECEPTORS (HYALADHERINS)

There are a number of cell surface receptors and large proteins that bind to hyaluronan in a physiologically significant manner. Cell surface receptors, large ECM proteins, and antibodies share similar characteristics in the binding of ligands, such as saturation, specificity, and reversibility.[94] In view of these similarities and sequence homology, Toole[95] has designated these hyaladherins. There has been considerable work on the binding of hyaluronan to C44 receptor.[96–98]

3.4.1 CD44

CD44 (the Hermes antigen; a lymphocyte homing protein)[98,99] is a type-1 single-pass transmembrane glycoprotein that contains four functional domains.[100] The distal Link module interacts with hyaluronan.[101–104] The distal Link module is connected to a mucin-like domain ("stalk") that is heavily glycosylated, contains covalently bound chondroitin sulfate and heparan sulfate, and can contain a variable number of inserts, resulting in a large number of isoforms for the CD44 receptor. The mucin-like domain is connected to a transmembrane domain with a cytoplasmic tail that interacts with the cytoskeleton (actin filaments).[105,106] The function of CD44 is highly regulated, with surface expression requiring an activation process.[107]

CD44 is the primary ligand for hyaluronan on a variety of cells including endothelial cells, epithelial cells, T cells, and fibroblasts.[99] CD44 also interacts with other ligands such as collagen, fibronectin, laminin, and osteopontin.[108] Variable splicing of 19 exons in the stalk region (membrane proximal, below the Link module) results in the CD44 isoforms.[88] The CD44 isoforms are expressed in a cell-specific manner.[108,109]

Hyaluronan is cleared from the circulation quite rapidly ($t_{1/2} = 2.5$–4.5 min.) and catabolized in the liver.[110] The turnover rate of hyaluronan in tissues is considerably longer and varies with location.[111] In the tissues, hyaluronan is fragmented and passed into the lymph and hence to the blood stream, where it is rapidly taken up by the liver and degraded. While there are enzymes that can degrade hyaluronan, ROS could play a major role.[112] Approximately one-third of the total body hyaluronan is catabolized every 24 hours.[113] Stern[113] has suggested that the catabolism of hyaluronan may be a new metabolic pathway. CD44 has been suggested to be responsible for the internalization and degradation of hyaluronan in cartilage as a local mechanism for hyaluronan turnover.[8] The binding of aggrecan to hyaluronan inhibits the process of internalization and degradation.[114] However, proteolytic fragmentation of aggrecan eliminates the ability of aggrecan to protect hyaluronan from internalization.

The physical nature of the binding of hyaluronan to CD44 is dependent on the size of the hyaluronan.[115,116] The binding of fluorophore-labeled hyaluronan fragments to a transfected murine T cell lymphoma cell is time dependent.[116] Determination of binding by competitive inhibition showed that avidity increased with the size of the hyaluronan fragment. More recent work[117] on the binding of hyaluronan to CD44 on HK-2 cells or BT549 cells has shown that clustering of CD44 receptors occurs in the presence of high-molecular-weight hyaluronan, while clustering of receptors was not observed with low-molecular-weight hyaluronan. A cell requires "activation" to enable the surface expression of CD44 prior to the binding of hyaluronan.[118,119]

Rochman and coworkers[118] showed that lymphoma cells can be activated with phorbol ester (phorbol 12-myristate, 13-acetate) to express CD44, as measured by the binding of hyaluronan. Nandi and coworkers[119] showed that activation of endothelial cells with TNF-α resulted in CD44 expression as measured by hyaluronan binding. This binding is suggested to be tight enough ($k_d \approx 10^{-8}-10^{-9}$ M) to permit the binding of "activated" leukocytes to the bound hyaluronan. This is suggested as a mechanism to permit rolling on the endothelium in extravasation of leukocytes. This activation of CD44 is related to the conformational change in CD44[23,24] required for binding hyaluronan (3.1.2.1).

3.4.2   RHAMM

There has been less interest in RHAMM (CD168),[120–123] the acronym of which is derived from the phrase "receptor for hyaluronan-mediated motility."[120] While most attention has focused on CD44 as a receptor for hyaluronan, other cell surface receptors have also been described. RHAMM has been described as a hyaluronan receptor involved in cell motility during development.[124,125] However, it has been of recent interest in oncology, where the binding of low-molecular-weight hyaluronan to RHAMM mediates fibrosarcoma cell adhesion to fibronectin.[126] It has also been suggested that the binding of low-molecular-weight hyaluronan to RHAMM activates an ERK1/2 signaling pathway. The role of RHAMM in cancer has stimulated the development of hyaluronan–drug conjugates.[127] Measurement of the expression of RHAMM has also advanced as a prognostic biomarker for large-cell lung cancer.[128]

3.4.3   OTHER CELL SURFACE RECEPTORS FOR HYALURONAN

Hyaluronan receptor for endocytosis (HARE) is a receptor with at least several isotypes that can participate in the endocytosis of hyaluronan, heparin, advanced glycation end products, and acetylated and oxidized glycoproteins.[129,130] HARE receptors were described in 2000 on rat sinusoidal endothelial cells[131] as responsible for the endocytosis of hyaluronan in liver catabolism of hyaluronan. Two receptors were described: 175 and 200 kDa. Immunological assays established the presence of these receptors in other tissues. Subsequent work established HARE as a receptor distinct from CD44.[132] HARE seems to be identical with stabilin 2.[133] Inhibition of stabilin 2/HARE has been suggested as a therapeutic strategy in cancer.[134]

Lymphatic vessel endothelial hyaluronic acid (HA) receptor (LYVE-1) is found in lymphatic tissue and has approximately 50% sequence homology with the CD44 receptor,[135,136] and its function is poorly understood.[136] As with the other hyaluronan receptors, recent work[137] has focused on the role of LYVE-1 in oncology.

3.4.4 Hyaluronan Binding to Other Hyaladherins

Binding constants (either K_a or K_d) for hyaluronan have been reported for a variety of hyaladherins, including pig laryngeal cartilage fragments,[138] simian virus 40–3T3 cells,[139] fibrinogen,[140–142] a rat colon cancer cell line,[143] a brain-derived proteoglycan,[144] and versican, a chondroitin sulfate proteoglycan.[144] The binding of hyaluronan to most ligands is reversible, with the exception being the endocytosis of hyaluronan by CD44 receptors,[145] and of "high affinity," with estimates of K_d ranging from 10^{-7} [127] to 10^{-9} M.[139] High-molecular-weight hyaluronan appears to bind with higher affinity than smaller species. While there is not a large amount of data, there appears to be great specificity in hyaluronan binding. Hyaluronan binds to rat tumor cells to a much greater extent than either chondroitin sulfate or dextran sulfate.[143] The studies on the binding of hyaluronan to fibrinogen[140] is estimated to be "high affinity" ($K_d \approx 4.5 \times 10^{-8}$ M), as calculated for a 150-mer hyaluronan fragment. The avidity of hyaluronan binding to fibrinogen was dependent on the size of the hyaluronan fragment, with small fragments ($M_r \sim 3900$) about half as effective as native hyaluronan in displacing fibrinogen from a hyaluronan matrix. In subsequent work, Rinaudo[141] showed that the addition of fibrinogen to low-molecular-weight hyaluronan (195 kDa) induces non-Newtonian behavior, with viscosity increasing with fibrinogen concentration. The effect of fibrinogen on viscosity decreases with the increasing molecular weight of fibrinogen. High-molecular-weight hyaluronan is considered to exhibit non-Newtonian viscosity,[142] so an effect of fibrinogen would be less pronounced.

There was little binding of hyaluronan to fibronectin under these assay conditions (solution phase binding).[140] Previous work[146] has suggested that fibronectin binds hyaluronan in a solid-phase system; the hyaluronan–fibronectin complex binds epithelial cells. Fibronectin[147] and fibrinogen[148] undergo conformational change on binding to a surface. In the case of fibrinogen, binding to a surface exposes epitopes associated with fibrin. Very little binding was observed for lysozyme to hyaluronan,[140] which is surprising, since lysozyme is a basic protein. Studies by other investigators have shown that the binding of lysozyme to hyaluronan is remarkably sensitive to ionic strength.[149] Van Damme and coworkers[149] observed that there was no specific binding of lysozyme to hyaluronan at concentrations of NaCl above 100 mM. A careful examination of the effect of NaCl concentration showed that the binding of lysozyme to immobilized hyaluronan increased at 10–20 mM NaCl and then rapidly decreased with increasing ionic strength.[150] The studies with fibrinogen cited above[140] were performed in phosphate-buffered saline (PBS) with an NaCl well in excess of 60 mM NaCl, which totally obviates lysozyme binding to solid-phase hyaluronan. This would argue for considerable specificity for the interactions of fibrinogen with hyaluronan.

3.5 LOW-MOLECULAR-WEIGHT HYALURONAN

Hyaluronan is degraded during the process of inflammation,[151–156] resulting in the formation of low-molecular-weight hyaluronan fragments. Considering the physiological difference in the behavior of low- and high-molecular-weight hyaluronan, it is surprising that there is so little physical or chemical comparison of the two species. Mosely and coworkers[157] evaluated the differences between low- and high-molecular-weight hyaluronan in the inhibition of the effects of PMN-derived ROS. High-molecular-weight hyaluronan showed antioxidant properties, while low-molecular-weight hyaluronan had no effect. Ferguson and coworkers[158] compared some of the solution characteristics of hyaluronan as a function of molecular size. Size fractions of hyaluronan were obtained by limited acid hydrolysis (0.4 M HCl) under varied conditions of time and temperature. Hydrodynamic radius (Stokes radius) was a direct function of molecular weight for the several hyaluronan fractions, consistent with an extended, rod-like conformation for the various molecular size fractions. A rod-like structure such as a stiff random coil for hyaluronan has been previously suggested[13,159] and is based on a model with mobile hydrogen bonding between adjacent saccharides and the repulsion of carboxyl groups.[28,160] There is some question as to whether hyaluronan has a stable secondary or tertiary structure in solution.[161] The effect of ionic strength on hyaluronan in solution[26] must be considered in any conjecture about conformation. The conformation of hyaluronan and possible changes in conformation on binding to hyaladherins is discussed in Sections 3.1.2, 3.1.2.1, and 3.1.3.

Given that there are no apparent differences in basic chemical composition, it is remarkable that there are such differences in the physiological responses elicited by low- and high-molecular-weight hyaluronan on binding to cell surface receptors such as CD44. The binding studies[17–19] discussed in Section 3.1.2.1 suggest that a decamer (five disaccharide units) was the smallest fragment that could bind to a hyaladherin; these were physical binding studies, not measurements of biological activity. Tolg and coworkers[158] showed that 6-mer and 8-mer oligosaccharide fragments of hyaluronan could stimulate dermal fibroblast migration; 4 kDa and 40 kDa fragments of hyaluronan had no effect, while 500 kDa hyaluronan was inhibitory. These investigators also showed that the 6-mer stimulated scratch wound repair; the action of the 6-mer required both CD44 and RHAMM expression. Low-molecular-weight hyaluronan (six disaccharide units) induced endothelial cell differentiation and angiogenesis in a CD44-dependent process involving the upregulation of a cytokine gene.[88] Takahashi and coworkers[88] showed that the hyaluronan dodecasaccharide stimulation of endothelial cell morphogenesis involved the chemokine CXCL1/GRO1. There is a similarity between the mechanisms of endothelial cell stimulation by FGF-2 and the hyaluronan dodecasaccharide. David-Raoudi and coworkers[163] reported different effects of native hyaluronan and fragments on human dermal fibroblasts. Cell adhesion and proliferation were enhanced by both a dodecamer and native hyaluronan. There were some differences between fragments and native hyaluronan in their effect on collagen synthesis. It was suggested that native hyaluronan (and, to a lesser extent, the dodecamer) would favor fetal wound healing by stimulation of collagen III synthesis, while the dodecamer would favor fibrosis by stimulation of collagen I synthesis. Knockdown studies suggest that while binding to CD44 is responsible for some of the effects of hyaluronan, other receptors such as RHAMM may also be involved. These investigators do discuss the differences in their results as compared to other studies, suggesting issues such as cell type and culture conditions. Cell-based assay systems and animal assays are plagued by the issue of reproducibility,[164–166] so the comments of David-Raoudi and coworkers[163] regarding discrepancies between different laboratories are of merit. In general, there are marked differences in the cellular responses to low- and high-molecular-weight hyaluronan. Joddar and Ramamurthi[167] examined the effect of hyaluronan and hyaluronan fragments (high molecular weight, 2×10^3 kDa; low molecular weight, 2×10^2 kDa; very low molecular weight, 20 kDa) on rat vascular smooth muscle cells in culture. Low- and very-low-molecular-weight hyaluronan stimulated cell growth (DNA content), while high-molecular-weight hyaluronan had no effect. The low-molecular-weight fragments inhibited elastin synthesis, while there was a modest stimulation of elastin synthesis with high-molecular-weight hyaluronan; an exception was observed at high concentrations of low-molecular-weight hyaluronan, where elastin synthesis approached control values. The effect on collagen synthesis depended on the concentration of the hyaluronan species. At low concentrations, the high-molecular-weight species stimulated collagen synthesis, but less effect was observed with the low-molecular-weight hyaluronan fragments. At higher concentrations of the hyaluronan species, inhibition of collagen synthesis was observed with the high-molecular-weight species, while stimulation was observed with the low-molecular-weight hyaluronan fragments. Fuchs and coworkers[168] studied the effect of high-molecular-weight hyaluronan and a small fragment (6–10 disaccharide units; 12–20-mer) on CXCL12 signaling in hepG2iso cells (a CXCR4-positive hepatoma cell line). High-molecular-weight hyaluronan enhanced CXCL12 signaling in both hepG2iso and HUVEC cells, while the small hyaluronan inhibited CXCL12 signaling. CXCL12 is a chemokine and CXCR4 is the receptor for CXCL12.[169] A final example of the difference between native hyaluronan and hyaluronan fragments is provided by studies on the effect hyaluronan fragments on dendritic cells. Termeer and coworkers[156] showed that tetrasaccharide and hexasaccharide derivatives of hyaluronan induced maturation of dendritic cells derived from human monocytes (upregulation of HLA-DR and CD83 and downregulation of CD115), increasing production of IL-1β, TNF-α, and IL-12. High-molecular-weight (600–1000 kDa) and intermediate hyaluronan (80–200 kDa) had no effect on the maturation of dendritic cells, but high-molecular-weight hyaluronan produced a smaller production of IL-1β, TNF-α, and

IL-12. Subsequent work from this group[170] showed that the effect of hyaluronan oligosaccharides on dendritic cells involved Toll-like receptor 4 (TLR-4). More recently, Muto and coworkers[171] demonstrated that small hyaluronan fragments promoted the migration of dendritic cells from the skin, resulting in a lack of immune response.

While there is substantial literature on the differences in cellular response to native hyaluronan and hyaluronan fragments, there are few studies on differences in the nature of the binding. There is evidence[115,116] that high-molecular-weight hyaluronan binds tighter to cell surface receptors than do hyaluronan fragments. The strongest data comes from the work of Yang and coworkers,[117] who showed that the binding of high-molecular-weight hyaluronan resulted in the clustering of CD44 receptors.

3.6   HYALURONAN AS A THERAPEUTIC

Hyaluronan has been advanced for several therapeutic applications,[172] including dermal augmentation, arthritic joints, as an antiadhesive, and as a medium for drug delivery. Hyaluronan has a long history of use as an orthopedic therapeutic. It has been known for some time that the hyaluronan in joints is degraded in both osteoarthritis and rheumatoid arthritis.[173,174] As a result, a number of hyaluronate preparations have been developed for therapeutic use. However, there are questions as to the value of these products.[175,176] Hunter has presented a recent critical review of clinical usage suggesting that viscosupplementation is not an effective treatment for osteoarthritis. There is some suggestion that the possible effectiveness may be related to molecular size, but the data is inconclusive.

Hyaluronan has been suggested to be useful in promoting dermal protein drug delivery.[177] Earlier work by Brown and coworkers[178] has suggested that hyaluronan enhanced the partitioning of a drug through the epidermis with localization in superficial layer. Hyaluronan has been reported to be more effective than either heparin or dextran sulfate.

A particularly novel application is the use of microneedles fabricated from hyaluronan for protein drug delivery.[179] The ability to use such technology for transcutaneous immunization[180] would be a major advance in vaccination technology, as there are an abundance of immunocompetent (dendritic) cells in skin.[181] Given the broad biocompatibility of hyaluronan, there is considerable interest in hyaluronan-containing hydrogels for tissue regeneration[2] and drug delivery.[182]

3.7   HYALURONIDASE AND DRUG DELIVERY
IN INTERSTITIAL SPACE

Hyaluronidase is used to enhance drug delivery via subcutaneous administration by degrading hyaluronan, decreasing resistance to drug distribution (Table 3.1).[183] Hyaluronidase was originally described as spreading factor[184,185] involved in the pathogenicity of microorganisms.[186] There was some early use of spreading factor to improve the bacille Calmette–Guérin (BCG) vaccination efficiency.[187]

TABLE 3.1
Use of Hyaluronidase as Therapeutic

Use	Comment	Refs
Human immunoglobulin for primary immune deficiencies and other applications	Recombinant hyaluronidase is used for the subcutaneous delivery of human plasma–derived immunoglobulin (intravenous immunoglobulin G, IVIG).	1,2
Ondansetron hydrochloride (Zofran, a serotonin-blocking agent; MW 293)	Subcutaneous administration with recombinant hyaluronidase was equivalent to intramuscular or intravenous and superior to oral administration.	3
Rituximab (MabThera®) and trastuzumab (Herceptin®)	Subcutaneous administration with human recombinant hyaluronidase yielded efficacy comparable with intravenous administration.	4
N-(2-hydroxypropyl)methyl-acrylamide copolymer labeled with [111]In (HPMA copolymer radiolabel)	Recombinant hyaluronidase was used to degrade the stroma around a tumor to permit imaging with the HPMA copolymer radiolabel.	5
Use of hollow microneedles	The coadministration of hyaluronidase lowers microneedle injection pressure with reduction of pain associated with the injection procedure.	6
Off-label use to manage hyaluronan fillers, scleroderma lesions, keloids, lymphedema	There are three products for direct use as a therapeutic: a bovine product, a sheep product, and a recombinant human product.	7
Amlodipine besylate (Norvasc®; MW 567; $K_{OW}=2.7$)	Hyaluronidase enhanced the transdermal delivery of amlodipine besylate.	8
Ceftriaxone (Rochephin®; MW 662)	Subcutaneous coadministration of hyaluronidase with ceftriaxone had no effect on plasma area under the curve (AUC) compared to intravenous administration or subcutaneous administration in the absence of hyaluronidase; the peak concentration (C_{max}) was higher with hyaluronidase and time to maximum concentration (TMAX) shorter.	9
Morphine (MW 286; $K_{OW}=6$)	Subcutaneous administration of morphine with human recombinant hyaluronidase shortens TMAX and increases C_{max} compared to subcutaneous administration of morphine in the absence of hyaluronidase.	10
Nanoparticle drug carriers	Hyaluronidase and collagenase used to enhance the convection-driven delivery of nanoparticles to the brain.	11
Dexamethasone	Hyaluronidase was used to enhance the penetration of dexamethasone into the posterior segment of the eye with sub-Tenon's injection. An increase of dexamethasone concentration in ocular tissues and serum was observed.	12
Gene therapy	Hyaluronidase and collagenase are incorporated in the pericardial injection of a replication-deficient adenovirus containing a β-galactosidase in a rodent model. The use of hyaluronidase and collagenase enhanced the diffusion of the β-galactosidase-containing vector.	13

(Continued)

TABLE 3.1 (CONTINUED)
Use of Hyaluronidase as Therapeutic

Use	Comment	Refs
Trastuzumab (Herceptin)	Trastuzumab formulated with human recombinant hyaluronidase.	14
Rapid-acting insulin analogs	Recombinant human hyaluronidase (rHuPH20) enhances the efficacy of subcutaneous administration of insulin analogs. The use of rHuPH20 decreases intrasubject variability and increases insulin absorption.	15,16

REFERENCES FOR TABLE 3.1

1. Wasserman, R.L., Overview of recombinant human hyaluronidase-facilitated subcutaneous infusion of IgG in primary immunodeficiencies, *Immunotherapy* 6, 553–567, 2014.
2. Sanford, M., Human immunoglobulin 10% with recombinant human hyaluronidase: Replacement therapy in patients with primary immunodeficiency disorders, *BioDrugs* 28, 411–420, 2014.
3. Dychter, S.S., Harrigan, R., Bahn, J.D., et al., Tolerability and pharmacokinetic properties of ondansetron administered subcutaneously with recombinant human hyaluronidase in minipigs and healthy volunteers, *Clin. Ther.* 36, 211–224, 2014.
4. Shpilberg, O. and Jackisch, C., Subcutaneous administration of rituximab (MabThera) and trastuzumab (Herceptin) using hyaluronidase, *Br. J. Cancer* 109, 1556–1561, 2013.
5. Buckway, B., Wang, Y., Ray, A., and Ghanderhari, H., Overcoming the stromal barrier for targeted delivery of HPMA copolymer in pancreatic tumors, *Int. J. Pharm.* 456, 202–211, 2013.
6. Gupta, J., Park, S.S., Bondy, B., et al., Infusion pressure and pain during microneedle injection into skin of human subjects, *Biomaterials* 32, 6825–6831, 2011.
7. Lee, A., Grummer, S.E., Kriegel, D., and Marmur, E., Hyaluronidase, *Dermatol. Surg.* 36, 1071–1077, 2010.
8. Patel, H.J., Patel, J.S., Desai, B.G., and Patel, K.D, Permeability studies of anti hypertensive drug amlodipine besylate for transdermal delivery, *Asian J. Pharm. Clin. Res.* 3, 31–34, 2010.
9. Harb, G., Lebel, F., Battikha, J., and Thackara, J.W., Safety and pharmacokinetics of subcutaneous ceftriaxone administered with or without recombinant human hyaluronidase (rHuPH20) versus intravenous ceftriaxone administration in adult volunteers, *Curr. Med. Res. Opin.* 26, 279–288, 2010.
10. Thomas, J.R., Yocum, R.C., Haller, M.F., and Flament J., The INFUSE-morphine IIB study: Use of recombinant human hyaluronidase (rHuPH20) to enhance the absorption of subcutaneous morphine in healthy volunteers, *J. Pain Symptom Manage.* 38, 673–582, 2009.
11. Neeves, K.B., Sawyer, A.J., Foley, C.P., et al., Dilation and degradation of the brain extracellular matrix enhances penetration of infused polymer nanoparticles, *Brain Res.* 1180, 121–132, 2007.
12. Kozak, I., Kayikcioglu, O.R., Cheng, L., et al., The effect of recombinant hyaluronidase on dexamethasone penetration into the posterior segment of the eye after sub-Tenon's injection, *J. Ocular Pharm. Ther.* 22, 362–369, 2006.

13. Fromes, Y., Salmon, A., Wang, X., et al., Gene delivery to the myocardium by intraperi-cardial injection, *Gene Ther.* 6, 683–688, 1999.
14. Wynne, C.J., Ellis-Pegler, R.B., Waaka, D.S., et al., Comparative pharmacokinetics of subcutaneous trastuzumab administered via handheld syringe or proprietary single-use injection device in healthy males, *Cancer Chemother. Pharmacol.* 72, 1079–1087, 2013.
15. Vaughn, D.E. and Muchmore, D.B., Use of recombinant human hyaluronidase to accel-erate rapid insulin analogue absorption: Experience with subcutaneous injection and continuous infusion, *Endocr. Pract.* 17, 914–921, 2011.
16. Muchmore, D.B. and Vaughn, D.E., Accelerating and improving the consistency of rapid-acting analog insulin absorption and action for both subcutaneous injection and continuous subcutaneous infusion using recombinant human hyaluronidase, *J. Diabetes Sci. Technol.* 6, 764–772, 2012.

REFERENCES

1. Peattie, R.A., Release of growth factors, cytokines, and therapeutic molecules by hyal-uronan-based hydrogels, *Curr. Pharm. Biotechnol.* 13, 1299–1305, 2012.
2. Johnson, T.D. and Christman, K.L., Injectable hydrogel therapies and their delivery strategies for treating myocardial infarction, *Expert Opin. Drug. Deliv.* 10, 59–72, 2013.
3. Matricardi, P., Di Meo, C., Coviello, T., Hennink, W.E., and Alhaique, F., Interpenetrating polymer networks polysaccharide hydrogels for drug delivery and tissue engineering, *Adv. Drug Deliv. Rev.* 65, 1172–1187, 2013.
4. Sarkanen, J.R., Ruusuvuori, P., Kuokkanen, H., Paavonen, T., and Ylikomi, T., Bioactive acellular implant induces angiogenesis and adipogenesis and sustained soft tissue resto-ration *in vivo*, *Tissue Eng. Part A* 18, 2568–2580, 2012.
5. Kim, Z.H., Lee, Y., Kim, S.M., et al., A composite dermal filler comprising cross-linked hyaluronic acid and human collagen for tissue reconstruction, *J. Microbiol. Biotechnol.* 25, 399–406, 2015.
6. Yu, Y., Broullette, M.J., Seol, D., et al., Use of recombinant human stromal cell–derived factor 1α–loaded fibrin/hyaluronic acid hydrogel networks to achieve functional repair of full-thickness bovine articular cartilage via homing of chondrogenic progenitor cells, *Arthritis Rheumatol.* 67, 1274–1285, 2015.
7. Garg, H.G. and Hales, C.A. eds., *Chemistry and Biology of Hyaluronan*, Elsevier, Amsterdam, the Netherlands, 2004.
8. Knudson, W., Chow, G., and Knudson, C.B., CD44-mediated uptake and degradation of hyaluronan, *Matrix Biol.* 21, 15–23, 2002.
9. Day, A.J. and Prestwich, G.D., Hyaluronan-binding proteins: Tying up the giant, *J. Biol. Chem.* 277, 4585–4588, 2002.
10. Laurent, T.C., Structure of the extracellular matrix and the biology of hyaluronan, in *Interstitium, Connective Tissue and Lymphatics*, eds. R.K. Reed, N.G. Meltall, J.L. Bert, et al., Chapter 1, pp. 1–12, Portland Press, London, UK, 1995.
11. Laurent, T.C. and Fraser, J.R.E., Hyaluronan, *FASEB J.* 6, 237–2404, 1992.
12. Park, J.W. and Chakrabarti, B., Solvent induced changes in conformation of hyaluronic acid, *Biopolymers* 16, 2807–2809, 1977.
13. Morris, E.R., Rees, D.A., and Welsh, E.J., Conformation and dynamic interactions in hyaluronate solution, *J. Mol. Biol.* 138, 383–400, 1980.
14. Heatley, F. and Schot, J.E., A water molecule participates in the secondary structure of hyaluronan, *Biochem. J.* 254, 289–493, 1988.

15. Hargittai, I. and Hargittai, M., Molecular structure of hyaluronan: An introduction, *Struct. Chem.* 19, 697–717, 2008.

16. Yaffe, N.R., Almond, A., and Bianch, E.W., A new route to carbohydrate secondary and tertiary structure using Raman spectroscopy and Raman optical activity, *J. Am. Chem. Soc.* 132, 10654–10655, 2010.

17. Courel, M.-N., Maingonnat, C., Tranchepain, F., et al., Importance of hyaluronan length in a hyaladherin-based assay for hyaluronan, *Anal. Biochem.* 302, 285–290, 2002.

18. Hascall, V.C. and Heinegård, D., Aggregation of cartilage proteoglycans: II. Oligosaccharide competitors of the proteoglycan hyaluronic acid interaction, *J. Biol. Chem.* 249, 4242–4249, 1974.

19. Tamm, R., MacCallum, D., Hascall, V.C., et al., Hyaluronan bound to CD44 on keratinocytes is displaced by hyaluronan decasaccharides and not hexasaccharides, *J. Biol. Chem.* 273, 28878–28888, 1998.

20. Cowman, M.K., Spagnoli, C., Kudasheva, D., et al., Extended, relaxed, and condensed conformations of hyaluronan observed by atomic force microscopy, *Biophys. J.* 88, 590–602, 2005.

21. Banerji, S., Wright, A.J., Noble, M., et al., Structures of the CD44–hyaluronan complex provides insight into a fundamental carbohydrate–protein interaction, *Nat. Struct. Mol. Biol.* 14, 234–239, 2007.

22. Higman, V.A., Briggs, D.C., Mahoney, D.J., et al., A refined model for the TSG-6 link module in complex with hyaluronan: Use of defined oligosaccharides to probe structure and function, *J. Biol. Chem.* 289, 5619–5634, 2014.

23. Jamison, F.W., II, Foster, T.J., Baker, J.A., et al., Mechanism of binding site conformational switching in the CD44–hyaluronan protein–carbohydrate binding, *J. Mol. Biol.* 406, 631–647, 2011.

24. Plazinski, W. and Knys-Dzieciuch, A., The "order-to-disorder" conformational transition in CD44 protein: An umbrella sampling analysis, *J. Mol. Graph. Model.* 45, 122–127, 2013.

25. Sharon, N., Mucopolysaccharides (proteoglycans): I. Chemical structure, in *Complex Carbohydrates: Their Chemistry, Biosynthesis and Function*, Chapter 14, pp. 250–281, Addison-Wesley, Reading, MA, 1975.

26. Vincent, J., Sugars and fillers, in *Structural Biomaterials*, 3rd edn., Chapter 3, pp. 61–83, Princeton University Press, Princeton, NJ, 2012.

27. Gribbon, P., Heng, B.C., and Hardingham, T.E., The molecular basis of the solution properties of hyaluronan investigated by confocal fluorescence recovery after photobleaching, *Biophys. J.* 77, 2210–2216, 1999.

28. Hardingham, T., Solution properties of hyaluronan, in *Chemistry and Biology of Hyaluronan*, eds. H.G. Garg and C.H. Hales, Chapter 1, pp. 1–19, Elsevier, Amsterdam, the Netherlands, 2004.

29. Altman, P.L. and Ditman, D.S., *Blood and Other Body Fluids*, Federation of American Societies of Experimental Biology, Washington, DC, 1961.

30. Bretag, A.H., Synthetic interstitial fluid for isolated mammalian tissue, *Life Sci.* 8, 319–329, 1969.

31. Stridh, S., Palm, F., and Hansell, P., Renal interstitial hyaluronan: Functional aspects during normal and pathological conditions, *Am. J. Physiol. Regul. Integr. Comp. Physiol.* 302, R1235–1249, 2012.

32. Sakai, S., Yasuda, R., Sayo, T., Ishikawa, O., and Inoue, S., Hyaluronan exists in the normal stratum corneum, *J. Invest. Dermatol.* 114, 1184–1187, 2000.

33. Verdier-Sévrain, S. and Bonté, F., Skin hydration: A review on its molecular mechanisms, *J. Cosmet. Dermatol.* 6, 75–82, 2007.

34. Stern, R. and Maibach, H.I., Hyaluronan in skin: Aspects of aging and its pharmacologic modulation, *Clin. Dermatol.* 26, 106–122, 2008.

35. Brandt, F.S. and Cazzaniga, A., Hyaluronic acid gel fillers in the management of facial aging, *Clin. Interv. Aging* 3, 153–159, 2008.

36. Kawada, C., Yoshida, T., Yoshida, H., et al., Ingestion of hyaluronans (molecular weights 800 k and 300 k) improves dry skin conditions: A randomized, double blind, controlled study, *J. Clin. Biochem. Nutr.* 56, 66–73, 2015.

37. Ping, L., Huang, L., Cardinali, B., et al., Substitution of the human αC region with the analogous chicken domain generates a fibrinogen with severely impaired lateral aggregation: Fibrin monomers assemble into protofibrils but protofibrils do not assemble into fibers, *Biochemistry* 50, 9066–9075, 2011.

38. Wilkins, D.K., Grimshaw, S.B., Receveur, V., et al., Hydrodynamic radii of native and denatured proteins measured by pulse field gradient NMR techniques, *Biochemistry* 38, 16424–16431. 1999.

39. Clasen, C., Plog, J.P., Kulicke, W.-M., et al., How dilute are dilute solutions in extensional flows?, *J. Rheol.* 50, 849–881, 2006.

40. Larson, R.G., Polymers, in *The Structure and Rheology of Complex Fluids*, Chapter 3, pp. 107–188, Oxford University Press, Oxford, UK, 1999.

41. Scott, D., Coleman, P.J., Mason, R.M., and Levick, J.R., Concentration dependence of interstitial flow buffering by hyaluronan in synovial joints, *Microvasc. Res.* 59, 345–353, 2000.

42. Szarpak, A., Pignot-Paintrand, I., Nicholas, C., Picart, C., and Auzely-Velty, R., Multilayer assembly of hyaluronic acid/poly(allylamine): Control of the buildup for the production of hollow capsules, *Langmuir* 24, 9767–9774, 2008.

43. Pires, A.M. and Santana, M.H.A., Rheological aspects of microbial hyaluronic acid, *J. Appl. Polym. Sci.* 122, 126–133, 2011.

44. Hellstrom, M., Engstrom-Laurent, A., Morner, S., and Johansson, B., Hyaluronan and collagen in human hypertrophic cardiomyopathy: A morphological analysis, *Cardiol. Res. Pract.* 2012, 5, 2012.

45. Pitcock, J.A., Lyons, H., Brown, P.S., et al., Glycosaminoglycans of the rat renomedullary interstitium: Ultrastructural and biochemical observations, *Exp. Mol. Pathol.* 49, 373–387, 1988.

46. Dwyer, T.M., Banks, S.A., Alonso-Galicia, M., et al., Distribution of renal medullary hyaluronan in lean and obese rabbits, *Kidney Int.* 58, 721–729, 2000.

47. Knepper, M.A., Saidel, G.M., Hascall, V.C., and Dwyer, T., Concentration of solutes in the renal inner medulla: Interstitial hyaluronan as a mechano-osmotic transducer, *Am. J. Physiol. Renal. Physiol.* 284, F433–F446, 2003.

48. Pinter, G.G. and Shohet, J.L., Two fluid compartments in the renal inner medulla: A view through the keyhole of the concentrating process, *Philos. Trans. A Math. Phys. Eng. Sci.* 304, 1551–1561, 2006.

49. Rügheimer, L., Olerud, J., Johnsson, C., et al., Hyaluronan synthases and hyaluronidases in the kidney during changes in hydration status, *Matrix Biol.* 28, 390–395, 2009.

50. Declèves, A.E., Caron, N., Nonclercq, D., et al., Dynamics of hyaluronan, CD44, and inflammatory cells in the rat kidney after ischemia/reperfusion injury, *Int. J. Mol. Med.* 18, 83–94, 2006.

51. Adembri, C., Selmi, V., Vitali, L., et al., Expression and characterization of anionic components in the tubulointerstitial compartment of the rat kidney during polymicrobial sepsis, *Acta Histochem.* 116, 94–105, 2014.

52. Schweinfurth, J.M. and Thieault, S.L., Does hyaluronic acid distribution in the larynx relate to the newborn's capacity for crying?, *Laryngoscope* 118, 1692–1699, 2008.

53. Jia, X., Yeo, Y., Clifton, R.J., et al., Hyaluronic acid–based microgels and microgel networks for vocal fold regeneration, *Biomacromolecules* 7, 3336–3344, 2006.

54. Chockalingam, P.S., Zeng, W., Morris, E.A., and Flannery, C.R, Release of hyaluronan and hyaladherins (aggrecan G1 domain and link proteins) from articular cartilage exposed to ADAMTS-4 (aggrecanase 1) or ADAMTS-5 (aggrecanase 2), *Arthritis
Rheum.* 50, 2839–2848, 2004.

55. Melrose, J. and Smith, S., Histochemical visualization of the cartilage hyaladherins
using a biotinylated hyaluronan oligosaccharide bioaffinity probe, *Methods Mol. Biol.*
101, 65–78, 2004.

56. Webber, J., Jenkins, R.H., Meran, S., et al., Modulation of TGFβ1-dependent myofibroblast differentiation by hyaluronan, *Am. J. Pathol.* 175, 148–160, 2009.

57. Young, R.A., The ground substance of connective tissue, *J. Physiol.* 16, 325–350,
1984.

58. Øien, A.H., Justad, S.R., Tenstad, O., and Wiig, H., Effects of hydration on steric and
electric charge–induced interstitial volume exclusion: A model, *Biophys. J.* 105, 1276–
1284, 2013.

59. Wiig, H., Gyenge, C., Iversen, P.O., et al., The role of the extracellular matrix in tissue
distribution of macromolecules in normal and pathological tissues: Potential therapeutic consequences, *Microcirculation* 15, 283–296, 2008.

60. Wiig, H., Kayson, G.A., al-Bander, H.A., et al., Interstitial exclusion of IgG in rat tissues estimated by continuous infusion, *Am. J. Physiol.* 266, H212–H219, 1994.

61. Mormone, E., George, J., and Nieto, N., Molecular pathogenesis of hepatic fibrosis and
current therapeutic approaches, *Chem. Biol. Interact.* 193, 225–231, 2011.

62. Laurent, T.C., History of a theory, *J. Chromatogr.* 633, 1–8, 1993.

63. Watson, P.D., Bell, D.R., and Renkin, E.M., Early kinetics of large molecule transport
between plasma and lymph in dogs, *Am. J. Physiol.* 239, H525–H531, 1980.

64. Watson, P.D. and Grodin, F.S., An analysis of the effects of the interstitial matrix on
plasma–lymph transport, *Microvasc. Res.* 16, 19–41, 1978.

65. Parker, J.C., Falgout, H.J., Parker, R.E., Granger, D.N., and Taylor, A.E., The effect of
fluid volume loading on exclusion of interstitial albumin and lymph fluid in the dog
lung, *Circ. Res.* 45, 440–450, 1979.

66. Laurent, T.C., The interaction between polysaccharides and other macromolecules: 9.
The exclusion of molecules from hyaluronic acid gels and solutions, *Biochem. J.* 93,
106–112, 1964.

67. Laurent, T.C., History of a theory, *J. Chromatogr.* 633, 1–8, 1993.

68. Shaw, M. and Schy, A., Diffusion coefficient measurement by the "stop-flow" method
in a 5% collagen gel, *Biophys. J.* 34, 375–381, 1981.

69. Sagstad, S.J., Oveland, E., Karlsen, T.V., et al., Age-related changes in rat dermal extracellular matrix composition affect the distribution of plasma proteins as a function of
size and charge, *Am. J. Physiol. Heart Circ. Physiol.* 308, H29–H38, 2015.

70. Gandhi, R.R. and Bell, D.R., Importance of charge on transvascular albumin transport
in skin and skeletal muscle, *Am. J. Physiol. Heart Circ. Physiol.* 262, H999–H1008,
1992.

71. Wiig, H., Kolmannskog, O., Tenstad, O., and Bert, J.L., Effect of charge on interstitial
distribution of albumin in rat dermis *in vitro*, *J. Physiol.* 550, 505–514, 2003.

72. Glazer, A.N. and Wellner, D., Adsorption of proteins on "Sephadex," *Nature* 194, 862–
863, 1962.

73. Gelotte, B., Studies on gel filtration: Sorption properties of the bed material Sephadex,
J. Chromatogr. 3, 330–342, 1960.

74. Albertsson, P.Å., Fractionation of particles and macromolecules in aqueous two-phase
systems, *Biochem. Pharmacol.* 5, 351–358, 1961.

75. Wiederhielm, C.A., Fox, J.R., and Lee, D.R., Ground substance mucopolysaccharide
and plasma proteins: Their role in capillary water balance, *Am. J. Physiol.* 230, 1121–
1125, 1976.

76. Sage, J., Mallèvre, F., Barbarin-Costes, F., et al., Binding of chondroitin 4-sulfate to cathepsin S regulates its enzymatic activity, *Biochemistry* 52, 6487–6498, 2013.
77. Iwanicki, J.L., Lu, K.W., and Taeusch, H.W., Reductions of phospholipase A_2 inhibition of pulmonary surfactant with hyaluronan, *Exp. Lung. Res.* 36, 167–174, 2010.
78. Li, Z., Hou, W.S., and Brömme, D., Collagenolytic activity of cathepsin K is specifically modulated by cartilage-resident chondroitin sulfates, *Biochemistry* 39, 529–536, 2000.
79. Bühling, F., Röcken, C., Brasch, F., et al., Pivotal role of cathepsin K in lung fibrosis, *Am. J. Pathol.* 164, 2203–2216, 2004.
80. Fields, G.B., Interstitial collagen catabolism, *J. Biol. Chem.* 288, 8785–8793, 2013.
81. Li, Z., Hou, W.S., Escalante-Torres, C.R., Gelb, B.D., and Bromme, D., Collagenase activity of cathepsin K depends on complex formation with chondroitin sulfate, *J. Biol. Chem.* 277, 28669–28676, 2002.
82. Forteza, R., Lauredo, I., Abraham, W.M., and Conner, G.E., Bronchial tissue kallikrein activity is regulated by hyaluronic acid binding, *Am. J. Respir. Cell. Mol. Biol.* 21, 666–674, 1999.
83. Casalino-Matsuda, S.M., Monzon, M.E., Conner, G.E., Salathe, M., and Forteza, R.M., Role of hyaluronan and reactive oxygen species in tissue kallikrein–mediated epidermal growth factor receptor activation in human airways, *J. Biol. Chem.* 279, 21606–21616, 2004.
84. Yu, H., Li, Q., Zhou, X., Kolosov, V.E., and Perelman, J.M., Role of hyaluronan and CD44 in reactive oxygen species–induced mucus hypersecretion, *Mol. Cell. Biochem.* 352, 65–75, 2011.
85. Meran, S., Lu, D.D., Simpson, R., et al., Hyaluronan facilitates transforming growth factor-β1–dependent proliferation via CD44 and epidermal growth factor receptor interaction, *J. Biol. Chem.* 286, 17618–17630, 2011.
86. David-Raoudi, M., Tranchepain, F., Deschrevel, B., et al., Differential effects of hyaluronan and its fragments on fibroblasts: Relation to wound healing, *Wound Repair Regen.* 16, 274–287, 2008.
87. Bradshaw, R.A. and Lundblad, R.L., Kallikrein, in *Encyclopedia of Cell Biology*, Vol. 1, eds. R. Bradshaw and P. Stahl, pp. 699–705, Academic Press, Waltham, MA, 2016.
88. ten Wolde, P.R. and Mugler, A., Importance of crowding in signaling, genetic, and metabolic networks, *Int. Rev. Cell. Mol. Biol.* 307, 419–442, 2014.
89. Laurent, T.C., An early look at macromolecular crowding, *Biophys. Chem.* 57, 7–14, 1995.
90. Aumiller, W.M., Jr., Davis, B.W., Hatzakis, E., and Keating, C.D., Interactions of macromolecular crowding agents and cosolutes with small-molecule substrates: Effect of horseradish peroxidase activity with two different substrates, *J. Phys. Chem. B.* 118, 10624–10632, 2014.
91. Balevicius, Z., Ignatjeva, D., Niaura, G., et al., Crowding enhances lipase turnover rate on surface-immobilized substrates, *Colloids Surf. B Biointerfaces* 131, 115–121, 2015.
92. Kim, Y.C., Best, R.B., and Mittal, J., Macromolecular crowding effects on protein–protein binding affinity and specificity, *J. Chem. Phys.* 133, 205101, 2010.
93. Feig, M. and Sugita, Y., Variable interactions between protein crowders and biomolecular solutes are important in understanding cellular crowding, *J. Phys. Chem. B.* 116, 599–605, 2012.
94. Englebienne, P., *Immune and Receptor Assays in Theory and Practice*, CRC Press, Boca Raton, FL, 2000.
95. Toole, B.P., Hyaluronan and its binding proteins, the hyaladherins, *Curr. Opin. Cell Biol.* 2, 839–844, 1990.
96. Barclay, A.N., Brown, M.H., Law, S.K.A., et al., *The Leucocyte Antigen FactBook*, 2nd edn., Academic Press, San Diego, CA, 1997.

97. Naor, D., CD44, in *Encyclopedia of Immunology*, Vol. 1, 2nd edn., eds. P.J. Delves and I.M. Raitt, pp. 488–491, Academic Press, San Diego, CA, 1998.

98. Cruse, J.M., Lewis, R.E., and Wang, H., *Immunology Guidebook*, Elsevier, Amsterdam, the Netherlands, 2004.

99. Underhill, C., CD44: The hyaluronan receptor, *J. Cell Sci.* 103, 293–298, 1992.

100. Knudson, W. and Peterson, R.S., The hyaluronan receptor CD44, in *Chemistry and Biology of Hyaluronan*, eds. H.G. Garg and C.H. Hales, pp. 83–123, Elsevier, Amsterdam, the Netherlands, 2004.

101. Kahmann, J.D., O'Brien, R., Werner, J.M., et al., Localization and characterization of the hyaluronan-binding site on the link module from human TSG-6, *Structure* 8, 763–774, 2000.

102. Bajorath, J., Molecular organization, structural features, and ligand binding characteristics of CD44, a highly variable cell surface glycoprotein with multiple functions, *Proteins* 39, 103–111, 2000.

103. Favreau, A.J., Faller, C.E., and Guvench, O., CD44 receptor unfolding enhances binding by freeing basic amino acids to contact carbohydrate ligand, *Biophysical J.* 105, 1217–1226, 2013.

104. Liu, L.K. and Finzel, B.C., Fragment-based identification of an inducible binding site on cell surface receptor CD44 for the design of protein–carbohydrate interaction inhibitors, *J. Med. Chem.* 57, 2714–2725, 2014.

105. Lacy, B.E. and Underhill, C.B., The hyaluronate receptor is associated with actin filaments, *J. Cell Biol.* 105, 1395–1404, 1987.

106. Bourguignon, L.Y., Hyaluronan-mediated CD44 activation of RhoGTPase signaling and cytoskeleton function promotes tumor progression, *Semin. Cancer Biol.* 18, 251–259, 2008.

107. Forster-Horváth, C., Bocsi, J., Rásó, E., et al., Constitutive intracellular expression and activation-induced cell surface up-regulation of CD44v3 in human T lymphocytes, *Eur. J. Immunol.* 31, 600–608, 2001.

108.. Lesley, J., Hyman, R., and Kincade, P.W., CD44 and its interaction with extracellular matrix, *Adv. Immunol.* 54, 271–335, 1993.

109. Stenson, W.F., Hyaluronic acid and interstitial inflammation, *Curr. Opin. Gastroenterol.* 26, 85–87, 2010.

110. Fraser, J.R., Laurent, T.C., Pertoft, H., and Baxter, E., Plasma clearance, tissue distribution and metabolism of hyaluronic acid injected intravenously in the rabbit, *Biochem. J.* 200, 415–424, 1981.

111. Lepperdinger, G., Fehrer, C., and Reitinger, S., Biodegradation of hyaluronan, in *Chemistry and Biology of Hyaluronan*, eds. H.G. Garg and C.A. Hales, Chapter 4, pp. 71–82, Elsevier, Amsterdam, the Netherlands, 2004.

112. Agren, U.M., Tammi, R.H., and Tammi, M.I., Reactive oxygen species contribute to epidermal hyaluronan catabolism in human skin organ culture, *Free Radic. Biol. Med.* 23, 996–1001, 1997.

113. Stern, R.L., Hyaluronan catabolism: A new metabolic pathway, *Eur. J. Cell Biol.* 83, 317–325, 2004.

114. Danielson, B.T., Knudson, C.B., and Knudson, W., Extracellular processing of the cartilage proteoglycan aggregate and its effect on CD44-mediated internalization of hyaluronan, *J. Biol. Chem.* 290, 9555–9570, 2015.

115. Lee-Sayer, S.S., Deng, Y., Arif, A.A., et al., The where, when, how, and why of hyaluronan binding by immune cells, *Front. Immunol.* 6, 150, 2015.

116. Lesley, J., Hascall, V.C., Tammi, M., and Hyman, R., Hyaluronan binding to cell surface CD44, *J. Biol. Chem.* 275, 26967–26975, 2000.

117. Yang, C., Cao, M., Liu, H., et al., The high and low molecular weight forms of hyaluronan have distinct effects on CD44 clustering, *J. Biol. Chem.* 287, 43094–43107, 2012.

118. Rochman, M., Moll, J., Herrich, P., et al., The CD44 receptor of lymphoma cells: Structure–function relationships and mechanism of activation, *Cell Adhes. Commun.* 7, 331–347, 2000.

119. Nandi, A., Estess, P., and Siegelman, M.H., Hyaluronan anchoring and regulation of the surface of vascular endothelial cells is mediated through the functionally active form of CD44, *J. Biol. Chem.* 275, 14939–14948, 2000.

120. Hardwick, C., Hoare, K., Owens, R., et al., Molecular cloning of a novel hyaluronan receptor that mediates tumor cell motility, *J. Cell Biol.* 117, 1343–1350, 1992.

121. Pilarski, L.M., Masellis-Smith, A., Belch, A.R., et al., RHAMM, a receptor for hyaluronan-mediated motility, on normal human lymphocytes, thymocytes and malignant B cells: A mediator in B cell malignancy? *Leuk. Lymphoma* 14, 363–374, 1994.

122. Sherman, L., Sleeman, J., Herrlich, P., and Ponta, H., Hyaluronate receptors: Key players in growth, differentiation, migration and tumor progression, *Curr. Opin. Cell Biol.* 6, 726–733, 1994.

123. Slevin, M., Krupinski, J., Gaffney, J., et al., Hyaluronan-mediated angiogenesis in vascular disease: Uncovering RHAMM and CD44 receptor signaling pathways, *Matrix Biol.* 26, 58–68, 2007.

124. Pilarski, L.M., Miszta, H., and Turley, E.A., Regulated expression of a receptor for hyaluronan-mediated motility on human thymocytes and T cells, *J. Immunol.* 150, 4292–4302, 1993.

125. Toole, B.P., Hyaluronan in morphogenesis, *J. Intern. Med.* 242, 35–40, 1997.

126. Kouvidi, K., Berdiaki, A., Nikitovic, D., et al., Role of the receptor for hyaluronic acid–mediated motility (RHAMM) in low molecular weight hyaluronan (LMWHA)–mediated fibrosarcoma adhesion, *J. Biol. Chem.* 280, 38509–38520, 2011.

127. Zhang, H., Huang, S., Yang, X., and Zhang, G., Current research on hyaluronic acid–drug bioconjugates, *Eur. J. Med. Chem.* 86, 310–317, 2014.

128. Augustin, F., Fiegl, M., Schmid, T., et al., Receptor for hyaluronic acid–mediated motility (RHAMM, CD168) expression is prognostically important in both nodal negative and nodal positive large cell lung cancer, *J. Clin. Pathol.* 68, 368–373, 2015.

129. Pandey, M.S. and Weigel, P.H., Hyaluronic acid receptors for endocytosis (HARE): Mediated endocytosis of hyaluronan, heparin, dermatan sulfate, and acetylated low density lipoprotein (AcLDL), but not chondroitin sulfate types A, C, D, or E, activated NF-κB-regulated gene expression, *J. Biol. Chem.* 289, 1756–1767, 2014.

130. Hare, A.K. and Harris, E.N., Tissue-specific splice variants of HARE/Stabilin-2 are expressed in bone marrow, lymph node, and spleen, *Biochem. Biophys. Res. Commun.* 456, 251–261, 2015.

131. Zhou, B., Weigel, J.A., Fauss L., and Weigel, P.H., Identification of the hyaluronan receptor for endocytosis (HARE), *J. Biol. Chem.* 275, 37733–37741, 2000.

132. Weigel, J.A., Raymond, R.C., and Weigel, P.H., The hyaluronan receptor for endocytosis (HARE) is not CD44 or CD54 (ICAM-1), *Biochem. Biophys. Res. Commun.* 294, 918–922, 2002.

133. Harris, E.N., Parry, S., Sutton-Smith. M., et al., *N*-Glycans on the link domain of human HARE/Stabilin-2 are needed for hyaluronan binding to purified ecto-domain but not for cellular endocytosis of hyaluronan, *Glycobiology* 20, 991–1001, 2010.

134. Hirose, Y., Saijou, E., Sugano, Y., et al., Inhibition of stabilin-2 elevates circulating hyaluronic acid levels and prevents tumor metastasis, *Proc. Natl. Acad. Sci. USA* 109, 4263–4268, 2012.

135. Banerji, S., Ni, J., Wang, S.-X., et al., LYVE-1, a new homologue of the CD44 glycoprotein, is a lymph-specific receptor for hyaluronan, *J. Cell. Biol.* 144, 789–801, 1999.

136. Jackson, D.G., Immunological functions of hyaluronan and its receptors in the lymphatics, *Immunol. Rev.* 230, 216–231, 2009.

137. Schledzewski, K., Falkowski, M., Moldehauer, G., et al., Lymphatic endothelium–specific hyaluronan receptor LYVE-1 is expressed by stabilin-1+, F4/80+, CD11b+ macrophages in malignant tumours and wound healing tissue *in vivo* and in bone marrow cultures *in vitro*: Implications for the assessment of lymphangiogenesis, *J. Pathol.* 209, 67–77, 2006.

138. Nieduszynski, I.A., Sheehan, J.K., Phelps, C.F., Hardingham, T.E. and Muir, H., Equilibrium binding studies of pig laryngeal cartilage proteoglycan to hyaluronan oligosaccharide fractions, *Biochem. J.* 185, 107–114, 1980.

139. Underhill, C.B. and Toole, B.P., Physical characteristics of hyaluronate binding to the surface of Simian 40: Transformed 3T3 cells, *J. Biol. Chem.* 255, 4544–4549, 1980.

140. LeBoeuf, R.D., Raja, R.H., Fuller, G.M., and Weigel, P.HW., Human fibrinogen specifically binds hyaluronic acid, *J. Biol. Chem.* 261, 12586–12592, 1986.

141. Rinauldo, M., Rheological investigation on hyaluronan–fibrinogen interaction, *Int. J. Biol. Macromol.* 43, 444–450, 2008.

142. Bray, B.A., The role of hyaluronan in the pulmonary alveolus, *J. Theoret. Biol.* 210, 121–130, 2001.

143. Samuelsson, C. and Gustafson, S., Studies on the interaction between hyaluronic acid and a rat colon cancer cell line, *Glycoconj. J.* 15, 169–175, 1996.

144. Iwata, M., Wright, T.N., and Carlson, S.J., A brain extracellular matrix proteoglycan forms aggregates with hyaluronan, *J. Biol. Chem.* 268, 15061–15069, 1993.

145. Culty, M., Shizan, M., Thompson, E.W., and Underhill, C.B., Binding and degradation of hyaluronan by human breast cancer cell lines expressing different forms of CD44: Correlation with invasive potential, *J. Cell Physiol.* 160, 275–286, 1994.

146. Nakamura, M., Mishima, H., Nishida, T., and Otori, T., Binding of hyaluronan to plasma fibronectin increases the attachment of corneal epithelial cells to a fibronectin matrix, *J. Cell. Physiol.* 159, 415–422, 1994.

147. Haas, R. and Culp, L.A., Binding of fibronectin to gelatin and heparin: Effect of surface denaturation and detergents, *FEBS Lett.* 174, 279–283, 1984.

148. Zamarron, C., Ginsberg, M.H., and Plow, E.F., Monoclonal antibodies specific for a conformationally altered state of fibrinogen, *Thromb. Haemost.* 64, 41–46, 1990.

149. Van Damme, M.P., Moss, J.M., Murphy, W.H., and Preston, B.N., Binding of hyaluronan to lysozyme at various pHs and salt concentrations, *Biochem. Int.* 24, 605–613, 1991.

150. Moss, J.M., Van Damme, M.P. I., Murphy, W.H., and Preston, B.N., Dependence of salt concentration on glycosaminoglycan–lysozyme interactions in cartilage, *Arch. Biochem. Biophys.* 348, 49–55, 1997.

151. Ormiston, M.L., Slaughter, G.R.D., Deng, Y., Stewart, D.J. and Courtman, D.W., The enzymatic degradation of hyaluronan is associated with disease progression in experimental hypertension, *Am. J. Physiol. Lung Cell. Mol. Physiol.* 298, L148–L157, 2010.

152. Gao, F., Koenitzer, J.R., Tobelewski, J.M., et al., Extracellular superoxide dismutase inhibits inflammation by preventing oxidative fragmentation of hyaluronan, *J. Biol. Chem.* 283, 6058–6066, 2008.

153. Hrabárova, E., Valachová, K., Juráncek, I., and Šoltés, L., Free-radical degradation of high-molar-mass hyaluronan induced by ascorbate *plus* cupric ions: Evaluation of anti-oxidative effect of cysteine-derived compounds, *Chem. Biodivers.* 9, 309–317, 2012.

154. Bourguignon, L.Y.W., Wong, G., Earle, C.A., and Xie, W., Interaction of low molecular weight hyaluronan with CD44 and Toll-like receptor promotes the actin filament-associated protein 110-actin binding and MyD88-NFκB signalling leading to proinflammatory cytokine/chemokine production and breast tumor invasion, *Cytoskeleton* 68, 671–693, 2011.

155. Vistejnova, L., Sofrankova, B., Nespanova, K., et al., Low molecular weight hyaluronan mediated CD44 induction of IL-6 and chemokines in human dermal fibroblasts potentiates innate immune response, *Cytokine* 70, 97–103, 2014.

156. Teermer, C., Hennies, J., Voith, U., et al., Oligosaccharides of hyaluronan are potent activators of dendritic cells, *J. Immunol.* 165, 1863–1870, 2000.

157. Mosely, R., Walker, M., Waddington, R.J., and Chen, W.Y.J., Comparison of the antioxidant properties of wound dressing materials: Carboxymethylcellulose, hyaluronan benzyl ester and hyaluronan, toward polymorphonuclear leukocyte-derived reactive oxygen species, *Biomaterials* 24, 1549–1557, 2003.

158. Ferguson, E.L., Roberts, J.L., Moseley, R., Griffiths, P.C., and Thomas, D.W., Evaluation of the physical and biological properties of hyaluronan and hyaluronan fragments, *Int. J. Pharm.* 420, 84–92, 2011.

159. Almond, A., DeAngelis, P.L., and Blundell, C.D., Hyaluronan: The local solution conformation determined by NMR and computer modeling is close to a contracted left-handed 4-fold helix, *J. Mol. Biol.* 358, 1256–1269, 2006.

160. Hardingham, T., Solution properties of hyaluronan, in *Chemistry and Biology of Hyaluronan*, eds. H.G. Garg and C.A. Hales, Chapter 1, pp. 1–19, Elsevier, Amsterdam, the Netherlands, 2004.

161. Blundell, C.D., Deangelis, P.L., and Almond, A., Hyaluronan: The absence of amide–carboxylate hydrogen bonds and the chain conformation in aqueous solution are incompatible with stable secondary and tertiary structure models, *Biochem. J.* 396, 487–498, 2006.

162. Tolg, C., Telmer, P., and Turley, E., Specific size of hyaluronan oligosaccharides stimulate fibroblast migration and excisional wound repair, *PLoS One* 9(2), e88479, 2014.

163. David-Raoudi, M., Tranchepain, E., Dreschrevel, B., et al., Differential effects of hyaluronan and its fragments on fibroblasts: Relation to wound healing, *Wound Repair Regen.* 16, 247–287, 2008.

164. Begley, C.G. and Ellis, L.M., Drug development: Raise standards for preclinical cancer research, *Nature* 483, 531–533, 2012.

165. Begley, C.G., Six red flags for suspect work, *Nature* 497, 433–434, 2013.

166. Freedman, L.P., Gibson, M.C., Ethier, S.P., et al., Reproducibility: Changing the policies and culture of cell line authentication, *Nat. Methods* 12, 493–497, 2015.

167. Joddar, B. and Ramamurthi, A., Fragment size- and dose-specific effects of hyaluronan on matrix synthesis by vascular smooth muscle cells, *Biomaterials* 27, 2994–3004, 2006.

168. Fuchs, K., Hippe, A., Schmaus, A., et al., Opposing effects of high- and low-molecular weight hyaluronan on CXCL12-induced CXCR4 signaling depend on CD44, *Cell Death Dis.* 4, e819, 2013.

169. Nagasawa, T., CXCL12/SDF-1 and CXCR4, *Front. Immunol.* 6, 301, 2015.

170. Termeer, C., Benedix, F., Sleeman, J., et al., Oligosaccharides of hyaluronan activate dendritic cells via Toll-like receptor 4, *J. Exp. Med.* 195, 99–111, 2002.

171. Muto, J., Morioka, Y., Yamasaki, K., et al., Hyaluronan digestion controls DC migration from the skin, *J. Clin. Invest.* 124, 1309–1319, 2014.

172. Falcone, J.J., Palmer, D.D., and Berg, R.A., Biomedical applications of hyaluronic acid, in *Polysaccharides for Drug Delivery and Pharmaceutical Applications*, eds. R.H. Marchessault, F. Ravenelle, and X.X. Zhu, Chapter 8, pp. 155–174, American Chemical Society, Washington, DC, 2006.

173. Fletcher, E., Jacobs, J.H., and Markham, R.L., Viscosity studies on hyaluronic acid of synovial fluid in rheumatoid arthritis and osteoarthritis, *Clin. Sci.* (London) 14, 653–660, 1955.

174. Egelius, N., Johsson, E., and Sunblad, L., Studies of hyaluronic acid in rheumatoid arthritis, *Ann. Rheum. Dis.* 15, 357–363, 1956.

175. Cheng, O.T., Souzdalnitski, D., Vrooman, B., and Cheng, J., Evidence-based knee injections for the management of arthritis, *Pain Med.* 13, 740–753, 2012.

176. Hunter, D.J., Viscosupplementation for osteoarthritis of the knee, *N. Engl. J. Med.* 372, 1040–1047, 2015.

177. Witting, M., Boreham, A., Brodwolf, R., et al., Interactions of hyaluronic acid with the skin and implication for the dermal delivery of biomacromolecules, *Mol. Pharm.* 12, 1391–1401, 2015.

178. Brown, M.B., Jones, S.A., He, W., and Martin, G.P., Hyaluronan: Investigations into the mode of action of hyaluronan in topical drug delivery, in *Polysaccharides for Drug Delivery and Pharmaceutical Applications*, eds. R.H. Marchessault, F. Ravenelle, and X.X. Zhu, Chapter 7, pp. 141–153, American Chemical Society, Washington, DC, 2006.

179. Lin, S., Jin, M.N., Quan, Y.S., et al., Transdermal delivery of relatively high molecular weight drugs using novel self-dissolving microneedle arrays fabricated from hyaluronic acid and their characteristics and safety after application to the skin, *Eur. J. Pharm. Biopharm.* 86, 267–176, 2014.

180. Hirobe, S., Azukizawa, H., Matsuo, K., et al., Development and clinical study of a self-dissolving microneedle patch for transcutaneous immunization device, *Pharm. Res.* 30, 2664–2674, 2013.

181. Weiss, R., Scheiblhofer, S., Machado, Y., and Thalhamer, J., New approaches to transcutaneous immunotherapy: Targeting dendritic cells with novel allergen conjugates, *Curr. Opin. Allergy Clin. Immunol.* 13, 669–676, 2013.

182. Johnson, T.D. and Christman, K.L., Injectable hydrogel therapies and their delivery strategies for treating myocardial infarction, *Expert Opin. Drug Deliv.* 10, 59–72, 2013.

183. Martanto, W., Moore, J.S., Kashlan, O., et al., Microinfusion using hollow microneedles, *Pharm. Res.* 23, 104–113, 2006.

184. Claude, A. and Reynals, F., Chemical properties of the purified spreading factor from testicle, *J. Exp. Med.* 65, 661–670, 1937.

185. Hobby, G.L., Dawson, M.H., Meyer, K., and Chaffee, E., The relationship between spreading factor and hyaluronidase, *J. Exp. Med.* 73, 109–123, 1941.

186. Duran-Reynals, F., Studies on a certain spreading factor existing in bacteria and its significance for bacterial invasiveness, *J. Exp. Med.* 58, 161–181, 1933.

187. Bergqvist, S., Attempts to heighten the effect of BCG vaccination with hyaluronidase, *Am. Rev. Tuberc.* 64, 442–447, 1951.

4 Proteolysis in the Interstitium

4.1 PROTEOLYTIC ENZYMES IN INTERSTITIAL SPACE

There is compelling evidence to suggest that there are a number of proteases in the interstitial space: either secreted proteases or zymogens, membrane-bound proteases, or shed membrane proteases. A select number of these are listed in Table 4.1. Some of these enzymes are discussed in the following chapters, while in the current chapter we focus on a disintegrin and metalloproteinase (ADAM) and a disintegrin and metalloprotease with thrombospondin motif (ADAMTS). Those readers searching for a comprehensive discussion of proteolytic enzymes, including those suggested to be present in the interstitial space, may consult the recent encyclopedic work edited by Neil Rawlings and Guy Salvesen.[1] In addition to the proteases discussed in the current work, there are a number of proteases expressed in the interstitial space during development and in tumors that are not normal constituents of the interstitial space. Many of the proteases suggested to be present in the interstitial space have not been physically isolated from a biological fluid or tissue but have rather been identified by cDNA technology. An example is provided by some members of the ADAM family described in Section 4.2.

We cannot think of a group of enzymes that are as diverse in function as proteases. Proteases may be broadly and somewhat artificially divided into digestive enzymes and regulatory enzymes.[2–4] Digestive enzymes such as trypsin usually have specificity for the structure of one of the amino acids in the scissile peptide bond; in the case of trypsin, specificity is derived from a positively charged amino acid such as arginine or lysine contributing to the carboxyl group in the peptide bond. Thrombin is a regulatory protease with tryptic-like specificity but which possesses inserts in the polypeptide chain, forming exosites that presumably add more constraints on the specificity of the cleaved peptide bond.[2,3] Other regulatory proteases have no defined specificity, and substrate availability is considered to define the cleaved peptide bond. Finally, while there are no data to support it, there is the possibility of substrate-assisted catalysis of peptide bond cleavage.[5] In substrate-assisted catalysis, catalytically functional groups are provided by both the *enzyme* and the *substrate*. The cleavage of the β1,4 linkage between N-acetylglucosamine and glucuronic acid in hyaluronan by human hyaluronidase has been suggested to involve substrate-assisted catalysis.[6]

We were surprised at the large number of enzymes that could be considered to have their primary function in the interstitial space. While some of these proteases have a digestive function in participating in the remodeling of the extracellular matrix (ECM), most of the enzymes can be considered to be regulatory in function. Some proteases, such as plasmin, can be considered to have both a regulatory and a

TABLE 4.1
Proteolytic Activities Described in the Interstitial Space

Enzyme	Comment
ADAM proteases	ADAM proteases are a group of metallproteinases[1,2] composed of a disintegrin domain and a metalloprotease domain.[1] ADAM proteases are members of the adamlysin family in the metzincin superfamily, which also includes MMPs.[3-] The disintegrin domain functions in binding to integrins on the cell membrane, possibly positioning the protease to act as a sheddase.[4] Not all of the members of the ADAM family have proteolytic activity, suggesting the importance of protein–ligand interactions in function.[5] ADAM proteases have a major role in development[6] and are of interest in oncology research.[7] The function of ADAM protease as a sheddase is of importance in inflammation, as shown by the release of TNF-α by ADAM-17.[8] See Section 4.2 for more detail.
ADAMTS (a disintegrin and metalloprotease with thrombospondin type-1 motif repeats)	ADAMTS proteases are a group of metalloproteinases consisting of an ADAM domain (see above) and thrombospondin motif repeats.[9–11] Unlike the ADAM proteases, which are membrane bound, the ADAMTS proteases are soluble proteins that are processed and secreted in a furin-mediated pathway.[12] Early work suggested that the thrombospondin domains in ADAMTS proteases enabled binding to the ECM.[13] ADAMTS proteases are best known for their degradation of proteoglycans, such as aggrecan,[14] and collagen processing.[15] One ADAMTS protease, ADAMTS[13], is involved in the processing of von Willebrand factor in endothelial cells.[16] See Section 4.3 for more detail.
Chymase	Chymase is a chymotrypsin-like serine protease that is a product of mast cells.[17,18] More specifically, chymase arising from mast cell degranulation in the arterial intimal fluid has been reported.[19–22] Chymase has biological activity in the interstitial space, such as stimulation of angiotensin II formation,[19] degradation of HDL,[30,21] and activation of MMPs.[23–25] Demonstrated to cleave nidogen but less effective than leucocyte elastase.[26] Also shown to increase glomerular permeability by cleavage of PAR-2 receptor.[27]
Factor VIIa	There is no direct measurement of factor VIIa in interstitial fluid, but indirect evidence supports the presence of this protease.[28,29] It is suggested that the formation of the thrombin in the interstitium occurs via the tissue factor pathway, which would require the conversion of factor VII to factor VIIa.[30,31] Perivascular tissue factor binds factor VIIa.[32] See Chapter 8 for more detail.
Factor Xa	There is no direct measurement of factor Xa in interstitial fluid, but indirect evidence supports the presence of this protease.[33,34] Factor Xa can activate cells via cleavage of the PAR-2 receptor.[35] See Chapter 8 for more detail.
Hepsin	A hepatic enzyme of unclear function.[36] There are studies with *in vitro* substrates, but *in vivo* substrates have not been described. Hepsin is a type II transmembrane serine protease (TTSP),[37] as is matripase.[38,39] Hepsin has been shown to activate factor VII.[40] Hepsin is involved in malignancy and is proposed as a therapeutic target.[41–45]

TABLE 4.1 (CONTINUED)
Proteolytic Activities Described in the Interstitial Space

Enzyme	Comment
Hyaluronan-binding serine protease	Hyaluronan-binding serine protease (HABP) was isolated from human plasma by affinity chromatography on hyaluronan conjugated to agarose.[46] Analysis of amino acid sequence derived from cDNA showed homology to hepatocyte growth factor activator. Further analysis of the gene for HABP showed some homology with coagulation factor XII, tPA, and urokinase.[47] HABP has been shown to undergo autocatalytic activation,[48,49] which was stimulated by the presence of either positively charged poly-lysine or negatively charged heparin.[48] Heparan sulfate and chondroitin sulfate have also been shown to stimulate the action of hyaluronan-binding serine protease on kininogens, forming kinins.[49] While a substrate in plasma has not been clearly identified,[50] hyaluronan-binding serine protease has been shown to upregulate ERK1/2 and P13K/Akt, signaling pathways in fibroblasts and stimulating cell proliferation and migration.[51] The conditioned media from HABP-treated fibroblasts had a growth-stimulating effect on quiescent fibroblasts.
Insulin-like growth factor binding protein-3 protease (IGFBP-3 protease)	IGFBP-3 protease is described more as an activity[52,53] than as a discrete molecular entity and the activity may be more a reflection of the susceptibility of IGFBP-3 to proteolysis by a wide variety of enzymes.[54–63] There is evidence to suggest that there is little proteolysis of IGFBP-3 in "normal" serum, but there is marked increase during pregancy.[64] Proteolysis of IGFBP-3 may increase IGF-1 bioavailability.[58,65] Proteolysis of IGFBP-3 occurs to a higher extent in interstitial fluid.[66–68]
Kallikrein-related peptidases[a]	A family of regulatory proteases related by structural homology and not biological function[69,70] (see Chapter 6).
Mastin	Mastin is a soluble tryptase-like enzyme[71] secreted by canine mast cells.[72] Mastin has a tryptic-like specificity with a preference for cleavage of arginine-containing peptide bonds.
Matriptase	Matriptase (MT-SP1, epitin, SNC19, TADG-15) was identified as a matrix-degrading serine protease in tumor cells.[73] Subsequent studies[74] demonstrated that matriptase was expressed on epithelial cells as a membrane-bound protease that could activate hepatocyte growth factor and urokinase plasminogen activator. Matriptase is inhibited by hepatocyte growth factor activator inhibitor 1 (HAI-1)[75] and antithrombin.[76,77] Matriptase can be detected by reaction with a biotinylated peptide chloromethyl ketone.[78] Matriptase occurs as a surface-bound zymogen that undergoes autocatalytic transactivation.[79] Matriptase is considered to part of a proteolytic cascade involving the activation of prostasin necessary for functionality of the stratum corneum barrier function.[80]
Matrix metalloproteinase	MMPs (matrixins)[81–83] are a group of proteolytic enzymes that are members of the metzincin superfamily[84,85] and involved in the degradation of ECM components.[86] MMPs vary considerably in structure and size but have a common mechanism involving a cysteine residue and a metal ion, usually zinc. MMPs are synthesized as precursor or zymogen forms that require activation.[87–90] Glycosaminoglycans may modulate MMP action.[91] MMPs are discussed in detail in Chapter 7.

(Continued)

TABLE 4.1 (CONTINUED)
Proteolytic Activities Described in the Interstitial Space

Enzyme	Comment
Meprin metalloproteases	Meprin A (meprin α) and meprin B (meprin β) are zinc metalloproteinases, which are astacins[92] in the metzincin superfamily.[84,85] Meprin A and Meprin B are transmembrane proteases that can be released (shed) into the interstitial space.[93,94] Meprin A may be secreted as a zymogen form. The functions of the meprin proteases are still being defined, but a number of potential substrates[95] have been identified, including amyloid protein,[96] procollagens,[97] and IL-6.[98]
Mesotrypsin[b]	Mesotrypsin has been described as a minor form of pancreatic trypsin derived from mesotrypsinogen by the action of enterokinase.[99,100] As with trypsin IV, mesotrypsin is resistant to inactivation by protein protease inhibitors.[99,101] It has been suggested that mesotrypsin is important for the degradation of trypsin inhibitors such as soybean trypsin inhibitor, permitting the digestion of food rich in natural trypsin inhibitors.[102]
	Mesotrypsin has been described in the upper epidermis as an enzyme responsible for the activation of epidermal kallikrein-like peptidases and for the degradation of lymphoepithelial Kazal-type-related inhibitor (LEKTI1), an inhibitor of the kallikrein-like peptidases.[103] As with the pancreatic proenzyme, epidermal mesotrypsinogen is activated by enterokinase, also found in the epidermis. These observations support a role for mesotrypsin in the desquamation process.
Neutrophil elastase	Neutrophil elastase has a chymotrypsin-like specificity and degrades elastin and collagen in the interstitial space.[104,105] Not to be confused with macrophage elastase (MMP-12; Chapter 8). The degradation of pulmonary elastin by neutrophil elastase is inhibited by hyaluronan.[106] Neutrophil elastase has been suggested to be important for the development of interstitial edema during pericardial inflammation.[107] Cleavage of E-cadherin by neutrophil elastase is suggested to result in loss of cell–cell contacts and adherens junctions in the development of experimental pancreatis.[108]
Neutrophil protease 3	A protease contained in neutrophils and expressed in the interstitial space after migration of the neutrophils from the vascular space.[109,110] Neutrophil protease 3, along with other neutrophil proteases such as neutrophil elastase, is synthesized as a zymogen, processed to a mature enzyme by dipeptidyl peptidase I,[111] and stored in azurophil granules.[110] A small amount of activated neutrophil protease 3 is expressed on the surface of resting neutrophils.[112] Neutrophil protease 3 cleaves the PAR-1 receptor at sites separate from the thrombin cleavage site.[113] However, the cleavage of PAR-1 receptor by neutrophil proteinase-3 does activate MAP-kinase. Antibodies against neutrophil protease 3 are observed in antineutrophil cytoplasmic antigens.[114,115] The surface presentation of neutrophil protease 3 is important for its role as an antineutrophil cytoplasmic antigen.[92] Neutrophil migration from the vascular space into the interstitial space is critical for the normal immune response,[116] and the expression of neutrophil proteinase 3 is critical for the defense response in the interstitial space.[117,118]

TABLE 4.1 (CONTINUED)
Proteolytic Activities Described in the Interstitial Space

Enzyme	Comment
Plasma kallikrein	The presence of plasma kallikrein in the interstitial space can be inferred from the presence of bradykinin and other kinin products released by plasma kallikrein from high-molecular-weight kininogen.[119–122] Plasma prekallikrein and high-molecular-weight kininogen have been found in cerebrospinal fluid.[123] Plasma kallikrein activates vascular smooth muscle cells by action on PAR receptors.[124] There is more extensive information on plasma kallikrein in Chapter 6.
Plasmin	A serine protease derived from plasminogen that has a specificity for the cleavage of peptide bonds where the carboxyl group is contributed by lysine.[125] Plasminogen is found in plasma and interstitial fluid;[126,127] plasmin can be found in serum,[128,129] urine,[130] and synovial fluid.[131–133] Plasmin is rapidly inhibited by α_2-antiplasmin, α_2-macroglobulin, and α_1-antitrypsin.[134–137] Cleavage of plasmin/plasminogen by a variety of proteolytic enzymes gives rise to angiostatin.[138–143] While best recognized for fibrinolytic activity, plasmin can directly interact with cells within the interstitium[144–146] and regulates the ECM and function.[147–152] See Chapter 5 for more detail.
Reelin	A large glycoprotein serine protease[153,154] associated with the ECM that is important for nervous system development and the regulation of synaptic transmission in the adult brain.[155] Reelin was identified as a product of the reeler gene,[156] which is a protein component of the ECM during early cortical development [157]
Thrombin	A serine protease derived from prothrombin[158,159] that has specificity for the cleavage of peptide bonds where the carboxyl group is contributed by basic amino acids (arginine and lysine).[160,161] Thrombin is important in the development of interstitial fibrosis.[162–164] While thrombin can form fibrin in the interstitial space,[165] the majority of interest is directed toward the interaction of thrombin with cells.[162,163,166] Thrombin may have a direct role in ECM degradation through the degradation of fibronectin[167] and proteoglycans[168] but also activates MMPs.[169,170] There are data to suggest that antithrombin can inactivate thrombin in the interstitial space[171] but there is no direct evidence for the formation of a thrombin–antithrombin complex. Thrombin can also activate hepatocyte growth factor activator.[172] See Chapter 8 for more detail.
Tissue kallikrein (KLK-1)[b]	A tryptic-like serine protease best known for the formation of kinins from kininogens.[173] It is suggested that tissue kallikrein is released into the interstitial space during inflammation[22,174] or is secondary to tissue damage[175,176] (see Chapter 6).
Tissue plasminogen activator (tPA)	tPA is a specific activator of plasminogen that is found in a variety of tissues,[177,178] with some emphasis on nervous tissue[179,180] and eye.[181] There is major interest in tPA expression in endothelial cells.[182] tPA is thought to bind to endothelial cell surfaces following secretion, with such binding important for fibrinolytic activity.[183] tPA is present in interstitial fluid[184,185] but is rapidly inactivated by PAI-1.[186] tPA is also found on macrophage surfaces.[128] tPA is active in a bound phase but poorly active in free solution.[187,188] The formation of plasmin on the melanoma cell surface, mediated by tPA activation of plasminogen bound on the cell surface, is considered important for invasiveness.[189]

(Continued)

TABLE 4.1 (CONTINUED)
Proteolytic Activities Described in the Interstitial Space

Enzyme	Comment
Tryptase	Tryptases are tryptic-like serine proteases that are products of mass cells.[18,190] There are several isoforms of tryptase[191] arising from variation in the tetramer structure of this protein.[192,193] Cleavage of PAR-2 on epithelial cells by tryptase may be of importance in the interstitium.[194,195] Tryptase activates TGF-β in airway smooth muscle cells in a PAR2-independent mechanism.[196] Heparin and other macropolyanions are involved in the storage and modulation of tryptase activity.[197–201] Human tryptase loses activity via a process described as spontaneous inactivation; the process of spontaneous inactivation is slowed/reversed by sulfated polyanions such as heparin or dextran sulfate.[202–205]
Trypsin IV[b]	Trypsin IV is an extrapancreatic isoform of trypsin found in the brain and is derived from trypsinogen IV, which may be a splice variant of mesotrypsinogen.[206,207] Trypsin IV may also be secreted by other extrahepatic sources, including certain epithelial cells.[208] Trypsin IV differs from classic pancreatic trypsin in being resistant to inhibition by protein trypsin inhibitors.[209] Trypsin IV has the ability to activate PAR receptors and may have a role in inflammation.[210]
Urokinase plasminogen activator (urokinase)	Urokinase plasminogen activator (uPA) is an enzyme synthesized in the kidney.[211,212] In addition to proteolysis, urokinase acts through binding to a specific cell surface receptor (urokinase plasminogen activator receptor; uPAR).[213] Urokinase and uPAR together with plasminogen activator inhibitor 1 (PAI-1) are important in inflammation[127] and VEGF-stimulated angiogenesis.[214] uPA is important in the programmed degradation of the ECM during development.[215] uPA is distinct from tissue plasminogen activator (tPA).[216,217] See Chapter 5 for more detail.

Note: These proteins are not unique to the interstitial space but are found in other fluid compartments, including the vascular bed. See Chapter 1 for a discussion of the origin of proteins in the interstitium.

[a] There are some issues with the nomenclature in this area and there are studies where mesotrypsin and trypsin IV are considered interchangeable. Trypsin IV and mesotrypsin do appear to be different enzymes but share some unusual properties, such as the resistance to inactivation by protein protease inhibitors.

REFERENCES FOR TABLE 4.1

1. Yamamoto, S., Higuchi, Y., Yoshiyama, K., et al., ADAM family proteins in the immune systems, *Immunol. Today* 20, 278–284, 1999.
2. Kleiin, T. and Bischoff, R., Active metalloproteases of the A Disintegrin and Metalloproteinases (ADAM) family: Biological function and structure, *J. Proteome Res.* 10, 17–33, 2011.
3. Rawlings, N.D., Protease families, evolution and mechanism of action, in *Proteases: Structure and Function*, eds. K. Brix and W. Stöcker, Chapter 1, pp. 1–35, Springer, Vienna, Austria, 2013.
4. White, J.M., ADAMS: Modulators of cell–cell and cell–matrix interactions, *Curr. Opin. Cell Biol.* 15, 598–606, 2003.

5. Edwards, D.R., Handsley, M.M., and Pennington, C.J., The ADAM metalloproteinases, *Mol. Aspects Med.* 29, 258–289, 2008.

6. Christian, L., Bahudhanapati, H., and Wei, S., Extracellular metalloproteinases in neural crest development and craniofacial morphogenesis, *Crit. Rev. Biochem. Mol. Biol.* 48, 544–560, 2013.

7. Moro, N., Mauch, C., and Zigrino, P., Metalloproteinases in melanoma, *Eur. J. Cell Biol.* 93. 23–29, 2014.

8. Lisi, S., D'Amore, M., and Sisto, M., ADAM17 at the interface between inflammation and autoimmunity, *Immunol. Lett.* 162, 159–169, 2014.

9. Kuno, K., Kanada, N., Nakashima, E., et al., Molecular cloning of a gene encoding a new type of metalloproteinase-disintegrin family protein with thrombospondin motifs as an inflammatory associated gene, *J. Biol. Chem.* 272, 556–562, 1997.

10. Tang, B.L. and Hong, W., ADAMTS: A novel family of proteases with an ADAM protease domain and thrombospondin 1 repeats, *FEBS Lett.* 445, 223–225, 1999.

11. Apte, S.S., The ADAMTS endopeptidases, in *The Handbook of Proteolytic Enzymes*, eds. N.D. Rawlings and G.S. Salvesen, Chapter 259, pp. 1149–1155, Academic Press/Elsevier, Amsterdam, the Netherlands, 2013.

12. Kuno, K., Terashima, Y., and Matsushima, K., ADAMTS-1 is an active metalloproteinase associated with the extracellular matrix, *J. Biol. Chem.* 274, 18821–18826, 1999.

13. Kuno, K. and Matsushima, K., ADAMTS-1 protein anchors at the extracellular matrix through the thrombospondin type I motifs and its spacing region, *J. Biol. Chem.* 273, 13912–13917, 1998.

14. Stanton, H., Melrose, J., Little, C.B., and Fosang, A.J., Proteoglycan degradation by the ADAMTS family of proteinases, *Biochim. Biophys. Acta* 1812, 1616–1629, 2011.

15. Bekhouche, M. and Colige, A., The procollagen N-proteinases ADAMTS2, 3 and 14 in pathophysiology, *Matrix Biol.* 44–46, 46–53, 2015.

16. Shang, D., Zheng, X.W., Niiya, M., and Zheng, X.L., Apical sorting of ADAMTS13 in vascular endothelial cells and Madin-Darby canine kidney cells depends on the CUB domains and their association with lipid rafts, *Blood* 108, 2207–2215, 2006.

17. Craig, S.S. and Schwartz, L.B., Tryptase and chymase, markers of distinct types of human mast cells, *Immunol. Res.* 8, 130–148, 1989.

18. Caughey, G.H., Chymases, in *Handbook of Proteolytic Enzymes*, 3rd edn., eds. N.D. Rawlings and G. Salvesen, Chapter 590, pp. 2675–2683, Elsevier, Amsterdam, the Netherlands, 2013.

19. Wei, C.C., Meng, Q.C., Palmer, R., et al., Evidence for angiotensin-converting enzyme- and chymase-mediated angiotensin II formation in the interstitial fluid space of the dog heart *in vivo*, *Circulation* 99, 2583–2589, 1999.

20. Lindstedt, L., Lee, M., and Kovanen, P.T., Chymase bound to heparin is resistant to its natural inhibitors and capable of proteolyzing high density lipoproteins in aortic intimal fluid, *Atherosclerosis* 155, 87–97, 2001.

21. Lee-Rueckert, M. and Kovanen, P.T., Extracellular modifications of HDL *in vivo* and the emerging concept of proteolytic inactivation of preβ-HDL, *Curr. Opin. Lipidol.* 22, 394–402, 2011.

22. Wei, C.C., Chen., Y., Powell, L.C., et al., Cardiac kallikrein-kinin system is upregulated in chronic volume overload and mediates an inflammatory-induced collagen loss, *PLoS One* 7(6), e40110, 2012.

23. Suzuki, K., Lees, M., Newlands, G.F., et al., Activation of precursors for matrix metalloproteinase 1 (interstitial collagenase) and 3 (stromelysin) by rat mast-cell proteinase I and II, *Biochem. J.* 305, 301–306, 1995.

24. Lundequist, A., Aabrink, M., and Pejler, G., Mass cell-dependent activation of pro matrix metalloprotease 2: A role for serglycin proteoglycan–dependent mass cell proteases, *Biol. Chem.* 387, 1513–1519, 2006.

25. Saarinen, J., Kalkkinen, N., Welgus, H.G., and Kovanen, P.T., Activation of human interstitial procollagenase through direct cleavage of the Leu83–Thr84 bond by mast cell chymase, *J. Biol. Chem.* 269, 18134–18140, 1994.

26. Mayer, U., Mann, K., Timpl, R., and Murphy, G., Sites of nidogen cleavage by proteases involved in tissue homeostasis, *Eur. J. Biochem.* 217, 877–884, 1993.

27. Sharma, R., Prasad, V., McCarthy, E.T., et al., Chymase increases glomerular albumin permeability via protease-activated receptor-2, *Mol. Cell. Biochem.* 297, 161–169, 2007.

28. Cella, G., Cipriani, A., Tommasini, A., et al., Tissue factor pathway inhibitor (TFPI) antigen plasma level in patients with interstitial lung disease before and after heparin administration, *Semin. Thromb. Hemost.* 23, 45–49, 1998.

29. Wygrecka, M., Jablonska, E., Guenther, A., et al., Current view on alveolar coagulation and fibrinolysis in acute inflammatory and chronic interstitial lung diseases, *Thromb. Haemost.* 99, 494–501, 2008.

30. Zucker, S., Mirza, H., Conner, C.E., et al., Vascular endothelial growth factor induces tissue factor and matrix metalloproteinase production in endothelial cells: Conversion of prothrombin to thrombin results in progelatinase A activation and cell proliferation, *Int. J. Cancer* 75, 780–786, 1998.

31. Günther, A., Mosavi, P., Ruppert, C., et al., Enhanced tissue factor pathway activity and fibrin turnover in the alveolar compartment of patients with interstitial lung disease, *Thromb. Haemost.* 83, 853–860, 2000.

32. Hoffman, M., Collina, C.M., McDonald, A.G., et al., Tissue factor around dermal vessels has bound factor VII in the absence of injury, *J. Thromb. Haemost.* 5, 1403–1408, 2007.

33. Idell, S., Gonzalez, K., Bradford, H., et al., Procoagulant activity in bronchoalveolar lavage in the adult respiratory distress syndrome: Contribution of tissue factor associated with factor VII, *Am. Rev. Respir. Dis.* 136, 1466–1474, 1987.

34. Uhicha, M., Okajima, K., Murakami, K., et al., Effect of human urinary thrombomodulin on endotoxin-induced intravascular coagulation and pulmonary vascular injury in rats, *Am. J. Hematol.* 54, 118–123, 1997.

35. Grandaliano, G., Pontrelli, P., Cerullo, G., et al., Protease-activated receptor-2 expression in IgA nephropathy: A potential role in the pathogenesis of interstitial fibrosis, *J. Am. Soc. Nephrol.* 14, 2072–2083, 2003.

36. Wu, Q. and Peng, J., Hepsin, in *Handbook of Proteolytic Enzymes*, 3rd edn., eds. N.D. Rawlings and G. Salvesen, Chapter 652, pp. 2985–2989, Elsevier, Amsterdam, the Netherlands, 2013.

37. Wu, Q., Type II transmembrane serine proteases, *Curr. Top. Dev. Biol.* 54, 167–206, 2003.

38. Qiu, D., Owen, K., Gray, K., et al., Roles and regulation of membrane-associated serine proteases, *Biochem. Soc. Trans.* 35, 583–587, 2007.

39. Owen, K.A., Qiu, D., Alves, J., et al., Pericellular activation of hepatocyte growth factor by the transmembrane proteases matriptase and hepsin, but not by the membrane-associated protease uPA, *Biochem. J.* 426, 219–228, 2010.

40. Kazama, Y., Hamamoto, T., Foster, D.C., and Kisiel, W., Hepsin, a putative membrane-associated serine protease, activates human factor VII and initiates a pathway of blood coagulation on the cell surface leading to thrombin formation, *J. Biol. Chem.* 270, 66–72, 1995.

41. Koschubs, T., Dengl, S., Dürr, H., et al., Allosteric antibody inhibition of human hepsin protease, *Biochem. J.* 42, 483–494, 2012.

42. Kim, H.J., Han, J.H., Chang, I.H., et al., Variants in the HEPSIN gene are associated with susceptibility to prostate cancer, *Prostate Cancer Prostatic Dis.* 15, 353–358, 2012.

43. Hemstreet, G.P., III, Rossi, G.R., Pisarev, V.M., et al., Cellular immunotherapy study of prostate cancer patients and resulting IgG responses to peptide epitopes predicted from prostate tumor–associated autoantigens, *J. Immunother.* 36, 57–65, 2013.
44. Guo, J., Li, G., Tang, J., et al., HLA-A2-restricted cytotoxic T lymphocyte epitopes from human hepsin as novel targets for prostate cancer immunotherapy, *Scand. J. Immunol.* 78, 248–257, 2013.
45. Tang, X., Mahajan, S.S., Nguyen, L.T., et al., Targeted inhibition of cell-surface serine protease hepsin blacks prostate cancer bone metastasis, *Oncotarget* 5, 1352–1362, 2014.
46. Choi-Miura, N.-H., Tobe, T., Sumiya, J., et al., Purification and characterization of a novel hyaluronan-binding protein (PHBP) from human plasma: It has three EGF, a kringle and a serine protease domain, similar to hepatocyte growth factor activator, *J. Biochem.* 119, 1157–1165, 1996.
47. Sumiya, J., Asakawa, S., Tobe, T., et al., Isolation and characterization of the plasma hyaluronan-binding protein (PHBP) gene (HABP2), *J. Biochem.* 122, 983–990, 1997.
48. Etscheid, M., Hunfeld, A., Kőnig, H., Seitz, R., and Dodt, J., Activation of proPHBSP, the zymogen of a plasma hyaluronan binding serine protease, by an intermolecular autocatalytic mechanism, *Biol. Chem.* 381, 1223–1231, 2000.
49. Etscheid, M., Beer, M., Fink, E., Seitz, R., and Johannes, D., The hyaluronan-binding serine protease from human plasma cleaves HMW and LMW kininogen and releases bradykinin, *Biol. Chem.* 383, 1633–1643, 2002.
50. Mcvey, J.H., Factor VII activating protease: Does it do what it says on the tin? *J. Thromb. Haemost.* 10, 857–858, 2012.
51. Estascheid, M., Beer, N., and Dodt, J., The hyaluronan-binding protease upregulates ERK1/2 and P13K/Akt signalling pathways in fibroblasts and stimulates cell proliferation and migration, *Cell Signal.* 17, 1486–1494, 2005.
52. Davenport, M.L., Pucilowska, J., Clemmons, D.R., ct al., Tissue-specific expression of insulin-like growth factor binding protein-3 protease activity during rat pregnancy, *Endocrinology* 130, 2505–2512, 1992.
53. Maile, L.A. and Holly, J.M.P., Insulin-like growth factor binding protein (IGFBP) proteolysis: Occurrence, identification, role and regulation, *Growth Horm. IGF Res.* 9, 85–95, 1999.
54. Berg, U., Bang, P., and Carlsson-Skwirut, C., Calpain proteolysis of insulin-like growth factor binding protein (IGFBP)-2 and -3, but not of IGFBP-1, *Biol. Chem.* 388, 859–863, 2007.
55. Nwosu, B.U., Soyka, L.A., Angelescu, A., and Lee, M.M., Evidence of insulin-like growth factor binding protein-3 proteolysis during growth hormone stimulation testing, *J. Pediatr. Endocrinol. Metab.* 24, 163–167, 2011.
56. Elzi, D.J., Lai, Y., Song, M., et al., Plasminogen activator inhibitor 1-insulin-like growth factor binding protein 3 cascade regulates stress-induced senescence, *Proc. Natl. Acad. Sci. USA* 109, 12052–12057, 2012.
57. Mitui, Y., Mochizuki, S., Kodama, T., et al., ADAM28 is overexpressed in human breast carcinomas: Implications for carcinoma cell proliferation through cleavage of insulin-like growth factor binding protein-3, *Cancer Res.* 66, 9913–9920, 2006.
58. Miyamoto, S., Yano, K., Sugimoto, S., et al. Matrix metalloproteinase-7 facilitates insulin-like growth factor bioavailability through its proteinase activity on insulin-like growth factor binding protein 3, *Cancer Res.* 64, 665–671, 2004.
59. Sadowski, T., Dietrich, S., Kochinsky, F., and Sedlacek, R., Matrix metalloproteinase 19 regulates insulin-like growth factor-mediated proliferation, migration, and adhesion in human keratinocytes through proteolysis of insulin-like growth factor binding protein-3, *Mol. Biol. Cell,* 14, 4569–4580, 2003.

60. Koistinen, H., Paju, A., Koistinen, R., et al., Prostate-specific antigen and other prostate-derived proteases cleave IGFBP-3, but prostate cancer is not associated with proteolytically cleaved circulating IGFBP-3, *Prostate* 50, 112–118, 2002.
61. Loechel, F., Fox, J.W., Murphy, G., et al., ADAM 12-S cleaves IGFBP-3 and IGFBP-5 and is inhibited by TIMP-3, *Biochem. Biophys. Res. Commun.* 278, 511–515, 2000.
62. Kübler, B., Draeger, C., John, H., et al., Isolation and characterization of circulating fragments of the insulin-like growth factor binding protein-3, *FEBS Lett.* 518, 124–128, 2002.
63. Booth, B.A., Boes, M., Dake, B.L., et al., IGFBP-3 binding to endothelial cells inhibits plasmin and thrombin proteolysis, *Am. J. Physiol. Endocrinol. Metab.* 282, E52–E58, 2002.
64. Yan, X., Payet, L.D., Baxter, R.C., and Firth, S.M., Activity of human pregnancy insulin-like growth factor binding protein-3: Determination by reconstituting recombinant complexes, *Endocrinology* 150, 4968–4976, 2009.
65. Bhat, C., Villaudy, J., and Binoux, M., *In vivo* proteolysis of serum insulin-like growth factor (IGF) binding protein-3 results in increased availability of IGF to target cells, *J. Clin. Invest.* 93, 2286–2290, 1994.
66. Lalou, C. and Binoux, M., Evidence that limited proteolysis of insulin-like growth factor binding protein-3 (IGFBP-3) occurs in the normal state outside of the bloodstream, *Regul. Pept.* 48, 179–188, 1993.
67. Hughes, S.C., Xu, S., Fernihough, J., et al., Tissue IGFBP-3 proteolysis: Contrasting pathophysiology to that in the circulation, *Prog. Growth Factor Res.* 6, 293–299, 1995.
68. Xu, S., Savage, P., Burton, J.L., et al., Proteolysis of insulin-like growth factor-binding protein-3 by human skin keratinocytes in culture in comparison to that in skin interstitial fluid: The role and regulation of components of the plasmin system, *J. Clin. Endocrinol. Metab.* 82, 1863–1868, 1997.
69. Clements, J.A., Reflections on the tissue kallikrein and kallikrein-related peptidase family: From mice to men; What have we learnt in the last two decades? *Biol. Chem.* 389, 1447–1454, 2008.
70. Pampakalis, G. and Sotiropoulou, G., Pharmacological targeting of human tissue kallikrein-related peptidases, in *Proteinases as Drug Targets*, ed. B.M. Dunn, Chapter 9, pp. 199–228, RSC Publishing, Cambridge, UK, 2012.
71. Trivedi, N.N., Tong, Q., and Raman, K., Mast cell α and β tryptases changed rapidly during primate speciation and evolved from γ-like transmembrane peptidases in ancestral vertebrates, *J. Immunol.* 179, 6072–6079, 2007.
72. Raymond, W.W., Sommerhoff, C.P., and Caughey, G.H., Mastin is a gelatinolytic mast cell peptidase resembling mini-proteasome, *Arch. Biochem. Biophys.* 435, 311–322, 2005.
73. Lin, C.-Y., Anders, J., Johnson, M., et al., Molecular cloning of cDNA for matriptase, a matrix-degrading serine protease with trypsin-like activity, *J. Biol. Chem.* 274, 18231–18239, 1999.
74. Lee, S.L., Dickson, R.B., and Lin, C.Y., Activation of hepatocyte growth factor and urokinase/plasminogen activator by matriptase, an epithelial membrane serine protease, *J. Biol. Chem.* 275, 36720–36725, 2000.
75. Miller, G.S. and List, K., The matriptase-prostasin proteolytic cascade in epithelial development and pathology, *Cell Tissue Res.* 351, 245–253, 2013.
76. Chou, F.P., Xu, H., Lee, M.S., et al., Matriptase is inhibited by extravascular antithrombin in epithelial cells but not in most carcinoma cells, *Am. J. Physiol. Cell Physiol.* 301, C1093–C1103, 2011.
77. Chen, Y.-W., Xu, Z., Baksh, A.N.H., et al., Antithrombin regulates matriptase activity involved in plasmin generation, syndecan shedding, and HGF activation in keratinocytes, *PLoS One* 8(5), e62826, 2013.

78. Godiksen, S., Soendergaard, C., Friis, S., et al., Detection of active matriptase using a biotinylated chloromethyl ketone peptide, *PLoS One* 8(10), e77146, 2013.
79. Oberst, M.D., Williams, C.A., Dickson, R.B., Johnson, M.D., and Lin, C.Y., The activation of matriptase requires its noncatalytic domains, serine protease domain, and its cognate inhibitor, *J. Biol. Chem.* 278, 26773–26779, 2003.
80. Buzza, M.S., Martin, E.W., Driesbaugh, K.H., et al., Prostasin is required for matriptase activation in intestinal epithelial cells to regulate closure of the paracellular pathway, *J. Biol. Chem.* 288, 10328–10337, 2013.
81. Woessner, J.F., Jr., Matrix metalloproteinases and their inhibitors in connective tissue remodeling, *FASEB J.* 5, 2145–2154, 1991.
82. Woessner, J.F., Jr., Quantification of matrix metalloproteinase in tissue samples, *Methods Enzymol.* 248, 510–528, 1995.
83. Chase, A.J. and Newby, A.C., Regulation of matrix metalloproteinase (matrixin) genes in blood vessels: A multi-step recruitment model for pathological remodelling, *J. Vasc. Res.* 40, 329–343, 2003.
84. Yamamoto, K., Murphy, G., and Troeberg, L., Extracellular regulation of metalloproteinases, *Matrix Biol.* 44–46, 255–263, 2015.
85. Ricard-Blum, S. and Vallet, S.D., Proteases decode the extracellular matrix cryptome, *Biochemie* 122, 300–313, 2016.
86. Ugalde, A.P., Ordóñez, G.R., Quirós, P.M., et al., Metalloproteinases in the degradome, in *Matrix Metalloproteinases Protocols*, ed. I.M. Clark, Chapter 1, pp. 2–29, Springer/Humana, New York, 2010.
87. Kleiner, D.E., Jr. and Stetler-Stevenson, W.G., Structural biochemistry and activation of matrix metalloproteases, *Curr. Opin. Cell Biol.* 5, 891–897, 1993.
88. Ra, H.J. and Parks, W.C., Control of matrix metalloproteinase catalytic activity, *Matrix Biol.* 26, 587–596, 2007.
89. Piperi, C. and Papavasssiliou, A.G., Molecular mechanisms regulating matrix metalloproteases, *Curr. Top. Med. Chem.* 12, 1095–1112, 2012.
90. Jacob-Ferreira, A.L. and Schulz, R., Activation of intracellular matrix metalloproteinase-2 by reactive oxygen–nitrogen species: Consequences and therapeutic strategies in the heart, *Arch. Biochem. Biophys.* 540, 82–93, 2013.
91. Tocci, A. and Parks, W.C., Functional interactions between matrix metalloproteinase and glycosaminoglycans, *FEBS J.* 280, 2332–2341, 2013.
92. von Vietinghoff, S., Eulenberg, C., Wellner, M., et al., Neutrophil surface presentation of the anti-neutrophil cytoplasmic antibody-antigen proteinase 3 depends on N-terminal processing, *Clin. Exp. Immunol.* 152, 508–516, 2008.
93. Bond, J.S., and Beynon, R.J., Meprin: A membrane-bound metallo-endopeptidase, *Curr. Top. Cell. Regul.* 28, 263–290, 1986.
94. Villa, J.P., Bertenshaw, G.P., Bylander, J.E., and Bond, J.S., Meprin proteolytic complexes at the cell surfaces and in the extracellular spaces, *Biochem. Soc. Symp.* 70, 53–63, 2003.
95. Jefferson, T., auf dem Keller, U., Bellac, C., et al., The substrate degradome of meprin metalloproteases reveals an unexpected proteolytic link between meprin β and ADAM10, *Cell. Mol. Life Sci.* 70, 309–333, 2013.
96. Bien, J., Jefferson, T., Causević, M., et al., The metalloprotease meprin β generates amino terminal-truncated amyloid β peptide species, *J. Biol. Chem.* 287, 33304–33313, 2012.
97. Prox, J., Arnold, P., and Becker-Pauly, C., Meprin α and meprin: Procollagen proteinases in health and disease, *Matrix Biol.* 44–46, 7–13, 2015.
98. Keiffer, T.R. and Bond, J.S., Meprin metalloproteases inactivated interleukin-6, *J. Biol. Chem.* 289, 7580–7588, 2014.

99. Rinderknecht, H., Renner, I.G., Abramson, S.B., and Carmack, C., Mesotrypsin: A new inhibitor-resistant protease from a zymogen in human pancreatic tissue and fluid, *Gastroenterology* 86, 681–692, 1984.

100. Knecht, W., Cottrell, G.S., Amadesi, S., et al., Trypsin IV or mesotrypsin and 23 cleave protease-activated receptors 1 and 2 to induce inflammation and hyperalgesia, *J. Biol. Chem.* 282, 26089–26100, 2007.

101. Sabin-Tóth, M., Human mesotrypsin defies natural trypsin inhibitors: From passive resistance to active destruction, *Protein Pept. Lett.* 12, 457–464, 2005.

102. Szmola, R., Kukor, Z., and Sabin-Tóth, M., Human mesotrypsin is a unique digestive protease specialized for the degradation of trypsin inhibitors, *J. Biol. Chem.* 278, 48580–48589, 2003.

103. Miyai, M., Matsumoto, Y., Yamanishi, H., et al., Keratinocyte-specific mesotrypsin contributes to the desquamation process via kallikrein activation an LEKTI degradation, *J. Invest. Dermatol.* 134, 1665–1674, 2014.

104. Ohlsson, K. and Olsson, I., The extracellular release of granulocyte collagenase and elastase during phagocytosis and inflammatory processes, *Scand. J. Haematol.* 19, 145–152, 1977.

105. Averhoff, P., Kolbe, M., Zychlinsky, A., and Weinrauch, Y., Single residue determines the specificity of neutrophil elastase for *Shigella* virulence factors, *J. Mol. Biol.* 377, 1053–1066, 2008.

106. Cantor, J.O., Cerreta, J.M., Armand, G., et al., The pulmonary matrix glycosaminoglycans and pulmonary emphysema, *Connect. Tissue Res.* 40, 97–104, 1999.

107. Zawieja, D.C., Garcia, C., and Granger, H.J., Oxygen radicals, enzymes, and fluid transport through pericardial interstitium, *Am. J. Physiol.* 262, H136–H143, 1992.

108. Molayerle, J., Schnekenburger, J., Juergen, K., et al., Extracellular cleavage of E-cadherin by leukocyte elastase during acute experimental pancreatitis in rats, *Gastroenterology* 129, 1251–1267, 2005.

109. Rao, N.V., Wehner, N.B., Marshall, B.C., et al., Characterization of proteinase-3 (PR-3), a neutrophil serine proteinase: Structural and functional properties, *J. Biol. Chem.* 266, 9540–9548, 1991.

110. Rao, N.V., Rao, G.V., Marshall, B.C., and Hoidal, J.R., Biosynthesis and processing of proteinase 3 in U937 cells: Processing pathways are distinct from those of cathepsin G, *J. Biol. Chem.* 271, 2972–2976, 1996.

111. Adkison, A.M., Raptis, S.Z., Kelley, D.G., and Pham, C.T, Dipeptidyl peptidase I activates neutrophil-derived serine proteases and regulates the development of acute experimental arthritis, *J. Clin. Invest.* 109, 363–371, 2002.

112. Hinkofer, L.C., Seidel, S.A.I., Korkmaz, B., et al., A monoclonal antibody (MCPR3–7) interfering with the activity of proteinase 3 by an allosteric mechanism, *J. Biol. Chem.* 288, 26635–26648, 2013.

113. Mihara, K., Ramachandran, R., Renaux, B., et al., Neutrophil elastase and proteinase-3 trigger G protein-biased signaling through proteinase-activated receptor-1 (PAR-1), *J. Biol. Chem.* 288, 32979–32990, 2013.

114. Gaudin, P.B., Askin, F.B., Falk, R.J., and Jennette, J.C., The pathologic spectrum of pulmonary lesions in patients with anti-neutrophil cytoplasmic autoantibodies specific for anti-proteinase 3 and anti-myeloperoxidase, *Am. J. Clin. Pathol.* 104, 7–16, 1995.

115. Korkmaz, B., Lesner, A., Letast, S., et al., Neutrophil proteinase 3 and dipeptidyl peptidase I (cathepsin C) as pharmacological targets in granulomatosis with polyangilitis (Wegener granulomatosis), *Semin. Immunopathol.* 35, 411–421, 2013.

116. Weninger, W., Biro, M., and Jain, R., Leukocyte migration in the interstitial space of non-lymphoid organs, *Nat. Rev. Immunol.* 14, 232–246, 2014.

117. Ley, K., Molecular mechanisms of leukocyte recruitment in the inflammatory process, *Cardiovasc. Res.* 32, 733–742, 1996.

118. Ng, L.G., Qin, J.S., Roediger, B., et al., Visualizing the neutrophil response to sterile tissue injury in mouse dermis reveals a three-phase cascade of events, *J. Invest. Dermatol.* 131, 2058–2068, 2011.
119. Orce, G.G., Carretero, O.A., Scicli, G., and Scicli, A.G., Kinins contribute to the contractile effects of rat glandular kallikrein on the isolated rat uterus, *J. Pharmacol. Exp. Ther.* 249, 470–475, 1989.
120. Meini, S., Cucchi, P., Catalani, C., et al., Pharmacological characterization of the bradykinin B2 receptor antagonist MEN16132 in rat *in vitro* bioassays, *Eur. J. Pharmacol.* 615, 10–16, 2009.
121. Garbe, G. and Vogt, W., Zur Natur der in menschlichem Plasma durch Pancreakallikrein, Glaskontakt under Säurebehandlung gebildeten Kinine, *Naunyn-Schmiedebergs Arch. Pharmak. u. exp. Path.* 256, 119–126, 1967.
122. Andreasson, S., Smith, L., Aasen, A.O., Saldeen, T., and Risberg, B., Local pulmonary activation after *Escherichia coli*-induced lung injury in sheep, *Eur. J. Surg.* 20, 289–297, 1988.
123. Dellalibera-Joviliano, R., Dos Reis, M.L., Cunha Fde, Q., and Donadi, E.A., Kinins and cytokines in plasma and cerebrospinal fluid of patients with neuropsychiatric lupus, *J. Rheumatol.* 30, 485–492, 2003.
124. Addallah, R.T., Keum, J.S., El-Shewy, H.M., et al., Plasma kallikrein promotes epidermal growth factor receptor transactivation and signaling in vascular smooth muscle through direct activation of protease-activated receptors, *J. Biol. Chem.* 285, 35206–35215, 2010.
125. Castellino, F.J. and Ploplis, V.A., Structure and function of the plasminogen/plasmin system, *Thromb. Haemost.* 93, 647–654, 2005.
126. Gonzalez, J., Klein, J., Chauhan, S.D., et al., Delayed treatment with plasminogen activator inhibitor-1 decoys reduces tubulointerstitial fibrosis, *Exp. Biol. Med.* 234, 1511–1518, 2009.
127. Schuliga, M., Westall, F., Xia, Y., and Stewart, A.G., The plasminogen activation system: New targets in lung inflammation and remodeling, *Curr. Opin. Pharmacol.* 13, 386–393, 2013.
128. Zhang, W.Y., Ishii, I., and Kruth, H.S., Plasmin-mediated macrophage reversal of low density lipoprotein aggregation, *J. Biol. Chem.* 275, 33176–33183, 2000.
129. Ferreira, H.C., A simple rapid method for estimating serum plasmin activity with fibrin-coated latex particles, *Blood* 25, 258–260, 1965.
130. Navarrete, M., Ho, J., Krokhin, O., et al., Proteomic characterization of serine hydrolase activity and composition in normal urine, *Clin. Proteomics* 10(1), 17, 2013.
131. Inman, R.D. and Harpel, P.C., Alpha 2-plasmin inhibitor-plasmin complexes in synovial fluid, *J. Rheumatol.* 13, 535–357, 1986.
132. Sakamaki, H., Ogura, N., Kujiraoka, H., et al., Activities of plasminogen activator, plasmin and kallikrein in synovial fluid from patients with temporomandibular joint disorders, *Int. J. Oral Maxillofac. Surg.* 30, 323–328, 2001.
133. Sinz, A., Bantscheff, M., Mikkat, S., et al., Mass spectrometric proteome analyses of synovial fluids and plasmas from patients suffering from rheumatoid arthritis and comparison to reactive arthritis or osteoarthritis, *Electrophoresis* 23, 3445–3456, 2002.
134. Idell, S., James, K.K., Levin, E.G., et al., Local abnormalities in coagulation and fibrinolytic pathways predispose to alveolar fibrin deposition in the adult respiratory distress syndrome, *J. Clin. Invest.* 84, 695–705, 1989.
135. Favier, R., Aoki, N., and Moerloose, P., Congenital α_2-antiplasmin deficiencie: A review, *Brit. J. Haematol.* 114, 4–10, 2001.
136. Banbula, A., Zimmerman, T.P., and Novokhatny, V.V., Blood inhibitory capacity toward exogenous plasmin, *Blood Coagul. Fibrinolysis* 18, 241–246, 2007.

137. Lee, K.N., Jackson, K.W., Christiansen, V.J., et al., Enhancement of fibrinolysis by inhibiting enzymatic cleavage of precursor α_2-antiplasmin, *J. Thromb. Haemost.* 9, 987–996, 2011.

138. Patterson, B.C. and Sang, Q.A., Angiostatin-converting enzyme activities of human matrilysin (MMP-7) and gelatinase B/type IV collagenase (MMP-9), *J. Biol. Chem.* 272, 28823–28825, 1997.

139. Falcone, D.J., Khan, K.M., Layne, T., and Fernandes, L., Macrophage formation of angiostatin during inflammation: A byproduct of the activation of plasminogen, *J. Biol. Chem.* 273, 31480–31485, 1998.

140. Wareicka, D.J., Narayan, M., and Twining, S.S., Maspin increases extracellular plasminogen activator activity associated with corneal fibroblasts and myofibroblasts, *Exp. Eye Res.* 93, 618–627, 2011.

141. Simard, B., Bouamrani, A., Jourdes, P., et al., Induction of the fibrinolytic system by cartilage extract mediates its antiangiogenic effect in mouse glioma, *Microvasc. Res.* 82, 6–17, 2011.

142. Brauer, R., Beck, I.M., Roderfeld, M., et al., Matrix metalloproteinase-19 inhibits growth of endothelial cells by generating angiostatin-like fragments from plasminogen, *BMC Biochem.* 12, 38, 2011.

143. Butera, D., Wind, T., Lay, A.J., et al., Characterization of a reduced form of plasma plasminogen as the precursor for angiostatin formation, *J. Biol. Chem.* 289, 2992–3000, 2014.

144. Zhang, G., Kernan, K.A., Collins, S.J., et al., Plasmin(ogen) promotes renal interstitial fibrosis by promoting epithelial-to-mesenchymal transition: Role of plasmin-activated signals, *J. Am. Soc. Nephrol.* 18, 846–859, 2007.

145. Deryugina, E.L. and Quigley, J.P., Surface remodeling by plasmin: A new function for an old enzyme, *J. Biomed. Biotechnol.* 2012, 21, 2012.

146. Stewart, A.G., Xia, Y.C., Harris, T., et al., Plasminogen-stimulated airway smooth muscle cell proliferation is mediated by urokinase and annexin A2, involving plasmin-activated cell signalling, *Br. J. Pharmacol.* 170, 1421–1435, 2013.

147. Bogenmann, E. and Jones, P.A., Role of plasminogen in matrix breakdown by neoplastic cells, *J. Natl. Cancer Inst.* 71, 1177–1182, 1983.

148. Rao, J.S., Kahler, C.G., Baker, J.B., and Festoff, B.W., Protease nexin I, a serpin, inhibits plasminogen-dependent degradation of muscle extracellular matrix, *Muscle Nerve* 12, 640–646, 1989.

149. Chiangjong, W. and Thongboonkerd, V., A novel assay to evaluate promoting effects of proteins on calcium oxalate crystal invasion through extracellular matrix based on plasminogen/plasmin activity, *Talanta* 101, 240–245, 2012.

150. Yamamoto, H., Okada, R., Iguchi, K., et al., Involvement of plasmin-mediated extracellular activation of progalanin in angiogenesis, *Biochem. Biophys. Res. Commun.* 430, 990–1004, 2013.

151. Ingram, K.C., Curtis, C.D., Silasi-Mansat, R., et al., The NuRD chromatin-remodeling enzyme CHD4 promotes embryonic vascular integrity by transcriptionally regulating extracellular matrix proteolysis, *PLoS Genet.* 9(12), e1004031, 2013.

152. Atkinson, J.M., Pullen, N., and Johnson, T.S., An inhibitor of thrombin activated fibrinolysis inhibitor (TAFI) can reduce extracellular matrix accumulation in an *in vitro* model of glucose induced ECM expansion, *Matrix Biol.* 32, 277–287, 2013.

153. Levenson, J.M., Qiu, S., and Weeber, E.J., The role of reelin in adult synaptic function and the genetic and epigenetic regulation of the reelin gene, *Biochim. Biophys. Acta* 1779, 422–431, 2008.

154. Förster, E., Bock, H.H., Herz, J., et al., Emerging topics in reelin function, *Eur. J. Neurosci.* 31, 1511–1518, 2010.

155. Fatemi, S.H., Reelin glycoprotein: Structure, biology and roles in health and disease, *Mol. Psychiatry* 10, 251–257, 2005.
156. Hirotsune, S., Takahara, T., Sasaki, N., et al., The reeler gene encodes a protein with an EGF-like motif expressed by pioneer neurons, *Nat. Genet.* 10, 77–83, 1995.
157. Pearlman, A.L. and Sheppard, A.M., Extracellular matrix in early cortical development, *Progress Brain Res.* 108, 117–134, 1996.
158. Krishnaswamy, S., The transition of prothrombin to thrombin, *J. Thromb. Haemost.* 11(1), 265–276, 2013.
159. Le Bonniec, B.F., Thrombin, in *Handbook of Proteolytic Enzymes*, 3rd edn., eds. N.D. Rawlings and G. Salvesen, Chapter 643, pp. 2915–2932, Elsevier, Amsterdam, the Netherlands, 2013.
160. Chang, J.-Y., Thrombin specificity: Requirement for apolar amino acids adjacent to the thrombin cleavage site of polypeptide substrate, *Eur. J. Biochem.* 151, 217–224, 1985.
161. Violand, B.N., Takano, M., Curran, D.F., and Bentle, L.A., A novel concatenated dimer of recombinant bovine somatotropin, *J. Prot. Chem.* 8, 619–628, 1989.
162. Tani, K., Yasuoka, S., Ogushi, F., et al., Thrombin enhances lung fibroblast proliferation in bleomycin-induced pulmonary fibrosis, *Am. J. Respir. Cell Mol. Biol.* 5, 34–40, 1991.
163. Hewitson, T.D., Martic, M., Kelynack, K.J., et al., Thrombin is a pro-fibrotic factor for rat renal fibroblasts *in vitro*, *Nephron Exp. Nephrol.* 101, e42–e49, 2005.
164. Atanelishvili, I., Liang, J., Akter, T., et al., Thrombin increases lung fibroblast survival while promoting alveolar epithelial cell apoptosis via the ER stress marker CHOP, *Am. J. Respir. Cell Mol. Biol.* 50, 893–902, 2014.
165. Idell, S., Garcia, J.G., Gonzalez, K., et al., Fibrinopeptide A reactive peptides and pro-coagulant activity in bronchoalveolar lavage: Relationship to rheumatoid interstitial lung disease, *J. Rheumatol.* 16, 592–598, 1989.
166. Song, J.S., Kang, C.M., Park, C.K., and Yoon, H.K., Thrombin induces epithelial–mesenchymal transition via PAR-1, PKC, and ERK$_{1/2}$ pathways in A549 cells, *Exp. Lung Res.* 39, 336–348, 2013.
167. Goldfarb, R.H. and Liotta, L.A., Thrombin cleavage of extracellular matrix proteins, *Ann. N.Y. Acad. Sci.* 485, 288–292, 1986.
168. Richardson, M., Hatton, M.W.C., and Moore, S., The plasma proteinases, thrombin and plasmin, degrade the proteoglycan of rabbit aorta segments *in vitro*: An integrated ultrastructural and biochemical study, *Clin. Invest. Med.* 11, 139–150, 1988.
169. Tamburro, A., Zanni, M., Mariani, B., et al., Thrombin induces the synthesis of stromelysin 1 (MMP-3): A novel effect of thrombin on extracellular matrix degradation, *Fibrinolyis Proteol.* 11, 251–257, 1997.
170. Fang, Q., Liu, X., Al-Mugotir, M., et al., Thrombin and TNF-α/IL-1β synergistically induce fibroblast-mediated collagen gel degradation, *Am. J. Respir. Cell Mol. Biol.* 35, 714–721, 2006.
171. Chappell, D., Jacob, M., Hofmann-Kiefer, K., et al., Antithrombin reduces shedding of the endothelial glycocalyx following ischaemia/reperfusion, *Cardiovasc. Res.* 83, 388–396, 2009.
172. Shimomura, T., Kondo, J., Ochiai, M., et al., Activation of the zymogen of hepatocyte growth factor activator by thrombin, *J. Biol. Chem.* 268, 22927–22932, 1993.
173. Proud, D. and Kaplan, A.P., Kinin formation: Mechanisms and role in inflammatory disorders, *Annu. Rev. Immunol.* 6, 49–83, 1988.
174. Stadnicki, A., Intestinal tissue kallikrein-kinin system in inflammatory bowel disease, *Inflamm. Bowel Dis.* 17, 645–654, 2011.
175. Gautvik, K.M., Hilton, S.M., and Torres, S.H., Consumption of the plasma substrate for glandular kallikrein on activation of the submandibular gland, *J. Physiol.* 197, 22P–23P, 1968.

176. Maier, H., Adler, D., Menstell, S., and Lenarz, T., Glandular kallikrein in chronic recurrent parotitis, *Laryng. Rhino. Otol.* 63, 633–635, 1984.

177. Astrup, T., Tissue activators of plasminogen, *Fed. Proc.* 25, 42–51, 1966.

178. Lu, X.-g., Wu, X.-g., Xu, X.-h., et al., Novel distribution pattern of fibrinolytic components in rabbit tissue extracts: A preliminary study, *J. Zhejiang Univ. Science B* 8, 570–574, 2007.

179. O'Rourke, J., Jiang, X., Hao, Z., et al., Distribution of sympathetic tissue plasminogen activator (tPA) to a distant microvasculature, *J. Neurosci. Res.* 79, 727–733, 2005.

180. Parmer, R.J. and Miles, L.A., Targeting of tissue plasminogen activator to the regulated pathway of secretion, *Trends Cardiovas. Med.* 8, 306–312, 1998.

181. Tripathi, R.C., Tripathi, B.J., and Park, J.K., Localization of urokinase-type plasminogen activator in human eyes: An immunocytochemical study, *Exp. Eye Res.* 51, 545–552, 1990.

182. van Hinsbergh, V.W., Regulation of the synthesis and secretion of plasminogen activators by endothelial cells, *Haemostasis* 18, 307–327, 1988.

183. Suzuki, Y., Yasui, H., Brzoska, T., et al., Surface-retained tPA is essential for effective fibrinolysis on vascular endothelial cells, *Blood* 118, 3182–3185, 2011.

184. Kirsten, C.G., Tuttle, P.R., and Berger, H., Jr., Quantitative assessment of subcutaneous fibrinolysis in the rat, *J. Pharmacol. Methods* 16, 125–138, 1986.

185. Hatton, M.W.C., Southward, S.M.R., Ross, B.L., et al., Relationships among tumor burden, tumor size, and the changing concentrations of fibrin degradation products and fibrinolytic factors in the pleural effusions of rabbits with VX2 lung tumors, *J. Lab. Clin. Med.* 147, 27–35, 2006.

186. Laschinger, C.A., Johnston, M.G., Hay, J.B., and Wasi, S., Production of plasminogen activator and plasminogen activator inhibitor by bovine lymphatic endothelial cells: Modulation by TNF-α, *Thromb. Res.* 59, 567–579, 1990.

187. Silverstein, R.L., Nachman, R.L., Leung, L.L.K., and Harpel, P.C., Activation of immobilized plasminogen by tissue activator: Multimolecular complex formation, *J. Biol. Chem.* 260, 10346–10352, 1985.

188. Suenson, E. and Petersen, L.C., Fibrin and plasminogen structures essential to stimulation of plasmin formation by tissue-type plasminogen activator, *Biochim. Biophys. Acta* 870, 510–519, 1986.

189. Meissnauer, A., Kramer, M.D., Schirrmacher, V., and Brunner, G., Generation of cell surface–bound plasmin by cell-associated urokinase-type or secreted tissue-type plasminogen activator: A key event in melanoma cell invasiveness *in vitro*, *Exp. Cell Res.* 199, 179–190, 1992.

190. Trivedi, N.N. and Caughey, G.H., Human α-, β-, and γ-tryptases, in *Handbook of Proteolytic Enzymes*, 3rd edn., eds. N.D. Rawlings and G. Salvesen, Chapter 591, pp. 2683–2693, Elsevier, Amsterdam, the Netherlands, 2013.

191. Selwood, T., Wang, Z.M., McCaslin, D.R., and Schechter, N.M., Diverse stability and catalytic properties of human tryptase: Alpha and beta isoforms are mediated by residue differences at the S1 pocket, *Biochemistry* 41, 3329–3340, 2002.

192. Schwartz, L.B., Bradford, T.R., Lee, D.C., and Chlebowski, J.F., Immunologic and physicochemical evidence for conformational changes occurring on conversion of human mast cell tryptase from active tetramer to inactive monomer: Production of monoclonal antibodies recognizing active tryptase, *J. Immunol.* 144, 2304–2311, 1990.

193. Sommerhoff, C.P., Bode, W., Pereira, P.J.B., et al., The structure of the human βII-tryptase tetramer: Fo(u)r better or worse, *Proc. Natl. Acad. Sci. USA* 96, 10984–10991, 1999.

194. He, S., Aslam, A., Gaca, M.D., et al., Inhibitors of tryptase as mast cell–stabilizing agents in the human airways: Effects of tryptase and other agonists of proteinase-activated receptor 2 of histamine release, *J. Pharmacol. Exp. Ther.* 309, 119–126, 2004.

195. Jacob, C., Yang, P.C., Darmoul, D., et al., Mast cell tryptase controls paracellular permeability of the intestine: Role of protease-activated receptor 2 and β-arrestins, *J. Biol. Chem.* 280, 31936–31948, 2005.

196. Tatler, A.L., Porte, J., Knox, A., et al., Tryptase activates TGFβ in human airway smooth muscle cells via direct proteolysis, *Biochem. Biophys. Res. Commun.* 370, 239–242, 2008.

197. Stevens, R.L. and Adachi, R., Protease–proteoglycan complexes of mouse and human mast cells and importance of their β-tryptase-heparin complexes in inflammation and innate immunity, *Immunol. Rev.* 217, 155–167, 2007.

198. Fukuoka, Y., Xia, H.Z., Sanchez-Muñoz, L.B., et al., Generation of anaphylatoxins by human β-tryptase form C3, C4, and C5, *J. Immunol.* 180, 6307–6316, 2008.

199. Shin, K., Nigrovic, P.A., Crish, J., et al., Mast cells contribute to autoimmune inflammatory arthritis via their tryptase/heparin complexes, *J. Immunol.* 182, 647–656, 2009.

200. Nagyeri, G., Radacs, M., Ghassemi-Nejad, S., et al., TSG-6 protein, a negative regulator of inflammatory arthritis, forms a ternary complex with murine mast cell tryptases and heparin, *J. Biol. Chem.* 286, 23559–23569, 2011.

201. Anower-E-Khuda, M.R., Habuchi, H., Nagai, N., et al., Heparan sulfate 6-O-sulfotransferase isoform-dependent regulatory effects of heparin on the activities of various proteases in mast cells and the biosynthesis of 6-O-sulfated heparin, *J. Biol. Chem.* 288, 3705–3717, 2013.

202. Schechter, N.M., Eng, G.Y., Selwood, T., and McCaslin, D.R., Structural changes associated with the spontaneous inactivation of the serine proteinase human tryptase, *Biochemistry* 34, 10628–10638, 1995.

203. Selwood, T., McCaslin, D.R., and Schechter, N.M., Spontaneous inactivation of human tryptase involves conformational changes consistent with conversion of the active site to a zymogen-like structure, *Biochemistry* 37, 13174–13183, 1998.

204. Selwood, T., Smolensky, H., McCaslin, D.R., and Schechter, N.M., The interaction of tryptase-β with small molecule inhibitors provides new insights into the unusual functional instability and quaternary structure of the protease, *Biochemistry* 44, 3580–3590, 2005.

205. Schechter, N.M., Choi, E.J., Selwood, T., and McCaslin, D.R., Characterization of three distinct catalytic forms of human tryptase-β: Their interrelationships and relevance, *Biochemistry* 46, 9615–9629, 2007.

206. Wiegand, U., Corbach, S., Minn, A., Kang, J., and Müller-Hill, B., Cloning of the cDNA encoding human brain trypsinogen and characterization of its product, *Gene* 136, 167–175, 1993.

207. Tóth, J., Siklódi, E., Medveczky, P., et al., Regional distribution of human trypsinogen 4 in human brain at mRNA and protein level, *Neurochem. Res.* 32, 1423–1433, 2007.

208. Cottrell, G.S., Adamesi, S., Grady, E.F., and Bunnett, N.W., Trypsin IV, a novel agonist of protease-activated receptors 2 and 4, *J. Biol. Chem.* 279, 13532–13539, 2004.

209. Katona, G., Berglund, G.I., Hajdu, J., Graf, L., and Szilagyi, L., Crystal structure reveals basis for inhibitor resistance of human brain trypsin, *J. Mol. Biol.* 315, 1209–1218, 2002.

210. Fu, Q., Cheng, J., Gao, Y., et al., Protease-activated receptor 4: A critical participator in inflammatory response, *Inflammation* 38, 886–895, 2014.

211. White, W.F. and Barlow, G., Urinary plasminogen activator (urokinase), *Methods Enzymol.* 19, 665–672, 1970.

212. Barlow, G.H., Urinary and kidney cell plasminogen activator (urokinase), *Methods Enzymol.* 45, 239–244, 1976.

213. Eden, G., Archinti, M., Furlan, F., et al., The urokinase receptor interactome, *Curr. Pharm. Des.* 17, 1874–1889, 2011.

214. Breuss, J.M. and Uhrin, P., VEGF-initiated angiogenesis and the uPA/uPAR system, *Cell Adh. Migr.* 6, 535–615, 2012.
215. Liu, Y.X., Regulation of the plasminogen activator system in the ovary, *Biol. Signals Recept.* 8, 160–177, 1999.
216. Thorsen, S. and Astrup, T., Biphasic inhibition of urokinase-induced fibrinolysis by epsilon-aminocaproic acid: Distinction from tissue plasminogen activator, *Proc. Soc. Exp. Biol. Med.* 130, 811–813, 1969.
217. Thorsen, S. and Astrup, T., Differences in the reactivities of human urokinase and the porcine tissue plasminogen activator, *Haemostasis* 5, 295–305, 1976.

digestive function. Plasmin can digest many components of the ECM[7] and regulate cell function by extracellular proteolysis.[8] In a more complex system, a regulatory protease such as ADAM-12 can initiate a cascade process, resulting in the activation of digestive enzymes such as matrix metalloproteinase (MMP)-2 and MMP-14 (Figure 7.5).

Since interstitial proteases can have such potent effects either as digestive enzymes or regulatory enzymes, it is critical that they are subject to regulation. Interstitial proteases are regulated at several levels, starting with protein expression and ending with inactivation of the mature protease. Within the context of the current discussion, expression is used broadly to include intracellular synthesis (transcription and translation), intracellular post-translational processing, and transit to the cell surface as a membrane-bound protease or secretion of a protease. Certain cell surface proteases may be released by the process of ectodomain cleavage, resulting in a soluble enzyme, but this process is different from that of secretion.

Expression may be constitutive where there is a basal level of expression, while regulated expression is a change in expression in response to cellular stimulus. As discussed in Chapter 1, cell stimulation can influence the polarity of secretion. In addition to the measurement of enzyme activity, the measurement of mRNA can also serve as a measure of protein expression.[9] However, there are also studies where an increase in mRNA did not result in increased enzyme activity. In one such study,[10] an increase in ADAMTS-4 mRNA activity did not result in increased aggrecanase activity, which suggests that caution should be taken in the interpretation of mRNA measurement. Rogerson and coworkers[10] state that post-translational processing steps may be required for the expression of an active enzyme. This also suggests that our view of expression may be simplistic, but we have focused on studies that measure protein and/or enzyme activity.

A second level of regulation is provided by the activation of a zymogen form of the protease. This may be autocatalytic, as seen with some MMPs (Chapter 8) and with matriptase-2.[11] More often, the zymogen form of an enzyme (proenzyme) is converted to an active protease by the process of limited proteolysis catalyzed by another enzyme after secretion or transit to the luminal membrane surface. There are examples, however, of intracellular activation of proenzyme forms by furin or furin-like enzymes.[12–15] Stawowy and coworkers[13] reported that furin proprotein convertase activates MMP-14 prior to transit to the membrane surface, where it can activate pro-MMP-2 (see Chapter 7). Longpré and Leduc[14] have shown that pro-ADAMTS-1 is most efficiently processed by furin in Golgi apparatus prior to secretion. Cao and coworkers[16] described the intracellular processing of ADAM-12. These investigators showed that pro-ADAM-12 was glycosylated in the endoplasmic reticulum and processed in prodomain in the Golgi apparatus prior to transit to the cell surface. Other investigators[17] have suggested the prodomain remains bound to the 68 kDa ADAM-12, perhaps keeping the mature enzyme inactive by preventing disruption of the cysteine switch.

A different example is provided by the proprotein convertase–mediated processing of pro-ADAMTS-5.[15] Longpré and coworkers[15] showed that furin and PC7 were responsible for the processing of pro-ADAMTS-5 and that such processing occurred in the extracellular space.

The activation of some metalloproteinases can involve a *cysteine switch* mechanism,[18] where the catalytic zinc atom at the enzyme active site is sequestered by binding to a cysteine sulfhydryl group. Activation is accomplished by modification of the cysteine residue by oxidation or some other modification of cysteine, followed by autocatalytic removal of the prodomain. Both autolytic activation and activation by another protease involves limited proteolysis. Limited proteolysis refers to the cleavage of a small number of possible scissile peptide bonds in a protein and is the process by which proprotein or zymogen forms of proteases are activated.[19] It is possible that the zymogen forms of the protease have significant activity without activation.[19–21] A related issue is the presence of cryptic tissue factor in the interstitial space (Section 8.7.1).

A third level of regulation involves the modulation of proteolytic activity, achieved by the binding of another molecule by the protease. This binding does not occur at the enzyme's active site and thus can be considered an allosteric effect, which may be observed with small and large molecules.[22] One example is provided by the binding of thrombin to thrombomodulin, changing thrombin specificity from fibrinogen to protein C, thus changing thrombin from a coagulant to an anticoagulant.[23] While there is no evidence for the presence of thrombomodulin in the interstitium, there is evidence for extravascular synthesis of thrombomodulin by adherent synovial fluid cells.[24] In addition, there is ample reason to suspect the protein C pathway is involved in the etiology of fibrosis.[25,26] An example relevant to the interstitium is provided by the binding of thrombin to heparan sulfate, which accelerates the activation of pro-MMP-2.[27] Syndecan-2 binds to pro-MMP-7, promoting the autoactivation of pro-MMP-7.[28] Pro-MMP-7 binds to heparan sulfate and other heparinoids, and this binding is suggested to promote the formation of MMP-7 by a process of transactivation.[29] MMP-7 bound to epithelial cells retains activity and is protected from inactivation by tissue inhibitor of metalloproteinase (TIMP)-2.[30]

The presence of interstitial components such as hyaluronan or collagen also plays a role in the regulation of extracellular proteolysis. In the study by Choi-Miura and coworkers,[31] a hyaluronan-binding protease was isolated from human plasma and was shown to cleave both high-molecular-weight kininogen (HMWK) and low-molecular-weight kininogen (LMWK).[32] Subsequent work showed that this enzyme can upregulate ERK1/2 and P13k/Akt signaling pathways in fibroblasts simulating cell proliferation and migration.[33] These investigators noted the hyaluronan-binding protease was structurally related to plasminogen activators, blood coagulation factor XII, and hepatocyte growth factor activator.[32,33] While it is not clear that hyaluronan affects enzyme activity, binding to hyaluronan may provide a mechanism for concentrating and stabilizing enzyme activity. Other studies have shown that hyaluronan[34] and hyaluronan fragments[35] influence the expression of uPA and PAI-1 proteases.

A fourth level of regulation is provided by the inactivation of proteases by protein protease inhibitors (Chapter 9), autolysis, or, in the case of membrane-bound proteases, endocytosis. The best-known group of protein protease inhibitors with specific relevance to interstitial proteolysis are the serpins (serine protease inhibitors), which are discussed in Chapter 9. MMPs (Chapter 7) are not serine proteinases but rather have a zinc at the active site. The activity of MMPs is modulated by TIMPs; TIMPs also inhibit ADAM and ADAMTS proteases.[36] The interaction of proteases with protease inhibitors can also be regulated by interaction with other macromolecules; the effect of heparin on antithrombin is one of the better-known examples. TIMP-3 binds to heparan sulfate or chondroitin sulfate, inhibiting binding to lipoprotein receptor–related protein-1; binding of TIMP-3 to heparan sulfate or chondroitin sulfate also increases the affinity of TIMP-3 for ADAMTS-5.[37] DNA accelerates the inactivation of human cathepsin V[38] by myeloid and erythroid nuclear termination (MENT) protein or serpin B3 (squamous cell carcinoma antigen-1; SCCA 1). Extracellular DNA, not RNA, has also been reported to accelerate the activation of plasminogen by uPA or tPA, as well as the inactivation of tPA or uPA by PAI-1.[39] The acceleration was observed with synthetic DNA and DNA isolated from pleural fluid. Finally, the activity of a protease may be regulated by cleavage by other proteases, such the degradation of pro-uPA by granulocyte elastase[40] or by autolysis with loss of activity. An example of autolysis is given by membrane-type-1 MMP (MT1-MMP; MMP-14).[41,42] The autolysis of MMP-14 has been suggested to be regulated by O-glycosylation.[43] Remacle and coworkers[43] suggest that the presence of sialic acid prevents access of the catalytic site to the hinge region, while incomplete glycosylation enhances autocatalysis and loss of activity. MMP-14 activity is also regulated by endocytosis.[43,44] The regulation by endocytosis involves internalization and recycling back to the plasma membrane.

The regulation of protease activity in the interstitial spaces occur at multiple levels in response to external stimuli. MMP-14 (Chapter 7) provides an example of the complexity in the regulation of expression. It has been suggested by Albrechtsen and coworkers[45] that ADAM-12 (see Section 4.2) regulates the function of MMP-14. MMP-14 is a one-pass membrane protease with a number of functions, including the degradation of the ECM, the activation of other proteases, and the shedding of functional exodomain. First, Albrechtson and coworkers showed that increased expression of ADAM-12 (transfection of 293-VnR cells) increased the tumor cell surface expression of MMP-14. Knockdown of ADAM-12 did not affect MMP-14 mRNA levels. Subsequent work has shown that ADAM-12 and MMP-14 colocalize on the tumor cell surface; the link between ADAM-12 and MMP-14 is provided by the integrin $\alpha_v\beta_3$. The colocalization of ADAM-12 and MMP-14 results in the degradation of gelatin, but the catalytic activity of ADAM-12 is not required for the degradation of gelatin. The translocation of the mature ADAM-12 protease to the cell surface is enhanced by the phorbol ester effect on protein kinase C-epsilon (PKCε),[46] mediated by the upregulation of RACK-1.[47] The upregulation of the ADAM-12 protease by the

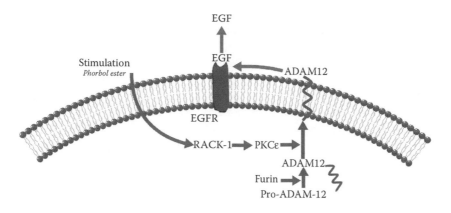

FIGURE 4.1 Control of HBEGF ectodomain release by cell simulation. Shown is the phorbol ester stimulation of RACK-1, which enhances protein kinase C. Protein kinase C in turn promotes the processing and transport of ADAM-12 to the cell surface, where it releases the HBEGF from the cell surface. Not shown is the potential transactivation of the cell by HBEGF. (From Shah, B.H., et al., *J. Biol. Chem,* 279, 414–420, 2004.)

PKC/RACK-1 pathway can also lead to the shedding of heparin-binding epidermal growth factor (EGF)-like growth factor (HBEGF; Figure 4.1), with possible transactivation of EGF receptors (EGFRs).[48]

4.2 ADAM PROTEASES

The ADAM protein family are characterized by the presence of a disintegrin domain and metalloproteinase domain,[50–54] thus having the ability to bind integrins to the cell surface and degrade proteins. ADAM proteins primarily function as membrane-bound proteases, distinguishing them from ADAMTS proteases, which are soluble. Several members of the ADAM protease family are soluble either from ectodomain cleavage or from secretion of the protein. ADAM proteases can be attached to a cell membrane with a transmembrane segment connected to a cytoplasmic tail. The ectodomain may contain an EGF domain in addition to a cysteine-rich domain, a disintegrin domain, a metalloproteinase domain with an amino-terminal prodomain, and a signal peptide. Several members of the ADAM protease family are present in soluble form (designated as *s* forms), as opposed to the membrane-bound form (designated as *m* forms).

Many of the members of the ADAM family have been identified by cloning rather than by classical methods of protein isolation from biological fluids or tissues.[50] A number of these ADAM family members do not exhibit proteolytic activity and are present in the ADAM family on the basis of sequence homology. In 2000, Primakoff and Myles[51] identified 29 members of the ADAM family, 17 of which had sequences consistent with active proteolytic function; 12 were defined as inactive proteases, but may possess the RGD sequence necessary for binding integrins. More recently, Cho[52] stated that there were at least 34 members of the ADAM family of membrane proteins in mice and 26 ADAM proteins in humans. Furthermore, there is tissue-specific expression, with more than half of these proteins located in the mammalian testes or epididymis. Once identified, the ADAM proteins have been suggested to have diverse functions.[49,51,55] The role of ADAM proteases as sheddases provides a process for the delivery of peptide growth factors such as EGF and other bioactive peptides into the interstitial space. Many of the ADAM proteases lack a consensus cleavage sequence, leading to the suggestion that substrate presentation is critical to ectoshedding. Hartmann and coworkers[56] make the case that the availability of substrate is a regulatory process to control specific ectodomain shedding. In subsequent work, Hartmann and coworkers[57] show that dimerization of CD44 driven by intracellular signaling is necessary for ectodomain cleavage by ADAM-10. These investigators also show the colocalization of proteases and substrate at the membrane surface prior to cellular stimulation of cleavage.

Membrane-bound ADAM-10 is involved in the processing of amyloid precursor protein. The soluble form of ADAM-10 likely produced by ADAM-9 has lost the capability to cleave the amyloid precursor protein.[58] It has been suggested that the cleavage of membrane-bound ADAM-10 is a regulatory process. ADAM-10 is widely expressed, with high concentrations in brain and muscle.[59] In addition to the processing of amyloid precursor protein, where it is referred to as an α-secretase,[60] ADAM 10 functions in the release of several EGFR ligands such as HBEGF.[61] ADAM-10 is also responsible for the shedding of meprin A.[62]

ADAM-12 was originally described as meltrin α, a metalloproteinase with a disintegrin sequence that participated in myoblast fusion during development.[63,64] Subsequent work from another laboratory[65] demonstrated the presence of a secreted form of ADAM-12 (ADAM-12s) as well as the canonical membrane form of ADAM-12 (ADAM-12m; ADAM-12-L), which arise from the splicing of a single gene product. mRNA expression of the membrane-bound form and secreted form could be detected by Northern blot analysis in placenta; mRNA for the membrane-bound form could also be detected at lower levels in skeletal, smooth, and cardiac muscle. Subsequent work by this group[16] demonstrated that ADAM-12s is an active protease based on a complex formation with α_2-macroglobulin.[66] Studies on the secreted ADAM-12[67] showed a lack of a consensus sequence in the cleavage of carboxymethylated transferrin, leading the authors to suggest that a substrate secondary structure is important in the specificity of ADAM-12s. The importance of a secondary structure of substrate in sites of limited proteolysis has been studied by other investigators.[68] These investigators also noted that physiological concentrations of NaCl resulted in almost total loss of catalytic activity. ADAM-12s also cleaves IGFBP-3 and IGFBP-5,[69] while ADAM-12m cleaves IGFBP-5 in osteoarthritic cartilage.[70] The cell adhesion activity of ADAM proteins is a property of the disintegrin domain, unrelated to the metalloprotease domain.[71] ADAM-12 is also important for the expression of MMP-14[2] as described in Section 4.1.

ADAM-17 was originally described as tumor necrosis factor α–converting enzyme (TACE).[72–75] ADAM-17 has received the most attention as a sheddase.[76–80] In 2012, Dreymuller and coworkers[81] listed 31 potential substrates for ADAM-17, including TNF-α, ICAM-1, L-selectin, HBEGF, CD44, and syndecans 1 and 4; 6 potential substrates for ADAM-12; 12 potential substrates for ADAM-10; and 1 for ADAM-28. The knockdown of ADAM-17 in nonsmall-cell lung cancer cells inhibited cell migration and cell invasion *in vitro* and tumor growth *in vivo*.[82] There has been long-term interest in ADAM-17 as a drug target in cancer.[75,83,84] A knockout of ADAM-17 has been shown to be lethal in embryonic development.[84]

ADAM-28 was first identified with recombinant DNA technology as eMCD II, a metalloprotease with a disintegrin species, in human epididymis[85] and subsequently enrolled as ADAM-28.[86] MDC-L was an ADAM protease expressed in human lymphocytes and enrolled as ADAM-23.[87] ADAM-23 and ADAM-28 are now considered to be the same protein[88] and the designation ADAM-23 is no longer used. Northern blot analysis suggested the presence of both membrane-bound and secreted forms of ADAM (MDC-L) in lymphoid tissue.[87] The membrane-bound form of ADAM-28, ADAM-28m, is activated by a combination of intracellular processing and autocatalytic removal of the prodomain.[88] The soluble form, ADAM-28s, can be activated by MMP-7 (matrilysin-1).[89] Enzymatically active ADAM-28s degrades IGFBP-3,[89] myelin basic protein,[90] and connective tissue growth factor.[91] The degradation reactions are relatively slow, occurring over hours instead of minutes at enzyme/substrate ratios of 1:10 to 1:50. However, it is not unreasonable to suggest that proteolysis in the interstitial space under conditions of normal homeostasis is a slow, carefully controlled process. It is possible to speculate with respect to the control of these proteases; such speculation with respect to ADAM-28s is shown in Figure 4.2, which illustrates the activation of pro-MMP-7 (see Chapter 7) by hypochlorite, arising from the reaction of hydrogen peroxide with chloride in a reaction catalyzed by myeloperoxidase. MMP-7 in turn can activate ADAM-28s,[89] which in turn can degrade insulin-like growth factor (IGF)-binding protein, releasing biologically active IGF (IGF-1), which may be involved in the development of fibrosis and the promotion of tumorogenesis.

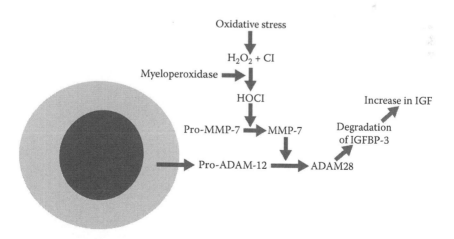

FIGURE 4.2 Interactions of ADAM-28. Shown is a cascade for ADAM-28, where MMP-7 is activated by oxidative stress. (From Fu, X., et al., *J. Biol. Chem.* 276, 41279–41287, 2001.) MMP-7 then activates pro-ADAM-28s. (From Mochizuki, S., et al., *Biochem. Biophys. Res. Commun.* 315, 79–84, 2004.)

The disintegrin domain of ADAM-29 binds to P-selectin glycoprotein ligand-1, enhancing adhesion of leukocytes to endothelial cells.[92] Other studies have shown that ADAM-28 binds the $\alpha_4\beta_1$ integrin, suggesting a mechanism for the interaction of lymphocytes with leukocytes.[93] As noted by Bridges and coworkers,[93] the binding of the disintegrin domain to cell surface integrins provides a mechanism for the localization of ADAM protease activity.

ADAM proteases are found in a number of cell types and may have apical or basolateral localization. A basolateral localization of ADAM proteases and substrates would permit the delivery of peptide growth factors such as EGF and cytokines such as TNF-α into the interstitial space. However, there are relatively few studies on the polarity of secretion and, as with other examples of polarity secretion (Chapter 1, Section 1.3), changes in cell status can influence the polarity of secretion. ADAM-10 is considered to be responsible for the shedding of meprin A,[62] and meprin A is shed from proximal tubule membranes on the basolateral side. ADAM-10 and ADAM-17 are shown to be responsible for the basolateral shedding of chemokine CX3CL1, promoting the movement of dendritic cells.[94] ADAM-10 has also been suggested to be responsible for the basolateral processing of E-cadherin.[95] ADAM-17 processes TGF-α on the basolateral surface of polarized MDCK cells.[96] Subsequently, ADAM-17 was shown to be localized on the basolateral surface of a polarized human colon cancer cell line (HCA-7), where it processed two EGF receptor ligands, TNF-α and amphiregulin.[97] Perivascular cells have been shown to express ADAM-12 and participate in scarring.[98] There is, however, evidence to support apical localization of ADAM proteases.[99,100] ADAM proteases are inhibited by TIMPs.[101,102]

4.3   ADAMTS PROTEASES

ADAMTS proteases are endopeptidases in a gene family distinct from the ADAM proteins.[103,104] There are 19 ADAMTS proteases (there is no ADAMTS-11, as it was found to be identical with ADAMTS-5) and 7 secreted ADAMTS-like glycoproteins of undefined function.[105,106] Kelwick and coworkers[107] emphasized the role of ADAMTS proteases in the regulation of the ECM as a primary function. There are only limited studies on the activation of the zymogen forms of the ADAMTS proteases, but it is likely that many are secreted as active enzymes with intracellular processing by furin-like enzymes, although further processing may occur after secretion.

As with many other proteases found in the interstitial space, ADAMTS proteases have been identified by cloning and largely characterized by recombinant protein production. An exception is provided by ADAMTS-2, which was initially purified from fetal calf skin[108] and subsequently cloned as bovine procollagen I N-proteinase.[109] This enzyme was designated as ADAMTS-2,[110] based on its domain similarities to ADAMTS-1, which had been cloned from a cachexigenic colon adenocarcinoma.[111] ADAMTS-2, -3, and -14 are responsible for the post-translation, extracellular processing of procollagen into fibrillar collagen.[110] The ADAMTS proteases ADAMTS-1, -4, and -5 are aggrecanases[111] defined by their ability to cleave the Glu_{333}–Ala_{374} peptide bond in the aggrecan core protein (Table 2.1). ADAMTS-4 and ADAMTS-5 have been shown to degrade reelin,[112] an extracellular signaling protein[113] suggested to be involved in Alzheimer's disease and other neurological disorders. While ADAMTS-4 is defined as an aggrecanase, it does degrade other chondroitin sulfate–containing proteoglycans, such as versican (Table 2.1).[114] Tissue-plasminogen activator activates the zymogen form of ADAMTS-4, which in turn results in the degradation of chondroitin sulfate proteoglycans, promoting neural regeneration.[115] Membrane type-4 matrix metalloproteinase (MT4-MMP; MMP-17) processes the C-terminal cleavage required for the activation of ADAMTS-4, permitting the canonical cleavage of aggrecan.[116] After activation, ADAMTS-4 is bound to sydecan-1 following activation.[116] Syndecan-1 is a cell surface proteoglycan containing both chondroitin sulfate and heparan sulfate.[117,118] There is one ADAMTS protease that functions outside of the interstitial space; ADAMTS-13 is responsible for the processing of pro–von Willebrand factor.[119,120]

4.4 COMMENT ON PROTEOLYTIC ENZYMES IN INTERSTITIAL SPACE

It is obvious that proteolytic enzymes have important functions in the interstitial space. It is also obvious that the various proteases described in this and the following chapters interact with each other. However, the majority of these putative interactions are posited from combining the results of several studies. It is also reasonable to assume that interstitial proteolysis is temporally and spatially specific and influenced by the microenvironment, including hyaluronan and components of the ECM.

There are real challenges in understanding proteolysis in the interstitial space, but such understanding is critical to advances in therapeutic approaches to fibrotic and inflammatory disease. We are skeptical that such understanding will come from *in vitro* studies but hope that advances in Raman spectroscopy and near-infrared (NIR) spectroscopy will permit further study of proteolysis in the interstitial space.

REFERENCES

1. Rawlings, N.D. and Salvesen, G.S., eds., *The Handbook of Regulatory Proteolysis*, 3rd edn., Academic Press/Elsevier, Amsterdam, the Netherlands, 2013.
2. Neurath, H., Proteolytic enzymes: Past and present, *Fed. Proc.* 44, 2907–2013, 1985.
3. Patthy, L., Evolution of blood coagulation and fibrinolysis, *Blood Coagul. Fibrinolysis* 1, 153–166, 1990.
4. Friedrich, P. and Bozóky, Z., Digestive versus regulatory proteases: On calpain action *in vivo*, *Biol. Chem.* 386, 609–612, 2005.
5. Dall'Acqua, W. and Carter, P., Substrate-assisted catalysis: Molecular basis and biological significance, *Protein Sci.* 9, 1–9, 2000.
6. Zhang, L., Bharadewaj, A.G., Casper, A., et al., Hyaluronidase activity of human Hyal1 requires active site acidic and tyrosine residues, *J. Biol. Chem.* 284, 9433–9442, 2009.
7. Liotta, L.A., Goldfarb, R.H., Brundage, R., et al., Effect of plasminogen activator (urokinase), plasmin, and thrombin on glycoprotein and collagenous components of basement membrane, *Cancer Res.* 41, 4629–4636, 1981.
8. Okunishi, K., Sisson, T.H., Huang, S.K., et al., Plasmin overcomes resistance to prostaglandin E2 in fibrotic lung fibroblasts by reorganizing protein kinase A signaling, *J. Biol. Chem.* 286, 32231–32243, 2011.

9. Okada, M., Suzuki, A., Yamawaki, H., and Hara, Y., Levosimendan inhibits interleukin-1β-induced cell migration and MMP-9 secretion in rat cardiac fibroblasts, *Eur. J. Pharmacol.* 718, 332–339, 2013.

10. Rogerson, F.M., Chung, Y.M., Deutscher, M.E., et al., Cytokine-induced increases in ADAMTS-4 messenger RNA expression do not lead to increased aggrecanase activity in ADAMTS-5-deficient mice, *Arthritis Rheum.* 62, 3365–3373, 2010.

11. Stirnberg, M., Mauer, E., Horstneyer, A., et al., Proteolytic processing of the serine protease matriptase-2: Identification of the cleavage sites required for its autocatalytic release from the cell surface, *Biochem. J.* 430, 87–95, 2010.

12. Seidah, N.G., Sadr, M.S., Crétien, M., and Mbikay, M., The multifaceted proprotein convertases: Their unique, redundant, complementary, and opposite functions, *J. Biol. Chem.* 288, 21473–21481, 2013.

13. Stawowy, P., Meyborg, H., Stilbenz, D., et al., Furin-like proprotein convertases are central regulators of the membrane type matrix metalloproteinase-pro-matrix metalloproteinase-2 proteolytic cascade in atherosclerosis, *Circulation* 111, 2820–2827, 2005.

14. Longpré, J.-M. and Leduc, R., Identification of prodomain determinants involved in ADAMTS-1 biosynthesis, *J. Biol. Chem.* 279, 33237–33245, 2004.

15. Longpré, J.-M., McCulloch, D.R., Koo, B.H., et al., Characterization of proADAMTS5 processing by propeptide convertases, *Int. J. Biochem. Cell Biol.* 41, 1116–1126, 2009.

16. Cao, Y., Kang, Q., Zhao, Z., and Zolkiewska, A., Intracellular processing of metalloproteinase disintegrin ADAM12, *J. Biol. Chem.* 277, 26403–26411, 2002.

17. Wewer, U.M., Mőrgelin, M., Holck, P., et al., ADAM12 is a four-leafed clover: The excised prodomain remains bound to the mature enzyme, *J. Biol. Chem.* 281, 9418–9422, 2006.

18. Springman, E.B., Angleton, E.L., Birkedal-Hansen, H., and Van Wart, H.E., Multiple modes of activation of latent human fibroblast collagenase: Evidence for the role of a Cys[73] active-site zinc complex in latency an a "cysteine switch" mechanism for activation, *Proc. Natl. Acad. Sci. USA* 87, 364–368, 1990.

19. Neurath, H., Limited proteolysis and zymogen activation, in *Protease and Biological Control*, eds. E. Reich, D.B. Rifkin, and E. Shaw, pp. 51–64, Cold Spring Harbor Laboratory, Cold Spring Harbor, NY, 1975.

20. Kassell, B. and Kay, J., Zymogens of proteolytic enzymes, *Science* 180, 1022–1027, 1973.

21. Yan, X., Chang, H.Y., and Baltimore, D., Autoproteolytic activation of pro-caspases by oligomerization, *Mol. Cell* 1, 319–325, 1998.

22. Merdanovic, M., Mőnig, T., Ehrmann, M., and Kaiser, M., Diversity of allosteric regulation in proteases, *ACS Chem. Biol.* 8, 19–26, 2013.

23. Yang, L., Manihody, C., Walston, T.D., Cooper, S.T., and Rezaie, A.R., Thrombomodulin enhances the reactivity of thrombin with protein C inhibitor by providing a binding site for the serpin and allosterically modulating the activity of thrombin, *J. Biol. Chem.* 278, 37465–37470, 2003.

24. Conway, E.M. and Nowkowski, B., Biologically active thrombomodulin is synthesized by adherent synovial fluid cells and is elevated in synovial fluid of patients with rheumatoid arthritis, *Blood* 81, 726–733, 1993.

25. Suzuki, K., Gabazza, E.C., Hayashi, T., et al., Protective role of activated protein C in lung and airway remodeling, *Crit. Care Med.* 32(5 Suppl.), S262–S265, 2004.

26. Anstee, Q.M., Dhar, A., and Thursz, M.R., The role of hypercoagulability in liver fibrogenesis, *Clin. Res. Hepatol. Gastroenterol.* 35, 526–533, 2011.

27. Koo, B.H., Han, J.H., Yeom, Y.L., and Kim, D.S., Thrombin-dependent MMP-2 activity is regulated by heparan sulfate, *J. Biol. Chem.* 285, 41270–41279, 2010.

28. Ryu, H.-Y., Lee, J., Yang, S., et al., Syndecan-2 functions as a docking receptor for pro-matrix metalloproteinase-7 in human colon cancer cells, *J. Biol. Chem.* 284, 35692–35701, 2009.

29. Fulcher, Y.G., Gari, R.R.S., Frey, N.C., et al., Heparinoids activate a protease, secreted by mucosa and tumors, via tethering supplemented by allostery, *ACS Chem. Biol.* 9, 957–966, 2014.

30. Berton, A., Selvais, C., Lemoine, P., et al., Binding of matrilysin-1 to human epithelial cells promotes its activity, *Cell. Mol. Life Sci.* 64, 610–620, 2007.

31. Choi-Miura, N.-H., Tobe, T., Sumiya, J., et al., Purification and characterization of a novel hyaluronan-binding protein (PHBP) from human plasma: It has three EGF, a kringle and a serine protease domain, similar to hepatocyte growth factor activator, *J. Biochem.* 119, 1157–1165, 1996.

32. Etscheid, M., Beer, N., Fink, E., Seitz, R., and Johannes, D., The hyaluronan-binding serine protease from human plasma cleaves HMW and LMW kininogen and releases bradykinin, *Biol. Chem.* 383, 1633–1643, 2002.

33. Etscheid, M., Beer, N., and Dodt, J., The hyaluronan-binding protease upregulates EFK1/2 and PI3K/Akt signalling pathways in fibroblasts and stimulates cell proliferation and migration, *Cell. Signal.* 17, 1486–1494, 2005.

34. Reijnen, M.M., van Goor, H., Falk, P., Hedgren, M., and Holmdahl, L., Sodium hyaluronate increases the fibrinolytic response of human peritoneal mesothelial cells exposed to tumor necrosis factor α, *Arch. Surg.* 136, 291–296, 2001.

35. Horton, M.R., Olman, M.A., Bao, C., et al., Regulation of plasminogen activator inhibitor-1 and urokinase by hyaluronan fragments in mouse macrophages, *Am. J. Physiol. Lung Cell. Mol. Physiol.* 279, L707–L715, 2000.

36. Murphy, G., Tissue inhibitors of metalloproteinases, *Genome Biol.* 12(11), 233, 2011.

37. Troeberg, L., Lazenbatt, C., Anower-E-Khuda, M.T., et al., Sulfated glycosaminoglycans control the extracellular trafficking and the activity of the metalloprotease inhibitor TIMP-3, *Chem. Biol.* 21, 1300–1309, 2014.

38. Ong, P.C., McGowan, S., Pearce, M.C., et al., DNA accelerates the inhibition of human cathepsin V by serpins, *J. Biol. Chem.* 282, 36980–36986, 2007.

39. Komissorov, A.A., Florova, G., and Idell, S., Effects of extracellular DNA on plasminogen activation and fibrinolysis, *J. Biol. Chem.* 286, 41949–41962, 2011.

40. Schmitt, M., Kanayama, N., Jänicke, F., Hafter, R., and Graeff, H., Human tumor cell urokinase-type plasminogen activator (uPA): Degradation of the proenzyme form (pro-uPA) by granulocyte elastase prevents subsequent activation by plasmin, *Adv. Exp. Med. Biol.* 297, 111–128, 1991.

41. Ellerbroek, S.M., Wu, Y.I., Overall, C.M., and Stack, M.S., Functional interplay between type I collagen and cell surface matrix metalloproteinase activity, *J. Biol. Chem.* 276, 24833–24842, 2001.

42. Cho, J.A., Osenkowski, P., Zhao, H., et al., The inactive 44-kDA processed form of membrane type 1 matrix metalloproteinase (MT1-MMP) enhances proteolytic activity via regulation of the endocytosis of active MT1-MMP, *J. Biol. Chem.* 283, 17391–17495, 2008.

43. Remacle, A.G., Chekanov, A.V., Golubkov, V.S., et al., *O*-Glycosylation regulated autolysis of cellular membrane type-1 matrix metalloproteinase (MT1-MMP), *J. Biol. Chem.* 281, 16897–16805, 2006.

44. Remacle, A.G., Shiryaev, S.A., Golubkov, V.S., et al., Non-destructive and selective imaging of the functionally active, pro-invasive membrane type-1 matrix metalloproteinase (MT1-MMP) enzyme in cancer cells, *J. Biol. Chem.* 288, 20568–20580, 2013.

45. Albrechtsen, R., Kvelborg, M., Stautz, D., et al., ADAM12 redistributes and activates MMP-14, resulting in gelatin degradation, reduced apoptosis and increased tumor growth, *J. Cell Sci.* 126, 4707–4720, 2013.

118 Proteolysis in the Interstitial Space

46. Sundberg, C., Thodet, C.K., Kveilborg, M., et al., Regulation of ADAM12 cell-surface expression by protein kinase C, *J. Biol. Chem.* 279, 51601–51611, 2004.
47. Bourd-Boittin, K., Le Pabic, H., Bonnier, D., L'Heigoualc'h, A., and Thére, N., RACK1, a new ADAM12 interacting protein: Contribution to liver fibrogenesis, *J. Biol. Chem.* 283, 26000–26009, 2008.
48. Asakura, M., Kitakaze, M., Takashima, S., et al., Cardiac hypertrophy is inhibited by antagonism of ADAM12 processing of HB-EGF: Metalloproteinase inhibitors as a new therapy, *Nat. Med.* 8, 35–40, 2002.
49. Wolfsberg, T.G., Bazan, J.F., Blobel, C.P., et al., The precursor region of a protein active in sperm–egg fusion containing a metalloproteinase and a disintegrin domain: Structural, functional, and evolutionary implications, *Proc. Natl. Acad. Sci. USA*, 90, 10783–10787, 1993.
50. Wolfsberg, T.G., Straight, P.D., Gerena, R.L., et al., ADAM, a widely distributed and developmentally regulated gene family encoding membrane proteins with a disintegrin and metalloprotease domain, *Dev. Biol.* 169, 378–383, 1995.
51. Primakoff, P. and Myles, D.C., The ADAM gene family: Surface proteins with adhesion and protease activity, *Trends Genet.* 16, 83–87, 2000.
52. Cho, C., Testicular and epididymal ADAMs: Expression and function during fertilization, *Nat. Rev. Urol.* 9, 550–560, 2012.
53. Hooper, N.M. and Lendeckel, U., eds., *The ADAM Family of Proteases*, Springer, Dordrecht, the Netherlands, 2005.
54. Wei, S., ADAM metalloproteinases, in *The Handbook of Proteolytic Enzymes*, eds. N.D. Rawlings and G.S. Salvesen, Chapter 248, pp. 1086–1194, Amsterdam, the Netherlands, 2013.
55. White, J., Bridges, L., DeSimone, D., Tamczuk, M., and Wolfsberg, T., Introduction to the ADAM family, in *The ADAM Family of Proteases*, eds. N.M. Hooper and U. Lendeckel, Chapter 1, pp. 1–18, Springer, Dordrecht, the Netherlands, 2005.
56. Hartmann, M., Herrlich, A., and Herrlich, P., Who decides when to cleave an ectodomain? *Trends Biochem. Sci.* 38, 111–120, 2013.
57. Hartmann, M., Parra, L.M., Ruschel, A., et al., Inside-out regulation of ectodomain cleavage of cluster-of-differentiation-44 (CD44) and of neuregulin-1 requires substrate dimerization, *J. Biol. Chem.* 290, 17041–17054, 2015.
58. Parkin, E. and Harris, B., A disintegrin and metalloproteinase (ADAM)–mediated ectodomain shedding of ADAM10, *J. Neurochem.* 2009, 1464–1479, 2009.
59. Postina, R. and Fahrenholz, F., ADAM 10, myelin-associated metalloproteinase, in *The Handbook of Proteolytic Enzymes*, eds. N.D. Rawlings and G.S. Salvesen, Chapter 251, pp. 1108–1114, Academic Press/Elsevier, Amsterdam, the Netherlands, 2013.
60. Endres, K. and Fahrenholz, F., Upregulation of the α-secretase ADAM10: Risk or reason for hope? *FEBS J.* 277, 1585–1596, 2010.
61. Bakken, A.M., Protack, C.D., Roztocil, E., Nicholl, S.M., and Davies, M.G., Cell migration in response to the amino-terminal fragment of urokinase requires epidermal growth factor receptor activation through an ADAM-mediated mechanism, *J. Vasc. Surg.* 49, 1296–1303, 2009.
62. Herzog, C., Haun, R.S., Ludwig, A., Shah, S.V., and Kaushal, G.P., ADAM10 is the major sheddase responsible for the release of membrane-associated meprin A, *J. Biol. Chem.* 289, 13308–13322, 2014.
63. Yagami-Hiromasa, T., Sato, T., Kurlsaki, T., et al., A metalloproteinase-disintegrin participating in myoblast fusion, *Nature* 377, 652–656, 1995.
64. Kveilborg, M., Frőhlich, C., Albrechtsen, R., and Wewer, U.M., ADAM12, in *The Handbook of Proteolytic Enzymes*, eds. N.D. Rawlings and G.S. Salvesen, Chapter 252, pp. 1114–1115, Academic Press/Elsevier, Amsterdam, the Netherlands, 2013.

65. Gilpin, B.J., Loechel, F., Mattei, M.-G., et al., A novel, secreted form of human ADAM12 (meltrin α) provokes myogenesis *in vivo*, *J. Biol. Chem.* 273, 157–166, 1995.
66. Nagase, H., Itoh, Y., and Binner, S., Interaction of α_2-macroglobulin with matrix metalloproteinases and its use for the identification of their active forms, *Ann. N.Y. Acad. Sci.* 732, 294–302, 1994.
67. Jacobsen, J., Visse, R., Sørensen, H.P., et al., Catalytic properties of ADAM12 and its domain deletion mutants, *Biochemistry* 47, 537–547, 2008.
68. Hubbard, S.J., Benyon, R.J., and Thornton, J.M., Assessment of conformational parameters as predictors of limited proteolytic sites in native protein structures, *Protein Eng.* 11, 349–359, 1998.
69. Loechl, F., Fox, J.W., Murphy, G., Albrechtsen, R., and Wewer, U.M., ADAM 12-C cleaves IGFBP-3 and IGFBP-5 and is inhibited by TIMP-3, *Biochem. Biophys. Res. Commun.* 278, 511–515, 2000.
70. Okada, A., Mochizuki, S., Yatabe, T., et al., ADAM-12 (Meltrin α) is involved in chondrocyte proliferation via cleavage of insulin-like growth factor binding protein 5 in osteoarthritic cartilage, *Arthritis Rheum.* 58, 778–789, 2008.
71. Jaconsen, J. and Wewe, U.M., Targeting ADAM12 in human disease: Head, body or tail? *Curr. Pharm. Des.* 15, 2300–2310, 2009.
72. Milla, M.E., Gonzales, P.E., and Leonard, J.D., The TACE zymogen, *Cell Biochem. Biophys.* 44, 342–348, 2006.
73. Murphy, G., ADAM17, Tumor necrosis factor α–convertase, in *The Handbook of Proteolytic Enzymes*, eds. N.D. Rawlings and G.S. Salvesen, Chapter 254, pp. 1126–1130, Academic Press/Elsevier, Amsterdam, the Netherlands, 2013.
74. Horiuchi, K., A brief history of tumor necrosis factor α–converting enzyme: An overview of ectodomain shedding, *Keio J. Med.* 62, 29–36, 2013.
75. Rose-John, S., ADAM17, shedding, TACE as therapeutic targets, *Pharmacol. Res.* 71, 19–22, 2013.
76. Kawahara, R., Lima, R.N., Domingues, R.R., et al., Deciphering the role the ADAM17-dependent secretome in cell signaling, *J. Proteome Res.* 13, 2080–2093, 2014.
77. Huang, Y., Benaich, N., Tape, C., Kwok, H.F., and Murphy, G., Targeting sheddase activity of ADAM17 by an anti-ADAM17 antibody D1(A12) inhibits head and neck squamous cell carcinoma cell proliferation and motility via blockage of bradykinin induced HERs transactivation, *Int. J. Biol. Sci.* 10, 702–714, 2014.
78. Uchikawa, S., Yoda, M., Tohmonda, T., et al., ADAM17 regulates IL-1 signaling by selectively releasing IL-1 receptor type 2 from the cell surface, *Cytokine* 71, 238–245, 2015.
79. Rios-Doria, J., Sabol, D., Chesebrough, I., et al., A monoclonal antibody to ADAM17 inhibits tumor growth by inhibiting EGFR and non-EGFR mediated pathways, *Mol. Cancer Ther.* 14, 1637–1649, 2015.
80. Mezyk-Kopeć, R., Wyroba, B., Stalińska, K., et al., ADAM17 promotes motility, invasion, and sprouting of lymphatic endothelial cells, *PLoS One* 10(7), e0132661, 2015.
81. Dreymueller, D., Pruessmeyer, J., Groth, E., et al., The role of ADAM-mediated shedding in vascular biology, *Eur. J. Cell Biol.* 91, 472–485, 2012.
82. Lv, X., Li, Y., Qian, M., et al., ADAM17 silencing suppresses the migration and invasion of non-small cell lung cancer, *Mol. Med. Rep.* 9, 1935–1940, 2014.
83. Arribas, J. and Esselens, C., ADAM17 as a therapeutic target in multiple diseases, *Curr. Pharm. Des.* 15, 2319–2335, 2009.
84. Scheller, J., Chalaris, A., Garbers, C., and Rose-John, S., ADAM17: A molecular switch to control inflammation and tissue regeneration, *Trends Immunol.* 32, 380–387, 2011.
85. Jury, J.A., Perry, A.C., and Hall, L., Identification, sequence analysis and expression of transcripts encoding a putative metalloproteinase, eMDC II, in human and macaque epididymis, *Mol. Hum. Reprod.* 5, 1127–1134, 1999.

86. Howard, L., Maciewicz, R.A., and Blobel, C.P., Cloning and characterization of ADAM28: Evidence for autocatalytic pro-domain removal and for cell surface localization of mature ADAM28, *Biochem. J.* 348, 21–27, 2000.
87. Roberts, C.M., Tani, P.H., Bridges, L.C., Laszik, Z., and Bowditch, R.D., MDC-L: A novel metalloprotease disintegrin cysteine–rich protein family member expressed by human lymphocytes, *J. Biol. Chem.* 274, 25251–25259, 1999.
88. Klein, T. and Bischoff, R., Active metalloproteases of the a disintegrin and metalloprotease (ADAM) family: Biological function and structure, *J. Proteome Res.* 10, 17–33, 2011.
89. Mochizuki, S., Shimoda, M., Shiomi, T., Fujii, Y., and Okada, Y., ADAM28 is activated by MMP-7 (matrilysin-1) and cleaves insulin-like growth factor binding protein-3, *Biochem. Biophys. Res. Commun.* 315, 79–84, 2004.
90. Howard, L., Zheng, Y., Horrocks, M., Maciewicz, R.A., and Blobel, C., Catalytic activity of ADAM28, *FEBS Lett.* 498, 82–86, 2001.
91. Mochizuki, S., Tanaka, R., Shimoda, M., et al., Connective tissue growth factor is a substrate of ADAM28, *Biochem. Biophys. Res. Commun.* 402, 651–657, 2010.
92. Shimoda, N., Hashimoto, G., Mochizuki, S., et al., Binding of ADAM28 to P-selectin glycoprotein ligand-1 enhances P-selectin-mediated leukocyte adhesion to endothelial cells, *J. Biol. Chem.* 282, 25864–25874, 2007.
93. Bridges, L.C., Tani, P.H., Hanson, K.R., et al., The lymphocyte metalloprotease MDC-L (ADAM28) is a ligand for the integrin $\alpha_4\beta_1$, *J. Biol. Chem.* 277, 3784–3792, 2002.
94. Johnson, L.A. and Jackson, D.G., The chemokine CX3CL1 promotes trafficking of dendritic cells through inflamed lymphatics, *J. Cell. Sci.* 126, 5259–5270, 2013.
95. Wild-Bode, C., Fellerer, K., Kugler, J., Haass, C., and Capell, A., A basolateral sorting signal directs ADAM10 to adherens junctions and is required for its function in cell migration, *J. Biol. Chem.* 281, 23824–23829, 2006.
96. Li, C., Franklin, J.L., Graves-Deal, R., et al., Myristoylated Naked2 escorts transforming growth factor alpha to the basolateral plasma membrane of polarized epithelial cells, *Proc. Natl. Acad. Sci. USA* 101, 5571–5576, 2004.
97. Merchant, N.B., Voskresensky, I., Rogers, C.M., et al., TACE/ADAM-17: A component of the epidermal growth factor receptor axis and a promising therapeutic target in colorectal cancer, *Clin. Cancer Res.* 14, 1182–1191, 2008.
98. Dulauroy, S., Di Carlo, S.E., Langa, F., Eberl, G., and Peduto, L., Lineage tracing and genetic ablation of ADAM12+ perivascular cells identify a major source of profibrotic cells during acute tissue injury, *Nature Med.* 18, 1262–1270, 2012.
99. Booth, B.W., Sandifer, T., Martin, E.L., and Martin, L.C., IL-13-induced proliferation of airway epithelial cells: Mediation by intracellular growth factor mobilization and ADAM17, *Respir. Res.* 8, 51, 2007.
100. van Loon, E.P., Pulskens, W.P., van der Hagen, E.A., et al., Shedding of klotho by ADAMs in the kidney, *Am. J. Physiol. Renal Physiol.* 309, F359–F368, 2015.
101. Murphy, G., Knäuper, V., Lee, M.H., et al., Role of TIMPs (tissue inhibitors of metalloproteinases) in pericellular proteolysis: The specificity is in the detail, *Biochem. Soc. Symp.* 70, 65–80, 2003.
102. Nakamura, H., Suenaga, N., Taniwaki, K., et al., Constitutive and induced CD44 shedding by ADAM-like proteases and membrane-type 1 matrix metalloproteinase, *Cancer Res.* 64, 876–882, 2004.
103. Kuno, K., Kanada, N., Nakashima, E., et al., Molecular cloning of a gene encoding a new type of metalloproteinase-disintegrin family protein with thrombospondin motifs as an inflammation associated gene, *J. Biol. Chem.* 272, 556–562, 1997.
104. Apte, S.S., The ADAMS endopeptidases, in *The Handbook of Proteolytic Enzymes*, eds. N.D. Rawlings and G.S. Salvesen, Chapter 259, pp. 1149–1155, Academic Press/Elsevier, Amsterdam, the Netherlands, 2013.

105. Hubmacher, D. and Apte, S.S., ADAMTS proteins as modulators of microfibril formation and function, *Matrix Biol.* 47, 34–43, 2015.

106. Duball, J. and Apte, S.S., Insights on ADAMTS proteases and ADAMTS-like proteins from mammalian genetics, *Matrix Biol.* 44–46, 24–37, 2015.

107. Kelwick, R., Desanis, I., Wheeler, G.N., and Edwards, D.R., The ADAMTS (a disintegrin and metalloproteinase with thrombospondin motifs) family, *Genome Biol.* 16, 113, 2015.

108. Colige, A., Beschin, A., Samyn, B., et al., Characterization and partial amino acid sequencing of a 107-kDa procollagen I *N*-proteinase purified by affinity chromatography on immobilized type XIV collagen, *J. Biol. Chem.* 270, 16724–16730, 1995.

109. Colige, A., Li, S.-W., Sieron, A.L., et al., cDNA cloning and expression of bovine procollagen I *N*-proteinase: A new member of the superfamily of zinc-metalloproteinases with binding sites for cells and other matrix components, *Proc. Natl. Acad. Sci. USA* 94, 2374–2379, 1997.

110. Bekhouche, M. and Colige, A., The procollagen N-proteinases ADAMTS2, 3, and 14 in pathophysiology, *Matrix Biol.* 44–46, 46–53, 2015.

111. Nagase, H. and Kashiwagi, M., Aggrecanases and cartilage matrix degradation, *Arthritis Res. Ther.* 5, 94–103, 2003.

112. Krytic, D., Rodriguez, M., and Knuesel, I., Regulated proteolytic processing of Reelin through interplay of tissue plasminogen activator (tPA), ADAMTS-4, and ADAMTS-5, and their modulators, *PLoS One* 7(10), e47793, 2012.

113. Sekine, K., Kubo, K., and Nakajima, K., How does Reelin control neuronal migration and layer formation in the developing mammalian neocortex? *Neurosci. Res.* 86, 50–58, 2014.

114. Stanton, H., Melrose, J., Little, C.B., and Fosang, A.J., Proteoglycan degradation by the ADAMTS family of proteinases, *Biochim. Biophys. Acta* 1812, 1616–1629, 2013.

115. Lemarchant, S., Pruvost, M., Hébert, M., et al., tPA promotes ADAMTS-4 induced CSPG degradation, thereby enhancing neuroplasticity following spinal cord injury, *Neurobiol. Dis.* 66, 28–42, 2014.

116. Gao, G., Plaas, A., Thompson, V.P., et al., ADAMTS4 (Aggrecanase-1) activation on the cell surface involves C-terminal cleavage by glycosylphosphatidyl inositol–anchored membrane type 4–matrix metalloproteinase and binding of the activated proteinase to chondroitin sulfate and heparan sulfate on syndecan-1, *J. Biol. Chem.* 279, 10042–10051, 2004.

117. Sanderson, R.D., Hinkes, M.T., and Bernfield, M., Syndecan-1, a cell-surface proteoglycan, changes in size and abundance when keratinocytes stratify, *J. Invest. Dermatol.* 99, 390–396, 1992.

118. Stepp, M.A., Pal-Ghosh, S., Tadvalkar, G., et al., Syndecan-1 and its expanding list of contacts, *Adv. Wound Care.* 4, 235–249, 2015.

119. Zheng, X.L., ADAMTS13 and von Willebrand factor in thrombotic thrombocytopenic purpura, *Annu. Rev. Med.* 66, 211–225, 2015.

120. Zander, C.B., Cao, W., and Zheng, X.L., ADAMTS13 and von Willebrand factor interactions, *Curr. Opin. Hematol.* 22, 452–459, 2015.

5 The Fibrinolytic System in the Interstitial Space

5.1 COMPONENTS OF FIBRINOLYTIC SYSTEM

The fibrinolytic system contains a number of proteins, including proenzyme/enzymes, inhibitors, modulators, and one biologically active peptide, angiostatin, derived from plasminogen/plasmin (see Table 5.1).[1,2] The canonical function of the fibrinolytic system in the vascular space is the orderly dissolution of fibrin clots in the process of wound healing and the dissolution of intravascular fibrin in the prevention of thrombosis. It is clear, however, that the components of the fibrinolytic system have considerable function beyond the dissolution of fibrin,[3] and it is likely that the majority of these functions occur in the interstitial space in tissues. Indeed, the "off-label" activity of the various components of the fibrinolytic system may well be the predominant function in the interstitial space. The actual process of fibrinolysis as demonstrated by the digestion of fibrin and fibronectin is likely limited to the resolution of fibrotic lesions formed by fibroblastic proliferation into provisional fibrin matrices. As an example, transforming growth factor (TGF)-β1 is suggested to enhance the expression of plasminogen activator inhibitor (PAI)-1, which is considered to be a profibrotic agent based on its inhibition of urokinase-type plasminogen activator (uPA).[4] In the study by Samarakoon and coworkers[4] and in reviews of uPA and its receptor (uPAR), the emphasis is not on the dissolution of fibrin in the interstitial space but rather on the activation of matrix metalloproteinases (MMPs) and action on cell surface receptors.[5,6] The effect of TGF-β on the components of fibrinolysis in pleural mesoepithelial cells and the subsequent effect on fibrosis is shown in Figure 5.1. Briefly, TGF-β enhances the release of PAI-1, resulting in the inhibition of plasmin formation, which in turn decreases production of MMP-1 and the resolution of fibrosis. Some of the plasminogen inhibitors may have pleomorphic functions that remain to be decscribed[7–9] but could be of great importance in the interstitial space.

5.2 FIBRINOLYTIC SYSTEM IN INTERSTITIAL SPACE

The great majority of work on the fibrinolytic system and the coagulation system (Chapter 8) is conceptually based on functions within the vascular space, where a response is required in a short period of time (i.e., seconds), such as for the formation of a clot; the time is likely longer for the dissolution of a clot and the start of the healing process. The putative actions of the various components of the fibrinolytic system within the interstitial space are likely to occur over a period of days; an example would be the remodeling of the extracellular matrix (ECM) and cell migration. Thus, the relatively low level of intrinsic activity of single-chain

TABLE 5.1
Components of the Fibrinolytic System in the Interstitial Space

Component	Description/Function	Presence in Interstitial Space
Plasminogen (Plg)	Plasminogen is a single-chain precursor of plasmin existing in several forms with molecular weights of approximately 90 kDa.[1-4] Activation of the single chain yields plasmin consisting of two polypeptide chains joined by disulfide bonds. Proteolytic digestion releases angiostatin, which is involved in angiogenesis. Plasminogen binds to cell surface receptors, such as α-enolase, that possess a C-terminal carboxyl group and to pro-uPA bound to uPAR. Plasminogen can also bind to cell surface receptors on bacteria, promoting activation by bacterial plasminogen activators.[5] Kringle domains were first described in plasminogen as 80 peptide regions with three disulfide bonds, with structural similarity to a Danish pastry; the kringle domains bind lysine-containing ligands and macromolecules such as fibrinogen. Plasminogen exists in multiple glycoforms,[6] which may have functional consequences.[7]	Presence in rat interstitial fluid at approximately 40% of plasma.[8] Presence in interstitial fluid is also inferred from analysis of peripheral lymph.[9] Plasminogen has been shown to be present in cerebrospinal fluid.[10] Degraded forms of plasminogen are found in synovial fluid.[11,12]
Plasmin (Pm)	Plasmin is a serine protease derived from plasminogen with a preference for cleavage at peptide bonds, where the carboxyl group is provided by lysine and, to lesser extent, arginine. The canonical function is digestion of fibrin, but plasmin is important in the interstitial space for the initiation of proteolytic cascades and digestion of fibronectin in the ECM. Thus, plasmin is an interesting protease that has both a digestive function in its action on fibrin and fibronectin and a regulatory function in the activation of pro-uPA and some MMPs.	It is likely that plasmin is generated from plasminogen in the interstitial space.[8] Plasmin does not appear to degrade fibrinogen or fibrin in the interstitial space as fibrinogen but not fibrin degradation products are present in lymph.[13] Plasmin that is generated in the interstitial space is probably inactivated rapidly by inhibitors such as α2-antiplasmin.
Urokinase-type plasminogen activator (uPA, urokinase)	uPA is responsible for the conversion of plasminogen to plasmin. The conversion of plasminogen to plasmin by uPA is most efficient on the cell surface in the presence of plasminogen and uPAR. Urokinase was a therapeutic product (Abbokinase®) originally isolated from urine for the lysis of fibrin clots; Abbokinase is now obtained from cell culture technology. Urokinase is a serine protease that can be isolated in several forms that differ in molecular weight.	No direct measurement of uPA in lymph. However, the presence of uPA in the interstitial/extravascular space is inferred from *in vitro* studies.[14,15]

TABLE 5.1 (CONTINUED)
Components of the Fibrinolytic System in the Interstitial Space

Component	Description/Function	Presence in Interstitial Space
Urokinase-type plasminogen activator receptor (uPAR)	uPAR is a highly glycosylated membrane protein with a molecular weight of approximately 60 kDa bound to the membrane by a glycosylphosphatidylinositol anchor.[16] As such, uPAR can initiate intracellular signaling but must rely on interaction with lateral partners such as integrins. It is best known for binding pro-uPA and uPA. uPAR also binds to vitronectin. There is considerable interest in the role of uPAR in oncology.[17]	uPAR has a wide tissue distribution including monocytes and fibroblasts. Distribution to various organs is increased with tissue remodeling.[18,19] There is increased expression in tumors and during inflammation. A soluble form is released during inflammation.
Streptokinase	A 45 kDa protease secreted by several strains of *Streptococcus* that converts plasminogen to plasmin on the surface of the bacteria.[20] It is an important factor in the virulence of the bacteria as it provides a mechanism for tissue destruction and concomitant bacterial invasion via either the direct action of plasmin or MMP. Streptokinase has use as a therapeutic for the lysis of fibrin clots.	The interstitial space is the area where bacterial invasion and ECM degradation takes place.
Staphylokinase	Somewhat less known is staphylokinase, a plasminogen activator secreted by lysogenic strains of *S. aureus*.[21] Staphylokinase is involved in the invasion of pathogenic bacteria by promotion of plasmin formation, which destroys the ECM.[22]	The interstitial space is the area where bacterial invasion and ECM degradation takes place.
Tissue plasminogen activator (tPA)	tPA is a serine protease expression on the luminal surface of endothelial cells and is responsible for initiation of intravascular fibrinolysis.[23] Recombinant tPA is used for the treatment of intravascular thrombosis.	Little evidence to support the presence of sufficient tPA in the interstitial space to activate plasminogen. Secretion of tPA by endothelial synthesis is apical (luminal).
Plasminogen activator inhibitor type 1 (PAI-1, serpinE1)	PAI-1 is a serpin that is considered to be the most important inhibitor of uPA in the interstitial space. PAI-1, as with certain other serpins, can adopt a latent conformation that is not effective as a protease inhibitor[24] but can be converted into an active form by treatment with chaotropic agents.[24,25] PAI-1 expressed in cell culture contains more than 90% latent material. In plasma and interstitial space, PAI-1 is stabilized by binding to vitronectin.[26,27] The complex of PAI-1 with target proteases such as uPA, tPA, and perhaps thrombin binds to lipoprotein receptor–related protein.	It was not possible to find information on the concentration of PAI-1 in interstitial fluid or lymph. The concentration of PAI-1 in serum has been determined in oncology patients. Much tissue measurement of PAI-1 is performed using immunohistochemistry, which measures PAI-1 associated with vitronectin.

(Continued)

TABLE 5.1 (CONTINUED)

Components of the Fibrinolytic System in the Interstitial Space

Component	Description/Function	Presence in Interstitial Space
Plasminogen activator inhibitor type 2 (PAI-2, serpinB2)	PAI-2 is a largely intracellular protein lacking a clearly defined function.[28] The intracellular form has a molecular weight of approximately 44 kDA, while the extracellular form has a molecular weight of approximately 60 kDa, reflecting the glycosylation of the intracellular protein prior to secretion.[29]	Keratinocytes secrete PAI-2 to control uPA in the interstitial space of skin.[30]
Plasminogen activator inhibitor type 3 (PAI-3, serpinA5)	PAI-3 was found to be identical with protein C inhibitor.[31]	Protein C inhibitor is present in bronchoalveolar lavage fluid and is associated with reduced fibrinolytic activity in interstitial lung disease.[32]
α_2-Antiplasmin (serpinF2)	α_2-Antiplasmin is a glycoprotein with a molecular weight of approximately 70 kDa and is considered to be the major inhibitor of plasmin in the vascular space.[33] α_2-Antiplasmin is best known for the inhibition of plasmin; it can also inhibit human kallikrein 5 (KLK-5) with modest affinity,[34] as well as trypsin and chymotrypsin. The reaction of α_2-plasmin inhibitor with trypsin is far more rapid than with either plasmin or chymotrypsin, which are in turn three orders of magnitude more rapid than the reaction with KLK-5. Oxidation of α_2-antiplasmin did not affect the rate of reaction with either trypsin, chymotrypsin, or plasmin.[35] Plasmin bound to uPAR after formation from plasminogen was resistant to inactivation by α_2-antiplasmin.[36] Plasminogen has an unusual structure consisting of three domains: the C-terminal region, which contains a cluster of basic amino acid residues and interacts with plasmin; the serpin domain, which contains the site that reacts with plasmin, resulting in inactivation; and an N-terminal extension that can be cross-linked to fibrin by factor XIIIa.[37]	Present in interstitial fluid at approximately 20% of the plasma concentration as shown in a rat model.[7]
Vitronectin	A protein component of the ECM that binds PAI-1. The binding is associated with the stabilization of PAI-1 and enhances the inactivation of tPA and uPA. Upon binding to vitronectin, PAI-1 also becomes a slow-acting thrombin inhibitor. The role of vitronectin is complicated by the viability of a vitronectin knockout mouse.[38]	Soluble monomeric vitronectin is thought to be transported from the vascular space into the interstitial space and deposited into the ECM.[39,40] There has been some suggestion of extravascular sites of synthesis.[40]

TABLE 5.1 (CONTINUED)
Components of the Fibrinolytic System in the Interstitial Space

Component	Description/Function	Presence in Interstitial Space
Angiostatin	A fragment derived from plasminogen via the limited proteolysis and reduction of two disulfide bonds. A reduced form of plasminogen can serve as a precursor for angiostatin with the participation of phosphoglycerate kinase.[41] The size of angiostatin fragments depends on the protease responsible for the fragmentation of plasminogen. While angiostatin formation is closely associated with tumor cells, it has also been shown to be derived from macrophages during inflammation. Angiostatin can exist in multiple glycoforms derived from plasminogen glycoforms.[6]	Though there is no evidence for the formation of angiostatins in the interstitial space, there is rapid transport of both angiostatin I and angiostatin II from the intravascular space to extravascular space.[42]

REFERENCES FOR TABLE 5.1

1. Castellino, F.J. and Ploplis, V.A., Structure and function of the plasminogen/plasmin system, *Thromb. Haemost.* 93, 647–654, 2005.
2. Robbins, K.C. and Summaria, L., Plasminogen and plasmin, *Methods Enzymol.* 45, 257–273, 1976.
3. Castellino, F.J. and Sodetz, J.M., Rabbit plasminogen and plasmin isozymes, *Methods Enzymol.* 45, 273–286, 1976.
4. Ponting, C.P., Marshall, J.M., and Cederholm-Williams, S.A., Plasminogen: A structural review, *Blood Coagul. Fibrinolysis* 3, 605–614, 1992.
5. Lähteenamäki, K., Kuusela, P., and Korhonen, T.K., Bacterial plasminogen activators and receptors, *FEMS Microbiol. Rev.* 25, 531–552, 2001.
6. Mori, K., Dwek, R.A., Downing, A.K., Oppenakker, G., and Rudd, P.M., The activation of type 1 and type 2 plasminogen by type I and type II tissue plasminogen activators, *J. Biol. Chem.* 270, 3261–3267, 1995.
7. Pirie-Shepherd, S.F., Jett, E.A., Andon, N.L., and Pizzo, S.V., Sialic acid content of plasminogen 2 glycoforms as a regulator of fibrinolytic activity: Isolation, carbohydrate analysis, and kinetic characterization of six glycoforms of plasminogen, *J. Biol. Chem.* 270, 5877–5881, 1995.
8. Kristen, C.G., Tuttle, P.R., and Berger, H., Jr., Quantitative assessment of subcutaneous fibrinolysis in the rat, *J. Pharmacol. Methods* 16, 125–138, 1986.
9. Hohage, R., Hilgard, P., and Hiemeyer, V., Lymphatic fibrinolysis in rats, *Experentia* 27, 328–329, 1971.
10. Priola, G.M., Foster, M.W., Deal, A.M., et al., Cerebrospinal fluid proteomics in children during induction for acute lymphoblastic leukemia: A pilot study, *Pediatr. Blood Cancer* 62, 1190–1194, 2015.
11. Moroz, L.A., Wing, S., and Lioté, F., Mini-plasminogen-like fragments of plasminogen in synovial fluid in acute inflammatory arthritis, *Thromb. Res.* 43, 417–424, 1986.

12. Shearin, T.V., Pizzo, S.V., and Growow, M., Molecular abnormality of human plasmino-gen isolated from synovial fluid of rheumatoid arthritis patients, *J. Mol. Med. (Berl.)* 75, 378–385, 1997.

13. Le, D.T., Borgs, P., Toneff, T.W., White, M.N., and Rapaport, S.I., Hemostatic factors in rabbit lymph: Relationship to mechanisms regulating extravascular coagulation, *Am. J. Physiol.* 274, H769–H778, 1998.

14. Idell, S., Endothelium and disordered fibrin turnover in the injured lung, *Crit. Care Med.* 30(5 Suppl), S274–S280, 2002.

15. Gardsvoll, H., Kjaergaard, M., Jacobsen, J., et al., Mimicry of the regulatory role of urokinase in lamellipodia formation by introduction of a non-native interdomain disul-fide bond in its receptor, *J. Biol. Chem.* 286, 43515–53526, 2011.

16. Behrendt, N., Ploug, M., Rønne, E., Høyer-Hansen, G., and Danø, C., Cellular receptor for urokinase-type plasminogen activator: L protein structure, *Methods Enzymol.* 223, 207–222, 1993.

17. Ngo, J.C., Jiang, L., Lin, Z., et al., Structural basis for therapeutic intervention of uPA/uPAR system, *Curr. Drug Targets* 12, 1729–1743, 2011.

18. Smith, H.W. and Marshall, C.J., Regulation of cell signalling by uPAR, *Nat. Rev. Mol. Cell Biol.* 11, 23–36, 2010.

19. Solberg, H., Ploug, M., Høyer-Hansen, G., Nielsen, B.S., and Lund, L.R., The murine receptor for urokinase-type plasminogen activator is primarily expressed in tissue actively undergoing remodeling, *J. Histochem. Cytochem.* 49, 237–246, 2001.

20. Chandrahas, V., Glinton, K., Liang, Z., et al., Direct host plasminogen binding to bacte-rial surface M-protein in pattern D strains of *Streptococcus pyogenes* is required for acti-vation by its natural coinherited SK2b protein, *J. Biol. Chem.* 290, 18833–18842, 2015.

21. Bokarewa, M.I., Jin, T., and Tarkowski, A., *Staphylococcus aureus*: Staphylokinase, *Int. J. Biochem. Cell Biol.* 38, 504–509, 2006.

22. Peetermans, M., Vanassche, T., Liesenborghs, L., et al., Plasminogen activation by staphylokinase enhances local spreading of *S. aureus* in skin infections, *BMC Microbiol.* 14, 302, 2014.

23. Murata, T., Nakashima, Y., Yasunaga, C., Maeda, K., and Sueishi, K., Extracellular and cell-associated localizations of plasminogen activators and plasminogen activator inhibitor-1 in cultured endothelium, *Exp. Mol. Pathol.* 55, 105–118, 1991.

24. Levin, E.G. and Santell, L., Conversion of the active to latent plasminogen activator inhibitor from human endothelial cells, *Blood* 70, 1090–1098, 1987.

25. Hekman, C.M. and Loskutoff, D.J., Endothelial cells produce a latent inhibitor of plas-minogen activators that can be activated by denaturants, *J. Biol. Chem.* 260, 11581–11587, 1985.

26. Ehrlich, H.J., Keijer, J., Preissner, K.T., Gebbink, R.K., and Pannekoek, H., Functional interaction of plasminogen activator inhibitor type 1 (PAI-1) and heparin, *Biochemistry* 30, 1021–1028, 1991.

27. Seifert, D., Mimuro, J., Schleef, R.R., and Loskutoff, D.J., Interactions between type 1 plasminogen activator inhibitor, extracellular matrix and vitronectin, *Cell Differ. Dev.* 32, 287–292, 1990.

28. Lee, J.A., Cochran, B.J., Lobov, S., and Ranson, M., Forty years later and the role of plasminogen activator inhibitor type 2/SerpinB2 is still an enigma, *Semin. Thromb. Hemost.* 37, 395–407, 2011.

29. Ye, R.D., Wun, T.-C., and Sadler, J.E., Mammalian protein secretion without signal peptide removal: Biosynthesis of plasminogen activator inhibitor-2 in U-937 cells, *J. Biol. Chem.* 263, 4869–4875, 1988.

30. Reinartz, J., Schaefer, B., Bechtel, M.J., and Kramer, M.D., Plasminogen activator inhibitor 2 (PAI-2) in human keratinocytes regulates pericellular urokinase-type plas-minogen activator, *Exp. Cell Res.* 223, 91–101, 1996.

31. Stief, T.W., Radtke, K.P., and Heimburger, N., Inhibition of urokinase by protein C-inhibitor (PCI): Evidence of identity of PCI and plasminogen activator inhibitor 3, *Biol. Chem. Hoppe Seyler* 368, 1427–1433, 1987.

32. Fujimoto, H., Gabazza, E.C., Hataji, O., et al., Thrombin-activatable fibrinolysis inhibitor and protein C inhibitor in interstitial lung disease, *Am. J. Respir. Crit. Care Med.* 167, 1687–1894, 2003.

33. Wiman, B., Human α_2-antiplasmin, *Methods Enzymol.* 80, 395–408, 1981.

34. Michael, I.P., Sotiropoulou, G., Pampalakis, G., et al., Biochemical and enzymatic characterization of human kallikrein 5 (hK5), a novel serine protease potentially involved in cancer progression, *J. Biol. Chem.* 280, 14628–14635, 2005.

35. Shieh, B.-H. and Travis, J., The reactive site of human α_2-antiplasmin, *J. Biol. Chem.* 262, 6055–6059, 1987.

36. Ellis, V., Behrendt, N., and Danø, K., Plasminogen activation by receptor-bound urokinase: A kinetic study with both cell-associated and isolated receptor, *J. Biol. Chem.* 266, 12752–12758, 1991.

37. Law, R.H., Sofian, T., Kan, W.T., et al., X-ray crystal structure of the fibrinolysis inhibitor, α_2-antiplasmin, *Blood* 111, 2049–2052, 2008.

38. Leavesley, D.I., Kashyap, A.S., Croll, T., et al., Vitronectin: Master controller or micromanager? *IUBMB Life* 65, 807–818, 2013.

39. Preissner, K.T. and Potzsch, B., Vessel wall–dependent metabolic pathways of the adhesive proteins, von-Willebrand-factor and vitronectin, *Histol. Histopathol.* 10, 239–251, 1995.

40. Seiffert, D., Bordin, G.M., and Loskutoff, D.J., Evidence that extrahepatic cells express vitronectin mRNA at rates approaching those of hepatocytes, *Histochem. Cell Biol.* 105, 195–201, 1996.

41. Butera, D., Wind, T., Lay, A.J., et al., Characterization of a reduced form of plasma plasminogen as the precursor for angiostatin formation, *J. Biol. Chem.* 289, 2992–3000, 2014.

42. Hatton, M.W., Day, S., Southward, S.M., et al., Metabolism of rabbit angiostatin glycoforms I and II in rabbits: Angiostatin-I leaves the intravascular space faster and appears to have greater anti-angiogenic activity than angiostatin-II, *J. Lab. Clin. Med.* 138, 83–93, 2001.

urokinase plasminogen activator (scuPA) or thrombin/uPA (see Section 5.3) may be significant in initiating matrix degradation; the physiological significance may depend on the respective venue. We also know little of the potential effects of interstitial components such as hyaluronan or collagen I on the components of the fibrinolytic system.

Several reviews have discussed the fibrinolytic system in the extravascular space with emphasis on the synovia and rheumatoid arthritis.[10–12] While these discussions might not have direct relevance to the interstitial space, the articles do contain interesting information. Carmassi and coworkers[11] report on the composition of synovial fluid from rheumatoid arthritis patients. The concentration of PAI-1 is markedly elevated in rheumatoid arthritis synovial fluid compared to patient plasma concentration, while plasminogen, tPA, and α_2-plasmin inhibitor are all markedly decreased. Chung and coworkers[10] remind the reader that fibrinolysis depends on the balance between the formation of enzymes that can dissolve fibrin, the cross-linking of fibrin by factor XIIIa, and inhibitors of fibrinolysis. In the circulation, factor XIII and plasminogen are tightly bound to fibrinogen. It is possible that these proteins would

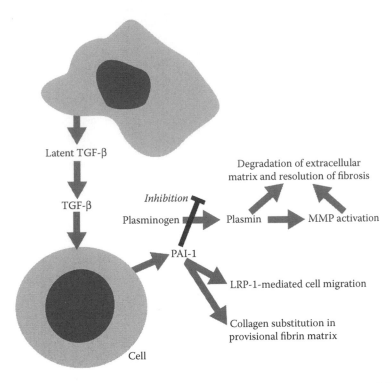

FIGURE 5.1 The role of the fibrinolytic system in TGF-β in the development of fibrosis. Activation of macrophages releases TGF-β in a latent form, which is activated by proteolysis. TGF-β enhances the release of PAI-1 from pleural mesothelial cells. (From Idell, S., et al., *In vivo, Am. J. Respir. Cell Mol. Biol.* 7, 414–426, 1992.) The net effect is the inhibition of plasmin, which prevents MMP activation and the subsequent resolution of fibrosis. (Adapted from Samarkoon, R., et al., *Cell. Signal.* 25, 264–268, 2013.) As can be observed, PAI-1 has additional profibrotic activities.

bind to fibrinogen in the interstitium, but it is likely that fibrinogen is present within the ECM (Chapter 2) and in interstitial fluid (Chapter 8). However, it is most likely that plasmin has functions other than the dissolution of fibrin in the interstitial space.

5.2.1 ORIGIN OF COMPONENTS OF FIBRINOLYTIC SYSTEM FOUND IN INTERSTITIUM

The components of the fibrinolytic system suggested to be present in the interstitial space are derived from a combination of extravasation from the vascular space and synthesis within the interstitial space. Basolateral secretion of proteins from endothelial and epithelial cells has been discussed in Chapter 1 as a process contributing to the composition of interstitial fluid. There is polarity in the secretion of tPA and uPA by epithelial cells, which contribute to the presence of these components in the interstitial space.[13] Apical secretion is the predominant pathway for tPA, while basolateral secretion is predominant for uPA in human epithelial cells (CaCo-2 cells) and apical secretion in Madin–Darby canine kidney (MDCK) cells. Other workers have found preferential basolateral secretion of tPA in cultured thyroid cells.[14]

Ragno and coworkers[15] reported that the polarity of secretion of uPA by epithelial cells depended on the cell line evaluated; the secretion of PAI-1 did not show polarity. Retinal pigmented epithelial cells have basolateral localization of uPAR.[16] It is suggested that the polarization of uPAR expression enhances the proteolytic degradation of the ECM and concomitant cell migration. The polarity of expression of PAI-1 can be influenced by systemic factors. *In vitro* studies with a two-chamber device showed that basolateral exposure to low-density lipoprotein (LDL) resulted in PAI-1 secretion into both the apical compartment and the basolateral (subendothelial) compartment; LDL on the apical side resulted in apical secretion. Exposure of both apical and basolateral surfaces to LDL resulted in enhanced secretion into both the apical and basolateral compartments.[17] Other work[18] using MDCK cells showed equal apical and basolateral secretion of PAI-1; antithrombin showed the same characteristics. Vogel and Larsen[18] also showed that α_1-antitrypsin and C1 inhibitor were found mostly in the apical secretion. uPAR is expressed by a number of different cell types[19] that can be found in the interstitial space and is increased in cancer[20] and inflammation.[21]

These studies suggest that there are physiologically significant concentrations of several components of the fibrinolytic system in the interstitial space. In addition, examinations suggest that there are components of the fibrinolytic system in lymph;[22–25] however, measurements such as euglobulin lysis time and the fibrin plate method tend to be indirect, and it is possible that lymph endothelial cells secrete components of the fibrinolytic system.[24,25] Thus, while it is reasonable that the components of the fibrinolytic system found in lymph are derived from the interstitium, it is possible that they are the products of secretion within the lymphatics. While it may not be possible to document the physical presence of some of the components of the fibrinolytic system in the interstitium, evidence of function may be present, as is noted with thrombin in the interstitial space (Chapter 8).

5.2.2   Effect of Hyaluronan On Components of Fibrinolytic System

As with the action of other interstitial proteases described elsewhere in this text, it is important to realize that these various activities are taking place within an environment that contains large amounts of hyaluronan, a structurally simple but functionally complex polysaccharide (Chapter 2), which is surrounded by the ECM (Chapter 3). Components of the ECM, such as heparan sulfate proteoglycans and vitronectin (Section 5.8), influence the expression of fibrinolytic activity in the interstitial space. Hyaluronan is a major component of the interstitial space that is often considered part of the ECM. There is some information on the effect of hyaluronan on components of the fibrinolytic system. Sitter and coworkers[26] showed the presence of hyaluronan at a concentration of 500 µg/mL decreased tPA expression in mesothelial cells, while lower concentrations (100 µg/mL) had no effect on the expression of either tPA or PAI-1. In earlier work, Olesen[27] showed that hyaluronan could stimulate the digestion of fibrin. Some stimulation was seen at lower concentrations of hyaluronan (125 µg/mL); maximal stimulation was observed at higher concentrations (250–1000 µg/mL). These experiments were performed with crude protein preparations (isoelectric precipitate from serum assay with unheated or heated fibrin plates). The comparison of heated and unheated fibrin plates allows one to distinguish between plasmin and a plasminogen activator. There was only a small difference between heated and unheated fibrin plates, suggesting the assays were measuring plasmin. No activity was observed in the absence of hyaluronan. In later studies with a different assay system, Scully and coworkers[28] showed that hyaluronan inhibited tPA-mediated fibrinolysis at a concentration of 2000 µg/mL. Marutsuka and coworkers[29] studied the effect of hyaluronan on the expression of PAI-1, tPA, and uPA in smooth muscle cells in culture. A significant increase in PAI-1 secretion was observed at physiologically relevant concentrations of hyaluronan (10–100 µg/mL), while a statistically significant increase in uPA secretion was observed only at high concentrations (1000 µg/mL) of hyaluronan. The expression of tPA in this system was an order of magnitude less than that observed for uPA and a statistically significant effect of hyaluronan was absent. Treatment of hyaluronan or the introduction of an antibody to CD44, a cell surface receptor for hyaluronan, attenuated the effect of hyaluronan on the expression of PAI-1 or uPA. Horton and coworkers[30] showed that fragments of hyaluronan (medium molecular mass of 200 kDa), such as that produced in inflammation, enhanced the mRNA expression and protein expression of PAI-1 in murine macrophages, while they reduced the mRNA expression and activity of uPA. The net effect of hyaluronan fragments would then be the reduction of pericellular fibrinolytic activity. While there is a lack of data and interpretation is complicated by the specific interaction of hyaluronan with fibrinogen (Chapter 3), the data suggest that hyaluronan inhibits fibrinolysis; it is not possible to predict the effect of hyaluronan on other activities of the fibrinolytic system.

5.3   UROKINASE-TYPE PLASMINOGEN ACTIVATOR

uPA (urokinase) is a two-chain protein linked by a disulfide bond formed by limited proteolysis of a single-chain protein, pro-urokinase-like plasminogen activator (pro-uPA, scuPA). The activation of pro-uPA occurs with pro-UPA bound to a cell surface receptor, uPAR. uPA activates plasminogen to plasmin and plasmin feeds back to activate pro-uPA bound to uPAR (Figure 5.2) in a process referred to as reciprocal activation. Petersen[31] showed that plasminogen bound to pro-uPA, which bound to uPAR, with both zymogens undergoing activation. In subsequent work, Liu and coworkers[32] used urokinase-activated anthrax toxin fusion protein, comprising a protective antigen of the anthrax toxin containing an amino acid sequence, which could be cleaved by uPA. The results demonstrated that both uPAR and plasminogen were required for the activation of this derivative. While there are questions about the precise mechanism, it is clear that both plasminogen and uPAR have important roles in the efficient activation of pro-uPA. It is possible that uPA and MMP are likely the best known of the various proteases within interstitial fluid, given their role in tissue remodeling. In its canonical function, uPA activates plasminogen to form plasmin, which digests insoluble fibrin to form soluble fibrin digestion products. However, as it is not clear that, except in disease states, plasmin digestion of fibrin occurs in the interstitial state, it is more likely that uPA is important as an initiator of regulatory proteolytic cascades[33] for the degradation of ECM than for the digestion of fibrin. An example is provided by the scheme shown in Figures 5.3 and 5.4, showing cascades

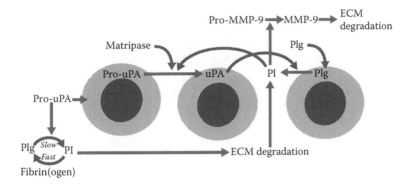

FIGURE 5.2 Reciprocal activation of urokinase plasminogen activator and plasminogen. Shown is the initial activation of pro-uPA to uPA by matriptase, which then activates plasminogen to plasmin. Plasmin can then activate uPA bound to uPAR. Also shown is the uPA-mediated activation of plasminogen bound to fibrin(ogen) in the ECM. (From Dejouvencel, T., et al., *Blood* 115, 2046–2056, 2010.)

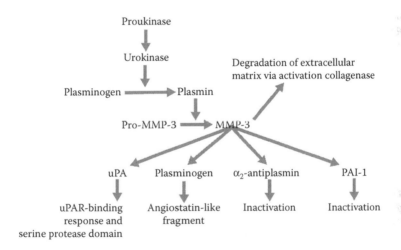

FIGURE 5.3 The interaction of MMP-3 with components of the fibrinolytic system. Shown is an hPA-initiated pathway resulting in plasmin formation, with the subsequent activation of MMP-3 (stromelysin-1). In addition to degradation of the ECM, MMP-3 acts on several components of the fibrinolytic system. (The concept is adapted, in part, from Lijnen, H.R., *Biochemistry* 67, 92–98, 2002.)

resulting in the activation of MMPs. Other enzymes that have been suggested to activate pro-uPA include hepsin,[34] stomelysin-1 (MMP-3),[35] glandular kallikrein,[36] plasma kallikrein,[37,38] prostase (human kallikrein 4, hK4),[39] plasma hyaluronan–binding protein,[40,41] and matriptase.[34,42] The activation of pro-uPA by hepsin was studied with pro-uPA in solution, not bound to uPAR.[42] The kinetic constants for activation of pro-uPA by hepsin were similar to those for plasmin, while matriptase was less efficient. Moran and coworkers[34] did show that a membrane-bound form of hepsin was effective in the activation of pro-uPA. While matriptase is less effective

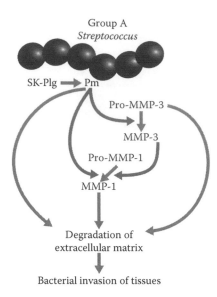

FIGURE 5.4 The role of bacterial surface activation of plasminogen. Shown is the activation of plasminogen on the bacterial surface, where there are specific receptors for plasminogen, such as enolase. Activation occurs via bacterial streptokinase, although uPA is also able to activate plasminogen bound to bacterial receptors. The plasmin may remain bound to the bacterial surface after activation, facilitating the bacterial invasion of tissues.

than hepsin, there is interest in this protease as an initiating factor in the uPA protease cascade[42] (Figure 5.2). Further support for the role of matriptase is provided from studies of matriptase expression in B-cell lymphoma.[43] Chou and coworkers[43] suggest that increased matriptase expression resulted from decreased expression of hepatocyte growth factor activator inhibitor type 1 (HAI-1). The increased matriptase expression results in shedding of active enzyme into the interstitial space with, in this case, activation of surface pro-uPA initiating the proteolytic cascade, resulting in ECM destruction. Chou and coworkers[43] suggested that the increase in soluble matriptase contributes to the growth of malignant B-cell lymphoma.

uPA is important in tumor development[44,45] and as a biomarker.[46,47] Harbeck and coworkers[47] note that the levels of uPA and/or PAI-1 are considered very useful prognostic biomarkers for breast cancer.

Pro-uPA, the single-chain precursor of uPA, has a low level of activity: 0.1%–0.4% of uPA.[48] While this rate is likely to be too slow for scuPA to be a factor in vascular fibrinolysis, it may be important in the interstitial space. Thrombin also cleaves scuPA, giving a two-chain form[49] cleaved at $Arg^{156.38}$ having very low activity[49] in the activation of plasminogen. Conversion to fully active uPA involves cleavage at Lys^{158}.[38,48] Cathepsin C (dipeptidyl peptidase I) converts thrombin-inactivated scuPA to uPA by removal of the amino-terminal dipeptide Phe^{157}–Lys^{158}.[50] Plasmin, which activates scuPA to uPA, also can convert the two-chain thrombin derivative by removing the above amino-terminal dipeptide; however, the rate is 500 times slower than the plasmin conversion of the native scuPA.[51] The inactivation of scuPA by thrombin is accelerated by the presence of thrombomodulin.[52] However, it is not clear that there is significant expression of thrombomodulin in the interstitial space.

5.4 UROKINASE-TYPE PLASMINOGEN ACTIVATOR RECEPTOR (CD87)

uPAR was first described on human monocytes but is found on other cell types.[53] uPA is bound to uPAR with nanomolar affinity as a single-chain precursor, pro-uPA.[19,54] It is suggested that the expression of uPAR on keratinocytes is coupled to cell migration. Pro-uPA is converted to an active, two-chain form by limited proteolysis by plasmin while bound to uPAR.[19,55] uPA then activates plasminogen to plasmin, which then activates bound pro-UPA in a process described as *reciprocal activation* (Figure 5.2).[55–57] The binding of pro-uPA to uPA enhances the rate of pro-uPA activation by plasmin.

There is a soluble form of uPAR (suPAR),[56–58] which is likely to be preferentially present in the interstitial space.[59] Chavakis and coworkers[60] showed that there is a polarized release of suPAR from cultured endothelial cells at the basolateral surface, while the membrane-bound urokinase receptor is found on the apical surface. These investigators showed that suPAR secreted from the basolateral surface lacked the GPI anchor associated with the membrane-bound form of uPAR; however, the mechanism of secretion is not clear. It is possible that the lack of a GPI anchor would result in movement of suPAR to the membrane surface, where it would be secreted. Murakami and coworkers[61] reported that a defect in GPI biosynthesis resulted in the secretion of alkaline phosphatase, a GPI-anchored protein that is normally found as a membrane protein. Electron microscope studies suggest that suPAR is associated with the ECM.[60] suPAR is elevated with inflammation.[62–64] Montuori and coworkers[59] note that suPAR and cleaved forms of uPAR could be degradation products or molecular entities with discrete functions. suPAR can bind some of the ligands, such as vitronectin, that bind to uPAR and could also bind uPA in the interstitial space. There are also differences between suPAR and cleaved forms of uPAR in the modulation of chemokine receptors. Proteolytic cleavage of suPAR unmasks a sequence that binds to the fMLP receptor, while this sequence is not available in suPAR. Regardless of fluid compartment distribution, there is considerable interest in the use of suPAR as a biomarker.[62–67]

Osteopontin has been reported to be associated with the increase in suPAR in septic shock patients.[68] Osteopontin has not been described in interstitial fluid but has a wide tissue distribution in addition to bone,[69] including synovial fluid from arthritic patients[70,71] and peritoneal fluid.[72] It is also possible that osteopontin expression in the interstitial space may be tissue specific and may be seen in central nervous system (CNS) tissue.[71]

uPAR interacts with a number of other proteins and this has been described as the uPAR *interactome*.[73] Eden and coworkers[73] describe the uPAR interactome as consisting of 42 proteins including 9 soluble proteins and 33 lateral partners. As uPAR is bound to the membrane by a glycerophosphatidylinositol anchor, there is no mechanism for interacting with the intracellular signaling pathways. Thus, intracellular signaling must be initiated by interaction with other membrane proteins described as *lateral partners*. Lateral partners include various integrins and L-selectin. uPAR also interacts with vitronectin as a soluble partner.[74] uPAR interaction with integrins and vitronectin is important for intracellular signaling, cell adhesion, and cell migration.[74,75] The various interactions of uPAR are shown in Figure 5.3.

Endo180 is a membrane glycoprotein of the macrophage mannose receptor family, which is associated with uPAR, and is associated with collagen degradation;[76–80] it is also referred to as urokinase plasminogen activator receptor–associated protein (uPARAP).[81,82] Endo180 combines with collagen and internalizes it for degradation during tissue remodeling. There is a preference for Endo180 to bind glycosylated collagens found in the basement membrane (BM), such as collagen IV.[83]

5.5 ACTIVATION OF PLASMINOGEN ON BACTERIAL SURFACES

Pathogenic bacteria can bind plasminogen to their surface, promoting activation by tPA and uPA,[84] enhancing the subsequent degradation of the ECM. Eberhard and coworkers evaluated the ability of 63 strains of bacteria to enhance plasminogen activation by tPA or uPA; enhancement of tPA activation of plasminogen was more significant than that observed with uPA. Battacharya and coworkers[85] have reviewed the role of bacterial surface receptors for plasminogen in the pathogenicity of these organisms. The binding of plasminogen to these cell surface receptors enhances the rate of activation of plasminogen to plasmin by plasminogen activators, including uPA, tPA, and bacterial plasminogen activators such as streptokinase. The bacterial surface receptors have been identified as specific proteins in a number of bacterial species,[85] including enolase in *Streptococci*.[86,87] Bergmann and coworkers[88] have examined the interaction of plasminogen with α-enolase in some detail. The binding of plasminogen to enolase enhances activation by uPA to greater extent than that observed with tPA. The combination of *Streptococci* bacteria, plasminogen, and uPA degrades the ECM from cultured epithelial cells or Matrigel®. These investigators were able to identify a nine-residue sequence in α-enolase from *Streptococcus pneumoniae*, which is responsible for the enhancement of plasminogen activation. The degradation of the ECM is necessary for bacterial cell invasion of tissue. Certain strains of *Streptococci* can bind plasminogen and secrete the enzyme streptokinase, which can convert plasminogen to plasmin.[89–91] Plasmin remains bound to the bacterial surface and participates either directly in the degradation of the ECM or by activation of MMPs such as MMP-3 (Figure 5.4).[91,92]

5.6 PLASMINOGEN RECEPTORS ON EUKARYOTIC CELLS

Eukaryotic cells such as macrophages, endothelial cells, and epithelial cells also have plasminogen receptors with a variety of functions.[93–95] The receptors are diverse in structure and function; the common characteristic is the structure displayed on the membrane surface, which is a C-terminal lysine or resembles a C-terminal lysine.[94] Plow and coworkers[94] list 12 plasminogen receptors, many of which will enhance plasminogen activation to plasmin and protect the formed plasmin from inactivation. Plow and coworkers do state that there are likely to be plasminogen receptors that they have not enumerated. Some cells, such as endothelial cells, macrophages, and neutrophils, express multiple plasminogen activators and many different cells express a plasminogen activator.[94] The binding of plasminogen to cell surface receptors can facilitate activation and protect plasmin from inactivation.[93,94] Annexin II (annexin A2) is a plasminogen receptor on endothelial cells that facilitates plasminogen activation by tPA.[96] This is important for intravascular fibrinolysis. We could not find any evidence for basolateral expression of annexin II in endothelial cells, while there is evidence for basolateral expression of a plasminogen receptor(s).[97] There is evidence for basolateral expression of annexin II in epithelial cells from a variety of tissue sources,[98] but we could not find any work on a possible role as a plasminogen receptor in any of the tissues. Dipeptidyl peptidase IV (CD26) is one of the more interesting plasminogen receptors.[99,100] Gonzalez-Gronow and coworkers[101] also showed that angiostatin bound to CD26 on human prostate tumor cells, blocking the expression of the MMP-9 required for invasion/metastasis. In a later study, Fleetwood and coworkers[102] showed that uPA was a regulator of macrophage migration and that MMP-9 is required for the uPA-mediated effect. The number of plasminogen receptors on macrophages suggests that the role of uPA is the activation of plasminogen.

The binding of plasminogen to cells can also facilitate cell adhesion and macrophage migration. Two plasminogen receptors, S100A10 (p11)[103] and Plg-RKT,[104] facilitate the activation of plasminogen to plasmin, which is likely responsible for cell stimulation. Glu-plasminogen, but not plasmin or Lys-plasminogen, has been shown to bind to ECM proteins such as fibrinogen and fibronectin and subsequently supports adhesion to cell surface integrins found on a variety of cells, including neutrophils.[105]

5.7 PLASMINOGEN AND PLASMIN

Plasminogen is a complex protein composed of several functional domains, including five kringle domains.[93] Kringle domains are disulfide-linked sequences forming functional domains in proteins; the descriptor *kringle* is derived from the similarity in appearance to a Danish pastry. Kringle domains bind to lysine ligands and functional groups resembling lysine,[106] as described in Section 5.6 for binding to plasminogen receptors on eukaryotic and bacterial cells and to proteins in the ECM such as fibrinogen.[107] It is important to note that the binding of fibrinogen to a matrix can result in conformational change such that the absorbed protein resembles fibrin.[108] The binding of plasminogen to fibrin has been the subject of study for some time[109] and involves the same kringle regions that are essential for the binding of plasminogen to other receptors. The binding of plasminogen to fibrin(ogen) is based on lysine-binding sites in kringles.[109,110] In this context, fibrin(ogen) is similar to other plasminogen receptors, as described in Sections 5.5 and 5.6.

A thorough consideration of the structure of plasminogen is beyond the scope of the current work and the reader is directed to several excellent reviews for more detail.[93,111,112] Glu-plasminogen is thought to be the native form of plasminogen and can be converted to Lys-plasminogen by the plasmin-catalyzed removal of an amino-terminal 77-residue peptide. Glu-plasminogen has more closed conformation than Lys-plasminogen and is less susceptible to activation. However, the binding of Glu-plasminogen to a receptor is suggested to stabilize the R-conformation, a more open conformation that is more susceptible to activation. Plasminogen also exists in several glycoforms, which affects the rate of plasmin formation,[113] likely resulting from the effect of glycosylation on plasminogen conformation.[114]

Plasmin is formed from precursor plasminogen by the action of uPA or tPA by the process of limited proteolysis.[115] Plasmin, while perhaps best known as a digestive enzyme in fragmenting fibrin and ECM proteins, has a variety of other activities[116–118] based on its functions as a regulatory protease.[119] He and coworkers[116] studied the activation of proenzymes of interstitial collagenase and interstitial stromelysin in a cell culture system consisting of dermal fibroblasts and epidermal keratinocytes (Figure 5.5). The activation is accomplished by a *cascade* comprised of uPA secreted by keratinocytes, which activates plasminogen to plasmin. The plasmin then converts pro-MMP-3 derived from dermal fibroblasts to MMP-3 (stromelysin), which then activates pro-MMP-1, also derived from dermal fibroblasts, to MMP-1 (interstitial collagenase), which can participate in tissue remodeling. Plasmin processes pro-MMP-1 to an active form by cleavage in the propeptide domain,[120] with full activity obtained by the removal of a carboxyl-terminal peptide. Full activation of MMP-1 requires the participation of MMP-3.[121,122] Plasmin bound to *Staphylococcus aureus* cells was as active as free plasmin in the partial activation of pro-MMP-1.[120] Van den Steen and coworkers[123] have described the action of plasmin, after the activation of plasminogen by uPA, in initiating a cascade, resulting in the activation of

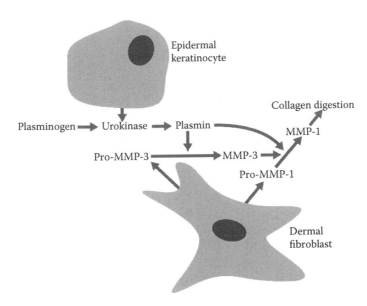

FIGURE 5.5   The role of plasmin in a proteolytic cascade, resulting in collagenolytic activity in skin. (This figure is adapted from He, C., et al., *Proc. Natl. Acad. Sci. USA* 86, 2632–2636, 1989.) Note that plasmin activation of pro-MMP-1 is required with MMP-3 for the efficient activation of pro-MMP-1.

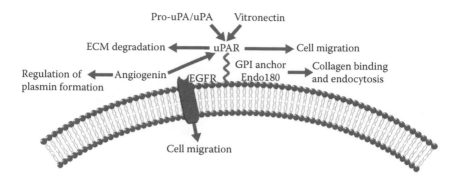

FIGURE 5.6 The urokinase-type plasminogen activator receptor (uPAR) interactome. uPAR is linked to the membrane by a glycosylphosphatidylinositol (GPI) anchor and thus has no mechanism for intracellular signaling. However, uPAR does interact with a number proteins, which have been described as the uPAR interactome. As shown, there are soluble components, such as vitronectin and pro-uPA, as well as membrane-bound or *lateral* partners, such as integrins, which provide uPAR with intracellular signaling capability.

pro-MMP-9 (progelatinase A). These investigators also note that plasmin can digest fibrin and fibronectin, but the various MMPs (MMP-1, MMP-3, and MMP-9) digest the bulk of the ECM components.

Remacle-Bonnet and coworkers[124] showed that cell-bound plasmin digested insulin-like growth factor binding protein (IGFBP)-4, increasing the availability of IGF-2 in colon cancer cells. Plasmin also degrades fibronectin with a variety of consequences.[125,126] Plasmin can degrade protein components in the BM[127] and has been used to remove such components from BM preparations for the study of collagen IV fibers.[128,129] The degradation of the BM by plasmin is considered important for tumor growth.[130,131] Plasmin can participate in a cascade with other proteases (Figure 5.6), resulting in multiple physiological responses. Plasmin formed by the action of uPA can alleviate pulmonary fibrosis but can also result in inflammation.[132–135] The balance between plasmin activity generated by uPA and PAI-1 is critical in the development of interstitial fibrosis.

5.8 VITRONECTIN

While not an active component of the fibrinolytic system, vitronectin (originally described as serum spreading factor), like uPAR, has an important role in the regulation of fibrinolysis in the interstitial space. Vitronectin is present in plasma and in the ECM.[136,137] Vitronectin plasma predominantly takes the 75 kDa monomer form, while multimers bind to endothelial cell surface receptors and pass to the subendothelial space, where the multimeric vitronectin is deposited into the ECM.[138–140] As with ECM proteins (Chapter 2), vitronectin contains several functional domains, including binding sites for PAI-1, α-β-integrins, the cell surface receptors for vitronectin, uPAR, plasminogen, and heparin. PAI-1 is stabilized on binding to a specific region in the amino-terminal region of vitronectin.[141] The binding of PAI-1 to vitronectin increases the rate of thrombin inactivation by vitronectin.[142] Vitronectin is subject to digestion by plasmin. Chain and coworkers[118] showed that plasmin cleavage of vitronectin also reduced the affinity for PAI-1, providing a mechanism for the increase of PAI-1 in the solution phase, which would result in increased fibrinolytic activity. Waltz and coworkers[143] reported that the plasmin digestion of vitronectin eliminated the binding of cells possessing urokinase receptors and promoted the dissociation of cells from a vitronectin matrix. Heparin also interacts with vitronectin at a specific site that also binds chondroitin sulfate.[144] There has been considerable interest in the binding of heparin to vitronectin, as shown by the following studies. However, it is most likely that heparan sulfate proteoglycan interacts with vitronectin in the ECM.[145] Sane and coworkers[117] showed that the cleavage of vitronectin by plasmin resulted in the formation of a 62 kD form that no longer binds heparin. Heparin also increases the rate of thrombin inactivation by PAI-1.[146,147] It is of interest that low-molecular-weight heparin was less effective than high-molecular-weight heparin in the acceleration of thrombin inactivation of PAI-1.[147] It has been suggested that the binding sites for heparin and PAI-1 on vitronectin are located adjacently in the primary structure.[146] In this study,[148] plasmin-digested vitronectin lost affinity for PAI-1 and heparin, but affinity for plasminogen was increased. Vitronectin modulates interstitial fibrinolysis by the stabilization of PAI-1;[149] a decrease in PAI-1 increases fibrinolytic activity and ECM degradation, while an increase in PAI-1 decreases fibrinolytic activity and ECM degradation.

5.9   PLASMINOGEN ACTIVATOR INHIBITOR 1 (SERPINE1)

PAI-1 is a single-chain glycoprotein with a molecular weight of approximately 50 kDa. The canonical function of PAI-1 is the inhibition of uPA in the interstitial space. In addition to the inhibition of uPA, PAI-1 has a variety of other functions.[2] Increased expression of PAI-1 is considered to be profibrotic,[38] associated with increased alveolar fibrin deposition.[150]

5.10   PLASMINOGEN ACTIVATOR INHIBITOR 2 (SERPINB2)

While PAI-2 does inhibit plasmin, it is not considered to be important in the vascular space, as only a small amount is secreted[7] and significant amounts are only found in plasma during pregancy.[8] PAI-2 may well be a significant factor in the interstitial space but there are no data to support this concept. A role in cellular immunity has been suggested.[9] PAI-2 is a poorly understood inhibitor of uPA, and while PAI-2 may well have important functions in the interstitial space, there are no studies in this area.

5.11   PLASMINOGEN ACTIVATOR INHIBITOR 3

PAI-3 was described as an unusual inhibitor of uPA purified from human urine.[151] This protein had a molecular weight of approximately 50 kDa and the rate of uPA inactivation was modestly enhanced by the presence of heparin. Subsequent work showed that this material was identical to protein C inhibitor.[152] Protein C inhibitor, as with the other serpins in the interstitial space, has diverse functions.[153] Protein C inhibitor inhibits matriptase-3.[154] Protein C inhibitor and thrombin-activated fibrinolysis inhibitor (TAFI) are elevated in pulmonary fibrosis, which is characterized by decreased fibrinolytic activity.[155]

5.12 α_2-PLASMIN INHIBITOR (SERPINF2)

α_2-Plasmin inhibitor is a serpin that is considered to be the major inhibitor of plasmin in the vascular space.[156] α_2-Plasmin inhibitor is a glycoprotein with a molecular weight of approximately 65 kDa and is characterized by a very rapid reaction with plasmin.[157] The designation of α_2-plasmin inhibitor is derived from the presence of the protein in the α_2-globulin fraction. Prior to the discovery of α_2-plasmin inhibitor, the plasmin inhibitory capacity of plasma was considered to be due to α_2-macroglobulin and, to a lesser extent, α_1-antitrypsin. Both of these inhibitors can be found in the interstitial space and are discussed in Chapter 9. α_2-Plasmin inhibitor has a latent form with no activity; however, the transition occurs at mildly acidic pH (4.9–5.8) at room temperature (assume 23°C).[158] The reaction is rapid at pH 4.9 ($t_{1/2} < 5$ min at 37°C), with marginal polymer formation. Very little reactivation could be obtained with the acid-inactivated material; latent material obtained by exposure to a chaotropic agent (3–4 M guanidine hydrochloride) could be reactivated to a greater extent (37% of potential α_2-plasmin inhibitor activity). α_2-Plasmin inhibitor has been suggested to be pleomorphic, with most of the possible functions occurring in the interstitial space. Kanno and coworkers[159] have suggested that α_2-plasmin inhibitor binds to fibroblasts, inducing the expression of TGF-β1 and collagen I, suggesting a function in the development of fibrosis other than the direct inhibition of plasmin. Experimentally induced perivascular fibrosis was reduced in α_2-plasmin inhibitor knockout mice, as was vascular remodeling.[160] The decrease in vascular remodeling observed in the absence of α_2-plasmin inhibitor is suggested to be due to increased expression of p53 and p21. There is only limited work in this area, which precludes a more complete evaluation of the possibility of pleomorphic function of α_2-plasmin inhibitor.

REFERENCES

1. Booth, N.A. and Bachman, F., Plasminogen-plasmin system, in *Thrombosis and Haemostasis*, eds. R.W. Colman, V.J. Marder, A.W. Clowes, J.N. George, and S.Z. Goldhaber, Chapter 18, pp. 335–364, Lippincott, Williams & Wilkins, Philadelphia, PA, 2006.
2. Zoria, E., Gilbert-Estellés., J., España, F., et al., Fibrinolysis: The key to new pathogenic mechanisms, *Curr. Med. Chem.* 15, 923–929, 2008.
3. Draxler, D.F. and Medcalf, R.L., The fibrinolytic system: More than fibrinolysis? *Transfus. Med. Rev.* 29, 182–189, 2015.
4. Samarakoon, R., Overstreet, J.M., and Higgins, P.J., TGF-β signaling in tissue fibroblasts: Redox controls, target genes and therapeutic opportunities, *Cell. Signal.* 25, 264–268, 2013.
5. Kuchawewicz, I., Kowal, K., Buczko, W., and Bodzenta-Lukaszyk, A., The plasmin system in airway remodeling, *Thromb. Res.* 112, 1–7, 2003.

6. Kang, L.I. and Mars, W.M., Fibrinolytic factors in liver fibrosis, *Curr. Pharm. Biotechnol.* 12, 1441–1446, 2011.
7. Medcalf, R.L. and Stasinopoulos, S.J., The undecided serpin: The ins and outs of plasminogen activator inhibitor type 2, *FEBS J.* 272, 4858–4867, 2005.
8. Lee, J.A., Cochran, B.J., Lobov, S., and Ranson, M., Forty years later and the role of plasminogen activator inhibitor type 2/SERPINB2 is still an enigma, *Semin. Thromb. Hemost.* 37, 395–407, 2011.
9. Schroder, W.A., Major, L., and Suhrbier, A., The role of SerpinB2 in immunity, *Crit. Rev. Immunol.* 31, 15–30, 2011.
10. Chung, S.I., Lee, S.Y., Uchino, R., and Carmassi, F., Factors that control extravascular fibrinolysis, *Sem. Thromb. Hemost.* 22, 479–488, 1996.
11. Carmassi, F., De Negri, F., Morale, M., Sung, K.Y., and Chung, S.I., Fibrin degradation in the synovial fluid of rheumatoid arthritis patients: A model for extravascular fibrinolysis, *Sem. Thromb. Hemost.* 22, 489–496, 1996.
12. Busso, N. and Hamilton, J.A., Extravascular coagulation and the plasminogen activator/plasmin system in rheumatoid arthritis, *Athritis Rheumat.* 46, 2268–2279, 2002.
13. Canipar, R., Zurzolo, C., Polistina, C., et al., Polarized secretion of plasminogen activators by epithelial cell monolayers, *Biochim. Biophys. Acta* 1175, 1–6, 1992.
14. Desruisseau-Gonzalvez, D., Delori, P., Gruffat, D., and Chabaud, O., Polarized secretion of tissue plasminogen activator in cultured thyroid cells, *In Vitro Cell. Dev. Biol.* 29A, 161–164, 1993.
15. Ragno, P., Estreicher, A., Gos, A., et al., Polarized secretion of urokinase-type plasminogen activator by epithelial cells, *Exp. Cell Res.* 203, 236–243, 1992.
16. Elner, S.G., Human retinal pigment epithelial lysis of extracellular matrix: Functional urokinase plasminogen activator receptor, collagenase, and elastase, *Trans. Am. Ophthalmol. Soc.* 100, 273–299, 2002.
17. Jovin, I.S., Willuweit, A., Taborski, U., et al., Low-density lipoproteins induce the polar secretion of PAI-1 by endothelial cells in culture, *Am. J. Hematol.* 73, 66–68, 2003.
18. Vogel, L.K. and Larsen, J.E., Apical and non-polarized secretion of serpins from MDCK cells, *FEBS Lett.* 473, 297–302, 2000.
19. Blasi, F., Stoppelli, M.P., and Cubellis, M.V., The receptor for urokinase-plasminogen activator, *J. Cell. Biochem.* 32, 179–186, 1986.
20. de Bock, C.E. and Wang, Y., Clinical significance of urokinase-type plasminogen activator receptor (uPAR) expression in cancer, *Med. Res. Rev.* 24(1), 13–39, 2004.
21. Nakayama, M., Yoshida, E., Sugiki, M., et al., Up-regulation of the urokinase-type plasminogen activator receptor by monotactic proteins, *Blood Coagul. Fibrinolysis* 13, 383–391, 2002.
22. Blomstrand, R., Nilsson, I.M., and Dahlbäck, O., Coagulation studies on human thoracic duct lymph, *Scandinav. J. Clin. Lab. Invest.* 15, 248–254, 1963.
23. Leandoer, L., Bergentz, S.-E., and Nilsson, I.M., Coagulation factors and components of the fibrinolytic system in lymph and blood in dogs, *Thromb. Diath. Haem.* 19, 129–135, 1968.
24. Lippi, G., Favalono, E.J., and Cervellin, G., Hemostatic properties of the lymph: Relationships with occlusion and thrombosis, *Semin. Thromb. Haemost.* 38, 213–221, 2012.
25. Vadas, P., Wasi, S., Movat, H.Z., and Hay, J.B., A novel, vasoactive product and plasminogen activator for afferent lymph cells draining chronic inflammatory lesions, *Proc. Soc. Exptl. Biol. Med.* 161, 82–85, 1979.
26. Sitter, T., Sauter, M., and Haslinger, B., Modulation of fibrinolytic system components in mesothelial cells by hyaluronan, *Perit. Dial. Int.* 23, 222–227, 2003.
27. Olesen, E.S., Fibrinolytic activity produced in guinea-pig serum by some human body fluids and hyaluronic acid, *Scand. J. Clin. Lab. Invest.* 13, 37–43, 1961.

28. Scully, M.F., Kakkar, V.V., Goodwin, C.A., and O'Regan, M., Inhibition of fibrinolytic activity by hyaluronan and its alcohol ester derivatives, *Thromb. Res.* 78, 255–258, 1995.
29. Marutsuka, K., Woodcock-Mitchell, J., Sakamoto, T., Sobel, B.E., and Fujii, S., Pathogenetic implications of hyaluronan-induced modification of vascular smooth muscle cell fibrinolysis in diabetes, *Coron. Artery Dis.* 9, 177–184, 1998.
30. Horton, M.R., Olman, M.A., Bao, C., et al., Regulation of plasminogen activator inhibitor-1 and urokinase by hyaluronan fragments in mouse macrophages, *Am. J. Physiol. Lung Cell. Mol. Physiol.* 279, L707–L715, 2000.
31. Petersen, L.C., Kinetics of reciprocal pro-urokinase/plasminogen activation: Stimulation by a template formed by the urokinase receptor bound to poly (D-lysine), *Eur. J. Biochem.* 245, 316–323, 1997.
32. Liu, S., Bugge, T.H., Frankel, A.E., and Leppla, S.H., Dissecting the urokinase activation pathway using urokinase-activated anthrax toxin, *Methods Mol. Biol.* 539, 175–190, 2007.
33. Berton, A., Lorimier, S., Emonard, H., et al., Contribution of the plasmin/matrix metalloproteinase cascade to the retraction of human fibroblast populated collagen lattices, *Molec. Cell Biol. Res. Commun.* 3, 173–180, 2000.
34. Moran, P., Li, W., Fan, B., et al., Pro-urokinase-type plasminogen activator is a substrate for hepsin, *J. Biol. Chem.* 281, 30439–30446, 2006.
35. Orgel, D., Schröder, W., Hecker-Kia, A., et al., The cleavage of pro-urokinase type plasminogen activator by stromelysin-1, *Clin. Chem. Lab. Med.* 35, 697–702, 1998.
36. List, K., Jensen, O.N., Bugge, T.H., et al., Plasminogen-independent initiation of the pro-urokinase activation cascade *in vivo*: Activation of pro-urokinase by glandular kallikrein (mGK-6) in plasminogen-deficient mice, *Biochemistry* 39, 508–415, 2000.
37. Hashimoto, M., Oiwa, K., Matsuo, O., et al., Suppression of argatroban-induced endogenous thrombolysis by PKSI-527, an antibodies to TPA and UPA, evaluated in a rat arterial thrombolysis model, *Thromb. Haemost.* 89, 820–825, 2003.
38. Ichinose, A., Fujikawa, K., and Suyama, T., The activation of pro-urokinase by plasma kallikrein and its inactivation by thrombin, *J. Biol. Chem.* 261, 3486–3489, 1986.
39. Beaufort, N., Debela, M., Creutzburg, S., et al., Interplay of human tissue kallikrein 4 (hK4) with the plasminogen activation system: hK4 regulates the structure and function of urokinase-type plasminogen activator receptor, *Biol. Chem.* 387, 217–222, 2006.
40. Choi-Miura, N.H., Yoda, M., Saito, K., Takahashi, K., and Tomita, M., Identification of the substrates for plasma hyaluronan binding protein, *Biol. Pharm. Bull.* 24, 140–143, 2001.
41. Choi-Miura, N.H., Novel human plasma proteins, IHRP (acute phase protein) and PHBP (serine protease), which bind to glycosaminoglycans, *Curr. Med. Chem. Cardiovasc. Hematol. Agents* 2, 239–248, 2004.
42. Kilpatrick, L.M., Harris, R.L., Owen, K.A., et al., Initiation of plasminogen activation on the surface of monocytes expressing the type II transmembrane serine protease matriptase, *Blood* 108, 2616–2623, 2006.
43. Chou, F.-P., Chen, Y.-W., Zhao, X.F., et al., Inbalanced matriptase pericellular proteolysis contributes to the pathogenesis of malignant B-cell lymphomas, *Am. J. Pathol.* 183, 1306–1317, 2013.
44. Demetriou, M.C., Pennington, M.E., Nagle, R.B., and Cress, A.E., Extracellular alpha 6 integrin cleavage by urokinase-type plasminogen activator in human prostate cancer, *Expt. Cell Res.* 294, 550–558, 2004.
45. Zorio, E., Gilabert-Estellés, J., España, F., et al., Fibrinolysis: The key to new pathogenetic mechanisms, *Curr. Med. Chem.* 15, 923–929, 2008.

46. Duffy, M.J., Maguire, T.M., McDermott, E.W., and O'Higgins, N., Urokinase plasminogen activator: A prognostic marker in multiple types of cancer, *J. Surg. Oncol.* 71, 130–135, 1999.

47. Harbeck, N., Schmitt, M., Meisner, C., et al., Ten-year analysis of the prospective multicenter Chemo-N0 trial validates American Society of Clinical Oncology (ASCO)-recommended biomarkers uPA and PAI-1 for therapy decision making in node-negative breast cancer patients, *Eur. J. Cancer* 49, 1825–1835, 2013.

48. Pannell, R. and Gurewich, V., Activation of plasminogen by single-chain urokinase or by two-chain urokinase: A demonstration that single-chain urokinase has a low catalytic activity (pro-urokinase), *Blood* 69, 22–26, 1987.

49. Braat, E.A., Levi, M., Bos, R., et al., Inactivation of single-chain urokinase-type plasminogen activator by thrombin in human subjects, *J. Lab. Clin. Med.* 134, 161–167, 1999.

50. Nauland, U. and Rijken, D.C., Activation of thrombin-inactivated single-chain urokinase-type plasminogen activator by dipeptidyl peptidase I (cathepsin C), *Eur. J. Biochem.* 223, 497–501, 1994.

51. Lijnen, H.R., Van Hoff, B., and Collen, D., Activation with plasmin of two-chain urokinase-type plasminogen activator derived from single-chain urokinase-type plasminogen activator by treatment with thrombin, *Eur. J. Biochem.* 169, 359–364, 1987.

52. Schenk-Braat, E.A., Morser, J., and Rijken, D.C., Identification of the epidermal growth factor-like domains of thrombomodulin essential for the acceleration of thrombin-mediated inactivation of single-chain urokinase-type plasminogen activator, *Eur. J. Biochem.* 268, 5562–5569, 2001.

53. Vassalli, J.D., Baccino, D., and Belin, D., A cellular binding site for the M_r 55,000 form of the human plasminogen activator, urokinase, *J. Cell. Biol.* 100, 86–92, 1985.

54. McNeill, H. and Jensen, P.J., A high-affinity receptor for urokinase plasminogen activator on human keratinocytes: Characterization and potential modulation during migration, *Cell Regul.* 1, 843–852, 1990.

55. Petersen, L.C., Kinetics of reciprocal pro-urokinase/plasminogen activation—stimulation by a template forme by the urokinase receptor bound to poly (D-lysine), *Eur. J. Biochem.* 245, 316–323, 1997.

56. Ellis, V., Functional analysis of the cellular receptor for urokinase in plasminogen activation: Receptor binding has no influence on the zymogenic nature of pro-urokinase, *J. Biol. Chem.* 271, 14779–14784, 1996.

57. Plesner, T., Behrendt, N., and Ploug, M., Structure, function and expression on blood and bone marrow cells of the urokinase-type plasminogen activator receptor, uPAR, *Stem Cells* 15, 398–408, 1997.

58. Stephens, R.W., Pedersen, A.N., Nielsen, H.J., et al., ELISA determination of soluble urokinase receptor in blood from health donors and cancer patients, *Clin. Chem.* 43, 1868–1876, 1997.

59. Montuori, N., Visconte, V., Rossi, G., and Ragno, P., Soluble and cleaved forms of the urokinase receptor: Degradation products on active molecules? *Thromb. Haemost.* 93, 192–198, 2005.

60. Chavakis, T., Willuweit, A.K., Lupu, F., Preissner, K.I., and Kanse, S.M., Release of soluble urokinase receptor from vascular cells, *Thromb. Haemost.* 86, 686–693, 2001.

61. Murakami, Y., Kanzawa, N., Saito, K., et al., Mechanism for release of alkaline phosphatase caused by glycosylphosphatidylinositol deficiency in patients with hyperphosphatasia metal retardation syndrome, *J. Biol. Chem.* 287, 6318–6325, 2012.

62. Toldi, G., Bekő, G., Kádár, G., et al., Soluble urokinase plasminogen activator receptor (suPAR) in the assessment of inflammatory activity of rheumatoid arthritis patients in remission, *Clin. Chem.* 51, 327–332, 2013.

63. Raggam, R.B., Wagner, J., and Prüller, F., Soluble urokinase plasminogen activator receptor predicts mortality in patients with systemic inflammatory response syndrome, *J. Intern. Med.* 276, 651–658, 2014.

64. Vasarheylyi, B., Soluble urokinase plasminogen activator receptor, the candidate prophetic biomarkers in severe inflammatory response syndrome, *J. Intern. Med.* 276, 645–647, 2014.

65. Skorecki, K.L. and Freedman, B.I., A suPAR biomarker for chronic kidney disease, *N. Engl. J. Med.* 373, 1971–1972, 2015.

66. Arbel, Y. and Strauss, B.H., suPAR: A cardiac biomarker with a future? *Can. J. Cardiol.* 31, 1223–1224, 2015.

67. Nayak, R.K., Allingstrup, M., Phanareth, K., and Kofoed-Enevoldsen, A., suPAR as a biomarker for risk of readmission and mortality in the acute medical setting, *Dan. Med. J.* 62, A5146, 2015.

68. Vaschetto, R., Navalesi, P., Clemente, N., et al., Osteopontin induces soluble urokinase-type plasminogen activator receptor production and release, *Minerva Anestesiol.* 81, 157–165, 2015.

69. Kunii, Y., Niwa, S., Hagiwara, Y., et al., The immunohistochemical expression profile of osteopontin in normal human tissues using two site-specific antibodies reveals a wide distribution of positive cells and extensive expression in the central and peripheral nervous systems, *Med. Mol. Morphol.* 42, 155–161, 2009.

70. Cheng, C., Gao, S., and Lei, G., Association of osteopontin with arthritis, *Rheumatol. Int.* 34, 1627–1631, 2014.

71. Zhang, F., Luo, W., Li, Y., Gao, S., and Lei, G., Role osteopontin in rheumatoid arthritis, *Rheumatol. Int.* 34, 1627–1631, 2014.

72. Nakae, M., Iwamoto, I., Fujino, T., et al., Preoperative plasma osteopontin levels as a biomarker complementary to carbohydrate antigen 125 in predicting ovarian cancer, *J. Obstet. Gynecol. Res.* 32, 309–314, 2006.

73. Eden, G., Archinti, M., Furlan, F., Murphy, R., and Degryse, B., The urokinase receptor interactome, *Curr. Pharm. Des.* 17, 1874–1889, 2011.

74. Madsen, C.D., Ferraris, G.M., Andolfo, A., Cunningham, O., and Sidenius, N., uPAR-induced cell adhesion and migration: Vitronectin provides the key, *J. Cell Biol.* 177, 927–939, 2007.

75. Smith, H.W. and Marshall, C.J., Regulation of cell signalling by uPAR, *Nature Rev. Mol. Cell Biol.* 11, 23–36, 2010.

76. Madsen, D.H., Engelholm, L.H., Ingvarsen, S., et al., Extracellular collagenases and the endocytic receptor, urokinase plasminogen activator receptor-associated protein/endo 180, cooperate in fibroblast-mediated collagen degradation, *J. Biol. Chem.* 282, 27037–27045, 2007.

77. Madsen, D.H., Ingvarsen, S., Jurgensen, H.J., et al., The non-phagocytic route of collagen uptake: A distinct pathway, *J. Biol. Chem.* 286, 26996–27020, 2011.

78. Jurgensen, H.J., Madsen, D.H., Ingvarsen, S., et al., A novel functional role of collagen glycosylation: Interaction with the endocytic collagen receptor, *J. Biol. Chem.* 286, 32736–32748, 2011.

79. Madsen, D.H., Leonard, D., Masedunskas, A., et al., M2-like macrophages are responsible for collagen degradation through a mannose receptor-mediated pathway, *J. Cell Biol.* 202, 951–966, 2013.

80. Sheikh, H., Yarwood, H., Ashworth, A., and Isacke, C.M., Endo180, an endocytic recycling glycoprotein related to the macrophage mannose receptor is expressed on fibroblasts, endothelial cells and macrophages and functions as a lectin receptor, *J. Cell Sci.* 113, 1021–1032, 2000.

81. Behrendt, N., Jensen, O.N., Engelholm, L.H., et al., A urokinase receptor–associated protein with specific collagen binding properties, *J. Biol. Chem.* 275, 1993–2002, 2000.

82. Behrendt, N., The urokinase receptor (uPAR) and the uPAR-associated protein (UPARAP/Endo180): Membrane proteins engaging in matrix turnover during tissue remodeling, *Biol. Chem.* 385, 103–136, 2004.

83. Jürgensen, H.J., Madsen, D.H., Ingvarsen, S., et al., A novel functional role of collagen glycosylation: Interaction with the endocytic collagen receptor uPARAP/Endo180, *J. Biol. Chem.* 32736–32746, 2011.

84. Eberhard, T., Ullberg, M., Sjöström, I., Kronvall, G., and Wiman, B., Enhancement of t-PA-mediated plasminogen activation by bacterial surface receptors, *Fibrinolysis* 9, 65–70, 1995.

85. Bhattacharya, S., Ploplis, V.A., and Castellino, F.J., Bacterial plasminogen receptors utilize host plasminogen system for effective invasion and dissemination, *J. Biomed. Biotechnol.* 2012, 482096, 2012.

86. Pancholi, V. and Fischetti, V.A., α-Enolase, a novel strong plasmin(ogen) binding protein on the surface of pathogenic streptococci, *J. Biol. Chem.* 273, 14503–14315, 1998.

87. Bergmann, S., Rohde, M., Chhatwal, G.S., and Hammerschmidt, S., α-Enolase of *Streptococcus pneumoniae* is a plasmin(ogen)-binding protein displayed on the bacterial cell surface, *Mol. Microbiol.* 40, 1273–1287, 2001.

88. Bergmann, S., Rohde, M., Preissner, K.T., and Hammerschmidt, S., The nine residue plasminogen-binding motif of the pneumococcal enolase is the major cofactor of plasmin-mediated degradation of extracellular matrix, dissolution of fibrin and transmigration, *Thromb. Haemost.* 94, 304–311, 2005.

89. Verhamme, I.M., Panizzi, P.R., and Bock, P.E., Pathogen activators of plasminogen, *J. Thromb. Haemost.* 13(Suppl. 1), S106–S114, 2015.

90. Magalhaes, V., Andrade, E.B., Alves, J., et al., Group B streptococcus hijacks the host plasminogen system to promote brain endothelial cell invasion, *PLoS One* 8(5), e63244, 2013.

91. Hollands, A., Gonzalez, D., and Leire, E., A bacterial pathogen co-opts plasmin to resist killing by cathelicidin antimicrobial peptides, *J. Biol. Chem.* 287, 40891–40897, 2012.

92. Chandrahas, V., Glinton, K., Liang, Z., et al., Direct host plasminogen binding to bacterial surface M-protein in pattern D strains of *Streptococcus pyogenes* is required for activation by its natural coinherited SK2b protein, *J. Biol. Chem.* 290, 18833–18842, 2015.

93. Castellino, F.J. and Ploplis, V.A., Structure and function of the plasminogen/plasmin system, *Thromb. Haemost.* 93, 647–654, 2005.

94. Plow, E.F., Doeuvre, L., and Das, R., So many plasminogen receptors: Why? *J. Biomed. Biotechnol.* 2012, 141806, 2012.

95. Miles, L.A. and Parmer, R.J., Plasminogen receptors: The first quarter century, *Semin. Thromb. Hemost.* 39, 329–337, 2011.

96. Hajjar, K.A., Jacovina, A.T., and Chacko, J., An endothelial cell receptor for plasminogen/tissue plasminogen activator: I. Identity with annexin II, *J. Biol. Chem.* 269, 21191–21197, 1994.

97. van Hinsbergh, V.W., Koolwijk, P., and Hanaemaaijer, R., Role of fibrin and plasminogen activators in repair-associated angiogenesis: *In vitro* studies with human endothelial cells, *EXS* 79, 391–411, 1997.

98. Massay-Harroche, D., Mayran, N., and Maroux, S., Polarized localizations of annexins I, II, VI, and XIII in epithelial cells of intestinal, hepatic and pancreatic tissues, *J. Cell Sci.* 111, 3007–3015, 1998.

99. Gonzalez-Gronow, M., Grenett, H.E., Weber, M.R., Gawdi, G., and Pizzo, S.V., Interaction of plasminogen with dipeptidyl peptidase IV initiates a signal transduction mechanism which regulates expression of matrix metalloproteinase-9 by prostate cancer cells, *Biochem. J.* 355, 397–407, 2001.

100. Gonzalez-Gronow, M., Kaczowka, A., Gawdi, G., and Pizzo, S.V., Dipeptidyl peptidase IV (DPP IV/CD26) is a cell-surface plasminogen receptor, *Front. Biosci.* 13, 1610–1618, 2008.

101. Gonzalez-Gronow, M., Grenett, H.E., Gawdi, G., and Pizzo, S.V., Angiostatin directly inhibits human prostate tumor cell invasion by blocking plasminogen binding to its cellular receptor, CD26, *Exp. Cell Res.* 303, 22–31, 2005.

102. Fleetwood, A.J., Achuthan, A., Scultz, H., et al., Urokinase plasminogen activator is a central regulator of macrophage three-dimensional invasion, matrix degradation, and adhesion, *J. Immunol.* 192, 3540–3547, 2014.

103. Phipps, K.D., Surette, A.P., O'Connell, P.A., and Waisman, D.M., Plasminogen receptor S100A10 is essential for migration of tumor-promoting macrophages into tumor sites, *Cancer Res.* 71, 6676–6683, 2011.

104. Lighvani, S., Balk, N., Diggs, J.E., et al., Regulation of macrophage migration by a novel plasminogen receptor Plg-RKT, *Blood* 118, 5622–5630, 2011.

105. Lishko, V.K., Novokhatry, V.V., Yakubenko, V.P., Skomorovska-Prokvolit, H.V., and Ugarova, T.P., Characterization of plasminogen as an adhesive ligand for integrins $\alpha_m\beta_2$ and $\alpha_5\beta_1$ (VLA-5), *Blood* 104, 719–726, 2004.

106. Winn, E.S., Hu, S.P., Hochschwender, S.M., and Laursen, R.A., Studies on the lysine-binding sites of human plasminogen: The effect of ligand structure on the binding of lysine analogs on plasminogen, *Eur. J. Biochem.* 104, 579–586, 1980.

107. Adelman, B. and Quynn, P., Plasminogen interactions with immobilized fibrinogen, *Thromb. Haemost.* 62, 1078–1082, 1989.

108. Zamarron, C., Ginsberg, M.H., and Plow, E.F., Monoclonal antibodies specific for a conformationally altered state of fibrinogen, *Thromb. Haemost.* 64, 41–46, 1990.

109. Bok, R.A. and Mangel, W.F., Quantitative characterization of the binding of plasminogen to intact fibrin clots, lysine-sepharose, and fibrin cleaved by plasmin, *Biochemistry* 24, 3279–3286, 1985.

110. Hoylaerts, M., Lijnen, H.R., and Collen, D., Studies on the mechanism of the antifibrinolytic action of tranexamic acid, *Biochim. Biophys. Acta* 673, 75–85, 1981.

111. Schaller, J. and Gerber, S.S., The plasmin-antiplasmin system: Structural and functional aspects, *Cell. Mol. Life Sci.* 68, 785–801, 2011.

112. Law, R.H., Abu-Ssaydeh, D., and Whisstock, J.C., New insights into the structure and function of the plasminogen/plasmin system, *Curr. Opin. Struct. Biol.* 23, 836–941, 2013.

113. Pirie-Shepard, S.R., Jett, E.A., Andon, N.L., and Pizzo, S.V., Sialic acid content of plasminogen 2 glycoforms as a regulator of fibrinolytic activity: Isolation, carbohydrate analysis, and kinetic characterization of six glycoforms of plasminogen, *J. Biol. Chem.* 270, 5877–5881, 1995.

114. Mølgaard, L., Ponting, C.P., and Christensen, U., Glycosylation at Asn-289 facilitates the ligand-induced conformational changes of human Glu-plasminogen, *FEBS Lett.* 405, 363–368, 1997.

115. Francis, C.W. and Marder, V.J., Physiologic regulation and pathologic disorders of fibrinolysis, *Hum. Pathol.* 18, 263–274, 1987.

116. He, C., Wilhelm, S.M., Pentland, A.P., et al., Tissue cooperation in a proteolytic cascade activating human interstitial collagenase, *Proc. Natl. Acad. Sci. USA* 86, 2632–2636, 1989.

117. Sane, D.C., Moser, T.L., and Greenberg, C.S., Limited proteolysis of vitronectin by plasmin destroys heparin binding activity, *Thromb. Haemost.* 66, 310–314, 1991.

118. Chain, D., Kreizman, T., Shapira, H., and Shaltiel, S., Plasmin cleavage of vitronectin: Identification of the site and consequent attenuation in binding plasminogen activator inhibitor-1, *FEBS Lett.* 285, 251–256, 1991.

119. Kazanov, M.D., Igarashi, Y., Eroshkin, A.M., et al., Structural determinants of limited proteolysis, *J. Proteome Res.* 10, 3642–3651, 2011.

120. Santana, A., Saarinen, I.J., Kovanen, P., and Kunsela, P., Activation of interstitial collagenase, MMP-1, by *Staphylococcus aureus* cells having surface-bound plasmin: A novel role of plasminogen receptors of bacteria, *FEBS Lett.* 461, 153–156, 1999.

121. Suzuki, K., Enghild, J.J., Morodomi, T., Salvesen, G., and Nagase, H., Mechanisms of activation of tissue procollagenase by matrix metalloproteinase 3 (stromelysin), *Biochemistry* 29, 10261–10270, 1990.

122. McLaughlin, B. and Weiss, J.B., Endothelial-cell-stimulating angiogenesis factor (ESAF) activates progelatinase A (72 Kd type IV collagenase), prostomelysin 1 and procollagenase and reactivates their complexes with tissue inhibitors of metalloproteinases: A role of ESAF in non-inflammatory angiogenesis, *Biochem. J.* 317, 739–745, 1996.

123. Van den Steen, P.E., Opdenakker, G., Wormald, M.R., Dwek, R.A., and Rudd, P.M., Matrix remodeling enzymes, the protease cascade and glycosylation, *Biochim. Biophys. Acta* 1528, 61–71, 2001.

124. Remacle-Bonnet, M.M., Garrouste, F.L., and Pommier, G.J., Surface-bound plasmin induces selective proteolysis of insulin-like-growth-factor (IGF)-binding protein-4 (IGFBP-4) and promotes autocrine IGF-II bio-availability in human colon-carcinoma cells, *Int. J. Cancer* 72, 835–843, 1997.

125. Horwitz, J.C., Rogers, D.S., Simon, R.H., Sisson, T.H., and Tahnnickal, V.J., Plasminogen activation–induced pericellular fibronectin proteolysis promotes fibroblast apoptosis, *Am. J. Respir. Cell Mol. Biol.* 38, 78–87, 2008.

126. Viera, M.L., Vasconcellos, S.A., Goncales, A.P., de Morais, Z.M., and Nascimento, A.L.T.O., Plasminogen acquisition and activation at the surface of *Leptospira* species lead to fibronectin degradation, *Infection. Immun.* 77, 4092–4101, 2009.

127. Liotta, L.A., Goldfarb, R.H., Brundage, R., et al., Effect of plasminogen activator (urokinase), plasmin, and thrombin on glycoprotein and collagenous components of basement membrane, *Cancer Res.* 41, 4629–4636, 1981.

128. Leblond, C.P. and Inoue, S., Structure, composition, and assembly of basement membrane, *Am. J. Anat.* 185, 367–390, 1989.

129. Inoue, S., Basic structure of basement membrane is a fine network of "cords," irregular anastomosing strands, *Microsc. Res. Tech.* 28, 29–47, 1994.

130. Jones, P.A. and De Clerk, Y.A., Extracellular matrix destruction by invasive tumor cells, *Cancer Metastasis Rev.* 1, 289–317, 1982.

131. Cohen, R.L., Xi, X.P., Crowlye, C.W., et al., Effects of urokinase receptor occupancy on plasmin generation and proteolysis of basement membrane by human tumor cells, *Blood* 78, 479–487, 1991.

132. Wygrecka, M., Jablonska, E., Guenther, A., et al., Current view on alveolar coagulation and fibrinolysis in acute inflammatory and chronic interstitial lung diseases, *Thromb. Haemost.* 99, 494–501, 2008.

133. Gharaee-Kermani, M., Hu, B., Phan, S.H., and Gyetko, M.R., The role of urokinase in idiopathic pulmonary fibrosis and implication for therapy, *Expert Opin. Investig. Drugs* 17, 905–916, 2008.

134. Eddy, A.A., Serine proteases, inhibitors and receptors in renal fibrosis, *Thromb. Haemost.* 101, 656–664, 2009.

135. Schuliga, M., Westall, G., Xia, Y., and Stewart, A.G., The plasminogen system: New targets in lung inflammation and remodeling, *Curr. Opin. Pharmacol.* 13, 386–393, 2013.

136. Preissner, K.T. and Seiffert, D., Role of vitronectin and its receptors in haemostasis and vascular remodeling, *Thromb. Res.* 89, 1–21, 1998.
137. Preissner, K.T. and Running, U., Vitronectin in vascular context: Facets of a multitalented matricellular protein, *Semin. Thromb. Hemost.* 37, 408–424, 2011.
138. Völker, W., Hess, S., Vischer, P., and Preissner, K.T., Binding and processing of multimeric vitronectin by vascular endothelial cells, *J. Histochem. Cytochem.* 41, 1823–1832, 1993.
139. Preissner, K.T. and Pötzsch, B., Vessel wall–dependent metabolic pathways of adhesive proteins, von-Willebrand-factor and vitronectin, *Histol. Histopathol.* 10, 239–251, 1995.
140. de Boer, H.C., Preissner, K.T., Bouma, B.N., and de Groot, P.G., Internalization of vitronectin–thrombin–antithrombin complex by endothelial cells leads to deposition of the complex into the subendothelial matrix, *J. Biol. Chem.* 270, 30733–30740, 1995.
141. Wun, T.C., Palmier, M.O., Siegel, N.R., and Smith, C.E., Affinity purification of active plasminogen activator inhibitor-1 (PAI-1) using immobilized anhydrourokinase: Demonstration of the binding, stabilization, and activation of PAI-1 by vitronectin, *J. Biol. Chem.* 264, 7862–7868, 1989.
142. Naski, M.C., Lawrence, D.A., Mosher, D.F., et al., Kinetics of inactivation of α-thrombin by plasminogen activator inhibitor-1: Comparison of the effects of native and urea-treated forms of vitronectin, *J. Biol. Chem.* 268, 12367–12372, 1993.
143. Waltz, D.A., Natkin, L.R., Fujita, R.M., et al., Plasmin and plasminogen activator inhibitor type 1 promote cellular motility by regulating the interaction between the urokinase receptor and vitronectin, *J. Clin. Invest.* 100, 58–67, 1997.
144. Suzuki, S., Pierschbacher, M.D., Hayman, E.G., et al., Domain structure of vitronectin: Alignment of active sites, *J. Biol. Chem.* 259, 15307–15314, 1984.
145. Wilkins-Port, C.E. and McKeown-Longo, P.J., Heparan sulfate proteoglycans functions in the binding and degradation of vitronectin by fibroblast monolayers, *Biochem. Cell. Biol.* 74, 887–897, 1996.
146. Ehrlich, H.J., Keijer, J., Preissner, K.T., et al., Functional interaction of plasminogen activator inhibitor type 1 (PAI-1) and heparin, *Biochemistry* 30, 1021–1028, 1991.
147. Nakamura, R., Umemura, K., Hashimmoto, H., and Urano, T., Less pronounced enhancement of thrombin-dependent inactivation of plasminogen activator inhibitor type 1 by low molecular weight heparin compared with unfractionated heparin, *Thromb. Haemost.* 95, 637–642, 2006.
148. Kost, C., Stüber, W., Ehrlich, H.J., et al., Mapping of binding sites for heparin, plasminogen activator inhibitor-1, and plasminogen to vitronectin's heparin-binding region reveals a novel vitronectin-dependent feedback mechanism for the control of plasmin formation, *J. Biol. Chem.* 267, 12098–12105, 1992.
149. Mesnard, L., Ratat, G., Vandermeesch, S., et al., Vitronectin dictates intraglomerular fibrinolysis in immune-mediated glomerulonephritis, *FASEB J.* 25, 3543–3543, 2011.
150. Idell, S., James, K.K., Gillies, C., Fair, D.S., and Thrall, R.S., Abnormalities of pathways of fibrin turnover in lung lavage of rats with oleic acid and bleomycin-induced lung injury support alveolar fibrin deposition, *Am. J. Pathol.* 135, 381–399, 1989.
151. Stump, D.C., Thienpot, M., and Collen, D., Purification and characterization of a novel inhibitor of urokinase from human urine: Quantification and preliminary characterization in plasma, *J. Biol. Chem.* 261, 12759–12766, 1986.
152. Heeb, M.J., España, F., Geiger, M., et al., Immunological identity of a heparin-dependent plasma and urinary protein C inhibitor and plasminogen activator inhibitor 3, *J. Biol. Chem.* 262, 15813–15816, 1987.
153. Suzuki, K., The multi-functional serpin, protein C inhibitor: Beyond thrombosis and hemostasis, *J. Thromb. Haemost.* 6, 2017–2026, 2008.

154. Szabo, R., Netzel-Arnett, S., Hobson, J.P., Anatlis, T.M., and Bugge, T.H., Matriptase-3 is a novel phylogenetically preserved membrane anchored serine protease with broad serpin reactivity, *Biochem. J.* 390, 231–242, 2005.
155. Fujimoto, H., Gabazza, E.C., Hataji, O., et al., Thrombin-activatable fibrinolysis inhibitor and protein C inhibitor in interstitial lung disease, *Am. J. Respir. Crit. Care Med.* 167, 1687–1694, 2003.
156. Aoki, N., Moroi, M., Matsuda, M., and Tachiya, K., The behavior of α_2-plasmin inhibitor in fibrinolytic states, *J. Clin. Invest.* 60, 361–369, 1977.
157. Moroi, M. and Aoki, N., Isolation and characterization of α_2-plasmin inhibitor from human plasma: A novel proteinase inhibitor which inhibits activator-induced clot lysis, *J. Biol. Chem.* 251, 5956–5965, 1976.
158. Wang, H., Pap, S., and Wiman, B., Inactivation of plasmin inhibitor at low pH: Evidence for the formation of latent molecules, *Thromb. Res.* 114, 301–306, 2004.
159. Kanno, Y., Kuroki, A., Okada, K., et al., α_2-Antiplasmin is involved in the production of transforming growth factor β_1 and fibosis, *J. Thromb. Haemost.* 5, 2266–2273, 2007.
160. Hou, Y.Z., Okada, K., Okamoto, C., Ueshima, S., and Mastuo, O., Alpha2-antiplasmin is a critical regulator of angiotensin II-mediated remodeling, *Arterioscler. Thromb. Vas. Biol.* 28, 1257–1262, 2008.

6 Kallikrein in the Interstitial Space

6.1 KALLIKREIN

Kallikrein is a functional activity defined by the ability of kallikreins (kininogenases) to form kinins (vasoactive peptides) from kininogens.[1] Early work defined two types of kallikrein, plasma kallikrein (KLK-B1) and tissue (glandular) kallikrein (KLK-1), which differed in distribution, size, and specificity. KLK-B1 (PK) is a plasma protein with a molecular weight of 80–90 kDa depending on the extent of glycosylation, while KLK-1 (TK) has a molecular weight of approximately 40 kDa.[2] More recent work has identified KLK-1 as a member of a family described as kallikrein-like peptidases (KLKs; Table 6.1).[3] Both KLK-B1 and KLK-1 are synthesized as precursor or zymogen forms—prekallikrein in the case of KLK-B1 and prokallikrein in the case of KLK-1—which require activation for full activity (Figure 6.1).

While KLK-B1 and KLK-1 have been suggested to have biologically important activity, there has been little consideration of their function in the interstitial space. Most of the work of KLK-B1 has focused on its synthesis in hepatocytes and secretion as prekallikrein into the vascular space. KLK-1 is primarily a protein secreted by the salivary glands and the pancreas and is also found in urine as a product of the kidney. KLK-1 has been looking for a function for a number of years, although it has had some interesting diagnostic and therapeutic applications. It is only recently that there has been some interest in the function of these enzymes in the interstitial space, and that interest seems to have been largely driven by the discovery of the various members of the KLK family of proteases. However, much of the work has been performed with little, if any, appreciation of the function of KLKs in the interstitial space. The following discussion will review studies supporting the presence and possible function of these enzymes in the interstitial space.

6.2 PLASMA KALLIKREIN

KLK-B1 will liberate kinin activity from high-molecular-weight kininogen (HMWK), while KLK-1 will liberate kinin activity from HMWK or low-molecular-weight kininogen (LMWK).[4] Plasma prekallikrein is known to participate in the contact phase of blood coagulation and is thought to circulate as a complex with HMWK.[5] While KLK-B1 is thought to have a primary role in blood coagulation, kinin generation, and complement in the vascular space, there is evidence to suggest that there is a considerable function for KLK-B1 in the interstitial space. Tsurata and coworkers[6] used immunohistochemistry to demonstrate the presence of factor XII and HMWK in the interstitial space of various organs, including the skin, liver, and kidney. These investigators suggested that synthesis of both factor XII and HMWK

TABLE 6.1

Kallikrein-Related Peptidases in the Interstitial Space

Kallikrein-Related Peptidase[a]	Specificity	Potential Substrates in the Interstitium[b]	Refs.
KLK-1 (classical tissue or glandular kallikrein; primary sites of synthesis in pancreas, kidney, and salivary glands; wide tissue distribution[1,2,3])	Cleavage of arginine–serine and methionine–lysine peptide bonds in kininogens; synthetic substrates include chromogenic arginine and lysine peptide nitroanilides[4,5]	Kininogen,[6,7] VEGF,[8] MMP zymogen,[9,10] IGFBP,[11] PAR,[12] pro-KLK-2,[13] pro-KLK-4,[13] pro-KLK-5,[13] pro-KLK-6,[13] pro-KLK-12,[13] pro-KLK-14[13]	1–13
KLK-2 (human glandular kallikrein 1; exclusive in the prostate[1])	Strict specificity for arginine-containing peptide bonds[14]	IGFBP-3,[15] fibronectin,[16,17] PSA,[16,18] semenogelin I,[17] semenogelin II,[17] uPA zymogen,[19] pro-KLK-2,[13] pro-KLK-4,[13] KLK-12,[13] KLK-14[13]	1,14–19
KLK-3 (prostate-specific antigen; exclusive in prostate[1])[c]	Cleavage at tyrosine-, phenylalanine-, and leucine-containing peptide bonds (chymotryptic-like specificity)[20,21]	May have antiangiogenic activity,[22,23] pro-KLK-2,[13] pro-KLK-4,[12] pro-KLK-5,[13] pro-KLK-6,[13] pro-KLK-7,[13] pro-KLK-12,[13] pro-KLK-14[13]	1,20–23
KLK-4 (prostase; wide distribution,[1] including prostate and enamel;[24,25] expressed in ovarian cancer[24,26])	Preference for arginine-containing peptide bonds[27,28]	PAR-1,[29] prourokinase,[30,31] pro-KLK-11,[30] pro-KLK-3,[31] uPAR,[32] enamelin,[33,d] amelogenin,[34] metalloproteinase meprin β[35]	1,24–35
KLK-5 (human stratum corneum tryptic enzyme [SCTE]; found in skin and breast tissue;[1,36] ovarian cancer[37])	Preference for cleavage of arginine peptide bonds; also cleavage of lysine peptide bonds[38]	Profilaggrin,[39] PAR-2,[40] plasminogen,[41] human-adapted influenza virus,[42] metalloproteinase meprin α and β,[35] pro-KLK-5,[13] pro-KLK-14[13]	1,36–42
KLK-6 (protease M; found in brain, pancreas;[1,43] proposed biomarker for ovarian cancer, brain trauma[44,45])	Preference for arginine peptide bonds; less for lysine in physiological substrates; broader specificity with peptide substrates[27,28]	Autoactivation,[46,47] fibrinogen,[47] collagen,[47,48] plasminogen,[47] vitronectin,[48] PAR-1,[49,50] PAR-2,[49] pro-KLK-4,[13] pro-KLK-5[13]	1,43–50
KLK-7 (human stratum corneum chymotryptic enzyme [SCCE]; found in skin, esophagus, heart, pancreas[1,51,52])	Preference for tyrosine peptide bonds (chymotryptic-like specificity);[27,28,53] activated by metalloproteinases meprin α or β[35]	Interleukin-1β,[54] E-cadherin,[55] fibronectin,[56] uPAR,[57] desmoglein 2,[58] pro-MMP-9,[59] caspase 14,[60] prochemerin,[61] pro-KLK-5[13]	1,51–61

TABLE 6.1 (CONTINUED)
Kallikrein-Related Peptidases in the Interstitial Space

Kallikrein-Related Peptidase[a]	Specificity	Potential Substrates in the Interstitium[b]	Refs.
KLK-8 (neuropsin; found in brain, skin, breast[1,62–66])	Preference for cleavage of arginine peptide bonds	PAR-1,[67,e] PAR-2,[67] fibronectin,[68] collagen IV,[68] fibrinogen,[68] HMWK,[68] single-chain tPA,[68] ephrin type-B receptor 2 (EphB2),[69] meprin β[35]	1,62–69
KLK-9 (wide tissue distribution;[1,70–72] ovarian tumors,[73] breast tumors[74])	Preference for arginine peptide bonds	pro-KLK-2,[13,75] pro-KLK-4,[13] pro-KLK-5,[13] pro-KLK-11,[13] pro-KLK-12,[13] pro-KLK-13,[13] pro-KLK-14[13]	1,70–75
KLK-10 (normal epithelial cell–specific 1 [NES1]; serine protease; wide tissue distribution[1,76–83])	Preference for arginine peptide bonds; cleavage also at lysine peptide bonds	pro-KLK-14,[13] measurement of expression is based on immunohistochemistry or nucleic acid technology (RT-PCR)[f]	1,76–83
KLK-11 (hippostasin; trypsin-like serine protease [TLSP]; wide tissue distribution[1] with various isoforms[–84–87])	Preference for arginine peptide bonds in physiological substrates; cleavage of methionine, lysine peptide bonds in combinatorial peptide library[27]	IGFBP-3,[88] pro-KLK-4,[13] pro-KLK-5,[13] pro-KLK-12,[13] pro-KLK-14[13]	1,84–88
KLK-12 (KLK-like 5; first identified by sequence analysis of the chromosomal region, encoding other members of the KLK family; may have isoforms showing wide tissue distribution[1,89–92])	Tryptic-like specificity for cleavage of arginine and lysine peptide bonds[93]	pro-KLK-12,[93,g] pro-KLK-11,[93] CCN family of matricellular proteins,[94,h] human-adapted influenza virus,[43] membrane-bound platelet-derived growth factor B,[95] HMWK[96,i]	1,89–96
KLK-13 (KLK-L4)[1,92,97–100]	Specificity for the cleavage of arginine and lysine peptide bonds;[97] activated by citrate, sulfate, and heparin[j]	Histatin C,[101,k] myelin basic proteins,[101,k] HMWK,[99,l] ECM proteins;[102,m] also inhibited by several members of the serpin family[103,104,n]	1,92,97–104
KLK-14 (KLK-L6; wide tissue distribution[1,105,106])	Specificity for the cleavage of arginine and lysine peptides bonds with preference for arginine peptide bonds;[107–110] proenzyme form activated by KLK-5[13,105]	PAR-2,[41,65,109] fibronectin,[107] collagen I,[107] collagen IV,[107] fibrinogen,[107] HMWK,[107] IGFBP-3,[107] pro-KLK-1,[111] pro-KLK-3,[111] pro-KLK-5,[112] pro-KLK-11,[111] latent TGF-β1,[113] complement factor C3[114]	1,105–114

(Continued)

TABLE 6.1 (CONTINUED)
Kallikrein-Related Peptidases in the Interstitial Space

Kallikrein-Related Peptidase[a]	Specificity	Potential Substrates in the Interstitium[b]	Refs.
KLK-15 (prostin; prostinogen; ACO protease; hK15; found in prostate, colon, thyroid[1,115–117])	Preference for cleavage of arginine and lysine peptide bonds;[75,115,117] presence of glutamic acid residue instead of aspartic acid residue at position 189[115] in amino acid sequence may promote preference for cleavage at lysine peptide bonds[75,119]	pro-KLK-3 (pro-PSA),[115,117] pro-KLK-1,[117] pro-KLK-2,[117] pro-KLK-7,[117] pro-KLK-8,[117] pro-KLK-9,[117] pro-KLK-14,[117] pro-KLK-15 (autocatalytic activation)[117,118]	1, 115–119
Plasma kallikrein (KLK-B1; formed from plasma prekallikrein [Fletcher factor]; primary site of synthesis in hepatocytes but found in a number of other tissues, including brain;[120,121] increased expression in monocytes suggested as biomarker for CLL[122])	Preference for arginine and lysine peptide bonds	Substrates include HMWK,[123,o] pro-uPA,[124] PK-120 glycoprotein,[125] ECM proteins contained in astrocyte secretome[126]	120–126

Note: This table is a listing of human KLKs. The rat and mouse KLK family is somewhat more complex (see Lundwall, A., et al., *Biol. Chem.* 387, 637–641, 2006). The reader is directed to several recent reviews for additional information on this family of proteases (Rawlings, N.D. and Barrett, A.J., Introduction: Serine peptidases and their clans, in *Handbook of Proteolytic Enzymes*, 3rd edn., eds. N.D. Rawlings and G. Salvesen, Chapter 559, pp. 2491–2525, Academic Press/Elsevier, Amsterdam, the Netherlands, 2013; Clements, J.A., et al., The human tissue kallikrein and kallikrein-related peptidase family, in *Handbook of Proteolytic Enzymes*, 3rd edn., eds. N.D. Rawlings and G. Salvesen, Chapter 606, pp. 2809–2813, Academic Press/Elsevier, Amsterdam, the Netherlands, 2013). It is noted that there has only been direct measurement of KLK-1 and KLK-B1 in lymph, presumably derived from interstitial fluid.

[a] This is a compilation of the various human KLKs (Lundwall, A. and Brattsand, M., Kallikrein-related peptidases, *Cell. Mol. Life. Sci.* 65, 2019–2038, 2008; Clements, J.A., et al., The human tissue kallikrein and kallikrein-related peptidase family, in *Handbook of Proteolytic Enzymes*, Vol. 3., eds. N.D. Rawlings and G. Salvesen, Chapter 606, pp. 2747–2756, Elsevier/Academic Press, Amsterdam, the Netherlands, 2013) as well as KLK-B1 (Björkqvist, J., et al., *Thromb. Haemost.* 110, 399–407, 2013).

TABLE 6.1 (CONTINUED)
Kallikrein-Related Peptidases in the Interstitial Space

[b] This is a listing of potential substrates for individual KLKs based on *in vitro* demonstration of cleavage(s). There is an absence of data supporting *in vivo* action. It should also be noted that the *in vitro* assays do not necessarily reflect the *in vivo* interstitial environment. For example, while hyaluronan is a major component of the interstitial space, we could not find any *in vitro* studies that included this anionic polymer, notwithstanding the several examples of an effect of polyvalent anions. A number of the cited studies suggest a cascade for the interaction of various kallikreins and prokallikreins, such as those proposed for blood coagulation and complement formation (Neurath, H. and Walsh, K.A., *Proc. Nal. Acad. Sci. USA* 73, 3825–3832, 1976). The formation of activation complexes that results in the removal of reactants from bulk solution to a local environment (e.g., Mann, K.G., et al., *Annu. Rev. Biochem.* 57, 915–956, 1988) greatly increases the catalytic efficiency of such processes. It is not unlikely that such complexes might function in the kallikrein cascades (Pampalakis, G. and Sotiropoulou, G., *Biochim. Biophys. Acta* 1776, 22–31, 2007). It is most likely that the physiological action of kallikrein(s) is at the local level in autocrine or paracrine action (Ma, J.X., et al., *Exp. Eye Res.* 63, 19–26, 1996).

[c] KLK-3 is better known as PSA, a diagnostic/prognostic biomarker for prostate cancer (Garg, V., et al., *Expert Rev. Pharmacoecon. Outcomes Res.* 13, 327–342, 2013).

[d] Only genetic evidence is available to support the importance of KLK-4 in humans; there are data on the processing of 32 kDa enamelin by KLK-4 (Yamakoshi, Y., et al., *Eur. J. Oral Sci.* 114[Suppl. 1], 45–51, 2006).

[e] PAR-1 on HEK cells is disarmed by KLK-8. Disarming refers to proteolysis of PAR-1, preventing its ability to activate following the cleavage of a specific peptide bond. The receptor can still be activated by a peptide but cannot be activated by a specific protease (see Dulon, S., et al., *Am. J. Respir. Cell Mol. Biol.* 28, 339–346, 2003).

[f] The presence of inhibitors in biological fluids might frustrate the measurement of KLKs (Oikonomopoulou, K., et al., *Biol. Chem.* 391, 381–390, 2010).

[g] KLK-12 undergoes autoactivation, as also seen with blood coagulation factor VII (Pedersen, A.H., et al., *Biochemistry* 28, 9331–9336, 1989). A factor VII–activating protease (FSAP) that binds hyaluronan has been described (Yamamichi, S., et al., *Biochem. Biophys. Res. Commun.* 489, 483–488, 2011). It should be noted that there is a recent study suggesting that FSAP does not activate factor VII (Stavenuiter, F., et al., *J. Thromb. Haemost.* 10, 859–866, 2012). The issue here is that the action of KLKs most likely occurs within the interstitial space, of which hyaluronan is a major component (Section 6.1). Thrombin also activates pro-KLK-12 (Yoon, H., et al., *Protein Sci.* 17, 1998–2007, 2008).

[h] The CCN family of proteins (CYR61; CTGF; NOV; Chen, C.C. and Lau, L.F., Functions and mechanisms of action of CCN matricellular proteins, *Int. J. Biochem. Cell Biol.* 41, 771–783, 2009) are matricellular proteins. Matricellular proteins are ECM proteins that may be involved in a variety of processes, including wound healing (Jun, J.I. and Lau, L.F., Taking aim at the extracellular matrix: CCN proteins as emerging therapeutic targets, *Nat. Rev. Drug Discov.* 10, 945–963, 2011). Cleavage of the CCN membrane proteins may influence the binding of various peptide growth factors.

[i] While there is facile cleavage of HMWK at the carboxyl-terminal end of the kinin sequence, liberation of kinin activity is poor because of poor cleavage at the amino-terminal end of the kinin sequence.

[j] Peptidase activity measured with a FRET peptide substrate (e.g., George, J., et al., Evaluation of an imaging platform during the development of a FRET protease assay, *J. Biomol. Screen.* 8, 72–80, 2003).

[k] Histatin C and myelin basic proteins were the only "protein" substrates evaluated in this study. The use of a matrix-bound peptide library as substrates for KLK-13 demonstrated cleavage of sequences consistent with a number of other proteins as potential substrates.

(Continued)

TABLE 6.1 (CONTINUED)
Kallikrein-Related Peptidases in the Interstitial Space

[l] HMWK was demonstrated to be a substrate for KLK-13, but there is only limited formation of kinin. See footnote j.

[m] Degradation of several ECM proteins by KLK-13 was evaluated by electrophoresis/Western blot. Rapid degradation of laminin was observed; degradation of collagen I, collagen II, collagen III, and fibronectin was also observed but less striking.

[n] Inhibition of KLK-13 was observed with α_2-antiplasmin, α_2-macroglobulin, α_1-antichymotrypin, protein C inhibitor, PAI-1, antithrombin, kallistatin, and C1-INH.

[o] See Section 6.2 for a more extensive discussion of KLK-B1 in the interstitial space.

REFERENCES FOR TABLE 6.1

1. Shaw, J.L.V. and Diamandis, E.P., Distribution of 15 human kallikreins in tissues and biological fluids, *Clin. Chem.* 53, 1423–1432, 2007.
2. Del Nery, F., Chagas, J.R., Juliano, M.A., et al., Evaluation of the binding site in human tissue kallikrein by synthetic substrates with sequences of human kininogen fragments, *Biochem. J.* 312, 233–238, 1995.
3. Chao, J., Human kallikrein 1, tissue kallikrein, in *Handbook of Proteolytic Enzymes*, eds. N.D.Rawlings and G. Salvesen, Vol. 3., Chapter 607, pp. 2751–2761, Elsevier, Amsterdam, Netherlands, 2013.
4. Del Nery, E., Chagas, J.R., Juliano, M.A., et al., Comparison of human and porcine tissue kallikrein substrate specificies, *Immunopharmacology* 45, 151–157, 1999.
5. Sousa, M.O., Miranda, T.L., Maia, C.N., et al., Kinetic peculiarities of human tissue kallikrein: 1-substrate activation in the catalyzed hydrolysis of H-D-valyl-L-arginine 4-nitroanilide and H-D-valyl-L-lysine 4-nitroanilide; 2-substrate inhibition in the catalyzed hydrolysis of Nα-*p*-tosyl-L-arginine methyl ester, *Arch. Biochem. Biophys.* 400, 7–14, 2002.
6. Proud, D. and Kaplan, A.P., Kinin formation: Mechanisms and role in inflammatory disorders, *Annu. Rev. Immunol.* 6, 49–83, 1988.
7. Cassim, B., Shaw, O.M., Mazur, M., et al., Kallikreins, kininogens and kinin receptors on circulating and synovial fluid neutrophils: Role in kinin generation in rheumatoid arthritis, *Rheumatology* (Oxford) 48, 490–496, 2009.
8. Nakamura, S., Morimoto, N., Tsuruma, K., et al., Tissue kallikrein inhibits retinal neovascularization via cleavage of vascular endothelial growth factor-165, *Arterioscler. Thromb. Vasc. Biol.* 31, 1041–1048, 2011.
9. Rosenblum, G., Meroueh, S., Toth, M., et al., Molecular structures and dynamics of the stepwise activation of mechanism of a matrix metalloproteinase zymogen: Challenging the cysteine switch dogma, *J. Am. Chem. Soc.* 129, 13566–13574, 2007.
10. Corthorn, J. Rey, S., Chacón, C., et al., Spatio-temporal expression of MMP-2, MMP-9 and tissue kallikrein in uteroplacental units of the pregnant guinea-pig (*Cavia porcellus*), *Reprod. Biol. Endocrinol.* 5:27, 2007.
11. Geisert, R.D., Chamberlain, C.S., Vonnahme, K.A., et al., Possible role of kallikrein in proteolysis of insulin-like growth factor binding proteins during the oestrous cycle and early pregnancy in pigs, *Reproduction* 121, 719–728, 2001.
12. Gao, L., Smith, R.S., Chen, L.M., et al., Tissue kallikrein promotes prostate cancer cell migration and invasion via a protease-activated receptor-1-dependent signaling pathway, *Biol. Chem.* 391, 803–812, 2010.

13. Yoon, H., Laxmikanthan, G., Lee, J., et al., Activation profiles and regulatory cascades of the human kallikrein-related peptidases, *J. Biol. Chem.* 282, 31852–31864, 2007.
14. Cloutier, S.M., Chagas, J.R., Mach, J.P., et al., Substrate specificity of human kallikrein 2 (hK2) as determined by phage display technology, *Eur. J. Biochem.* 269, 2747–2754, 2002.
15. Hekim, C., Riipi, T., Weisell, J., et al., Identification of IGFBP-3 fragments generated by KLK2 and prevention of fragmentation by KLK2-inhibiting peptides, *Biol. Chem.* 391, 4785–479, 2010.
16. Lövgren, J., Airas, K., and Lilja, H., Enzmatic action of human glandular kallikrein 2 (hK2). Substrate specificity and regulation by Zn^{2+} and extracellular protease inhibitors, *Eur. J. Biochem.* 262, 781–789, 1999.
17. Veneris-Lowe, T.L., Kruger, S.J., Walsh, T., et al., Seminal fluid characterization for male fertility and prostate cancer: Kallikrein-related serine proteases and whole proteome approaches, *Semin. Thromb. Hemost.* 33, 87–99, 2007.
18. Lövgren, J., Rajakoski, K., Karp, M., et al., Activation of the zymogen form of prostate-specific antigen by human glandular kallikrein 2, *Biochem. Biophys. Res. Commun.* 238, 549–555, 1997.
19. Frenette, G., Tremblay, R.R., Lazure, C., et al., Prostatic kallikrein hK2, but not prostate-specific antigen (hK3), activates single-chain urokinase-type plasminogen activator, *Int. J. Cancer.* 71, 897–899, 1997.
20. Andrade, D., Assis, D.M., Lima, A.R., et al., Substrate specificity and inhibition of human kallikrein-related peptidase 3 (KLK3 or PSA) activated with sodium citrate, *Arch. Biochem. Biophys.* 498, 74–82, 2010.
21. Härkönen, H.H., Mattsson, J.M., Määttä, J.A.E., et al., The discovery of compounds that stimulate the activity of kallikrein-related peptidase 3 (KLK3), *ChemMedChem* 6, 2170–2178, 2011.
22. Mattsson, J.M., Laakkonen, P., Klipinen, S., et al., Gene expression changes associated with the anti-angiogenic activity of kallikrcin-related peptidase 3 (KLK3) on human umbilical vein endothelial cells, *Biol. Chem.* 389, 765–771, 2008.
23. Mattsson, J.M., Naevaenen, A., Stenman, U.-H., and Koistinen, H., Peptide binding to prostate-specific antigen enhance its antiangiogenic activity, *Prostate* 72, 1586–1594, 2012.
24. Stephenson, S.A., Verity, K., Ashworth, L.K., et al., Localization of a new prostate-specific antigen-related serine protease gnee, KLK4, is evidence for an expanded human kallikrein gene family cluster on chromosome 19q13.3–13.4, *J. Biol. Chem.* 274, 23210–23214, 1999.
25. Lu, Y., Papagerakis, P., Yamakoshi, Y., et al., Functions of KLK4 and MMP-20 in dental enamel formation, *Biol. Chem.* 389, 695–700, 2008.
26. Dong, Y., Kaushal, A., Bui, L., et al., Human kallikrein 4 (hK4) is highly expressed in serous ovarian carcinomas, *Clin. Cancer Res.* 7, 2363–2371, 2001.
27. Debela, M., Magdolen, V., Schechter, N., et al., Specificity profiling of seven human tissue kallikreins reveals individual subsite preferences, *J. Biol. Chem.* 281, 25678–25688, 2006.
28. Debela, M., Beaufort, N., Magdolen, V., et al., Structures and specificity of the human kallikrein-related peptidases KLK 4, 5,6, and 7, *Biol. Chem.* 389, 623–632, 2008.
29. Wang, W., Mize, G.J., Zhang, X., and Takayama, T.K., Kallikrein-related peptidase-4 initiates tumor-stroma interactions in prostate cancer through protease-activated receptor 1, *Int. J. Cancer* 126, 599–610, 2010.
30. Beaufort, N., Plaza, K., Utzschneider, D., et al., Interdependence of kallikrein-related peptidases in proteolytic networks, *Biol. Chem.* 391, 581–587, 2010.

31. Takayama, T.K., McMullen, B.A., Nelson, P.S., et al., Characterization of hK4 (prostase), a prostate-specific serine protease: Activation of the precursor of prostate-specific antigen (pro-PSA), and single-chain urokinase plasminogen activator and degradation of prostatic acid phosphatase, *Biochemistry* 40, 15341–15348, 2001.
32. Beaufort, H., Debela, M., Creutzburg, S., et al., Interplay of human tissue kallikrein 4 (hK4) with the plasminogen activation system: HK4 regulates the structure and functions of the urokinase-type plasminogen activator receptor (uPAR), *Biol. Chem.* 387, 217–222, 2006.
33. Stephanopoulos, G., Garefalaki, M.E., and Lyroudia, K., Genes and related proteins involved in amelogenesis imperfecta, *J. Dent. Res.* 84, 1117–1126, 2005.
34. Sun, Z., Carpiaux, W., Fan, D., et al., Apatite reduces amelogenin proteolysis by MMP-20 and KLK4 *in vitro*, *J. Dent. Res.* 89, 344–348, 2010.
35. Ohler, A., Debela, M., Wagner, S., et al., Analyzing the protease web in skin: Mephrin metalloproteases are activated specifically by KLK4, 5, and B vice versa leading to processing of proKLK7 thereby triggering its activation, *Biol. Chem.* 391, 455–460, 2010.
36. Brattsand, M. and Egelrud, T., Purification, molecular cloning and expression of a human stratum corneum trypsin-like serine protease with possible function in desquamation, *J. Biol. Chem.* 274, 30033–30040, 1999.
37. Yousef, G.M., Kapadia, C., Polymeris, M.E., et al., The human kallikrein protein 5 (hK5) is enzymatically active, glycosylated and forms complexes with two protease inhibitors in ovarian cancer fluids, *Biochim. Biophys. Acta* 1628, 88–96, 2003.
38. Egelrud, T., Brattsand, M., Kreutzmann, P., et al., hK5 and hK7, two serine proteinases abundant in human skin, are inhibited by LEKTI domain 6, *Brit. J. Dermatol.* 153, 1200–1203, 2005.
39. Sakabe, J., Yamamoto, M., Hirakawa, S., et al., Kallikrein-related peptidase 5 functions in proteolytic processing of profillaggrin in culture human keratinocytes, *J. Biol. Chem.* 288, 17179–17189, 2013.
40. Stefansson, K., Brattsand, M., Roosterman, D., et al., Activation of proteinase-activated receptor-2 by human kallikrein-related peptidases, *J. Invest. Dermatol.* 128, 18–25, 2008.
41. de Souza, L.R., Melo, P.M., Paschoal, T., et al., Human tissue kallikreins 3 and 5 can act as plasmingen activator releasing active plasmin, *Biochem. Biophys. Res. Commun.* 433, 333–337, 2013.
42. Hamilton, B.S. and Whittaker, G.R., Cleavage activation of human-adapted influenza virus subtypes by kallikrein-related peptidases 5 and 12, *J. Biol. Chem.* 288, 17399–17407, 2013.
43. Bayani, J. and Diamandis, E.P., The physiology and pathobiology of human kallikrein-related peptidase 6 (KLK6), *Clin. Chem. Lab. Med.* 50, 211–233, 2011.
44. Scarisbrick, I.A., Radulovic, M., Burda, J.E., et al., Kallikrein 6 is a novel molecular trigger of reactive astrogliosis, *Biol. Chem.* 393, 355–367, 2012.
45. Murakami, K., Jiang, Y.P., Tanaka, T., et al., *In vivo* analysis of kallikrein-related peptidase 6 (KLK6) function in oligodendrocyte development and the expression of myelin proteins, *Neuroscience* 236, 1–11, 2013.
46. Bayés, A. Tsetsenis, T., Ventura, S., et al., Human kallikrein 6 activity is regulated via an autoproteolytic mechanism of activation/inactivation, *Biol. Chem.* 385, 517–524, 2004.
47. Magklara, A., Mellati, A.A., Wasney, G.A., et al., Characterization of the enzymatic activity of human kallikrein 6: Autoactivation, substrate specificity, and regulation by inhibitors, *Biochem. Biophys. Res. Commun.* 307, 948–955, 2003.

48. Ghosh, M.C., Grass, L., Soosaipillai, A., et al., Human kallikrein 6 degrades extracellular matrix proteins and may enhance the metastatic potential of tumour cells, *Tumour Biol.* 25, 193–199, 2004.

49. Yoon, H., Radulovic, M., Wu, J., et al., Kallikrein 6 signals through PAR1 and PAR2 to promote neuron injury and exacerbate glutamate neurotoxicity, *J. Neurochem.* 127, 283–298, 2013.

50. Burda, J.E., Radulovic, M., Yoon, H., and Scarisbrick, I.A., Critical roles of PAR1 in kallikrein 6-mediated oligodendrogliopathy, *Glia* 61, 1456–1470, 2013.

51. Ekholm, E. and Egelrud, T., Expression of stratum corneum chymotryptic enzyme in relation to other markers of epidermal differential in a skin explant model, *Exp. Dermatol.* 9, 65–70, 2000.

52. Yousef, G.M., Scorilas, A., Marklara, A., et al., The KLK7 (PRSS6) gene, encoding for the stratum corneum chymotryptic enzyme is a new member of the human kallikrein gene family—Genomic charaterization, mapping, tissue expression and hormonal regulation, *Gene* 254, 119–128, 2000.

53. Skytt, A., Strömqvist, M., and Egelrud, T., Primary substrate specificity of recombinant human stratum corneum chymotryptic enzyme, *Biochem. Biophys. Res. Commun.* 211, 586–589, 1995.

54. Nylander-Lundqvist, E. and Egelrud, T., Formation of active IL-1 beta from pro-IL-1 beta catalyzed by stratum corneum chymotryptic enzyme *in vitro*, *Acta Derm-Venereol.* 77, 203–206, 1997.

55. Johnson, S.K., Ramani, V.C., Hennings, L., and Haun, R.S., Kallikrein 7 enhances pancreatic cancer cell invasion by shedding E-cadherin, *Cancer* 109, 1811–1820, 2007.

56. Ramani, V.C. and Haun, R.S., The extracellular matrix protein fibronectin is a substrate for kallikrein 7, *Biochem. Biophys. Res. Commun.* 369, 1169–1173, 2008.

57. Ramani, V.C., and Haun, R.S., Expression of kallikrein 7 diminishes pancreatic cell adhesion to vitronectin and enhances urokinase-type plasminogen activator receptor shedding, *Pancreas* 37, 399–404, 2008.

58. Ramani, V.C., Hennings, L., and Haun, R.S., Desmoglein 2 is a substrate of kallikrein 7 in pancreatic cancer, *BMC Cancer* 8, 373, 2008.

59. Ramani, V.C., Kaushal, G.P., and Haun, R.S., Proteolytic action of kallikrein-related peptidase 7 produces unique active matrix metalloproteins-9 lacking the C-terminal hemopexin domains, *Biochim. Biophys. Acta* 1813, 1525–1531, 2011.

60. Yamamoto, M., Miyai, M., Matsumoto, Y., et al., Kallikrein-related peptidase-7 regulates caspase-14 maturation during keratinocyte terminal differentiation by generating an intermediate form, *J. Biol. Chem.* 287, 32825–23834, 2012.

61. Schultz, S., Saalbach, A., Heiker, J.T., et al., Proteolytic activation of prochemerin by kallikrein 7 breaks an ionic linkage and results in C-terminal rearrangement, *Biochem. J.* 452, 271–280, 2013.

62. Shimizu, C., Yoshida, S., Shibata, M., et al., Characterization of recombianant and brain neuropsin, a plasticity-related serine protease, *J. Biol. Chem.* 273, 11189–11196, 1998.

63. Komai, S., Matsuyama, T., Matsumoto, K., et al., Neuropsin regulates an early phase of schaffer-collateral long-term potentiation in the murine hipppocampus, *Eur. J. Neurosci.* 12, 1479–1486, 2000.

64. Tomimatsu, Y., Idemoto, S., Moriguchi, S., et al., Proteases involved in long-term potentiation, *Life Sci.* 72, 355–361, 2002.

65. Kishi, T., Grass, L., Soossalpillai, A., et al., Human kallikrein 8: Immunoassay development and identification in tissue extracts and biological fluids, *Clin. Chem.* 49, 87–96, 2003.

66. Eissa, A., Amodeo, V., Smith, C.R., and Diamandis, E.P., Kallikrein-related peptidase-8 (KLK8) is an active serine protease in human epidermis and sweat and is involved in a skin barrier proteolytic cascade, *J. Biol. Chem.* 286, 687–706, 2011.

67. Ramachandran, R., Eissa, A., Mihara, K., et al., Protease-activated receptors (PARs): Differential signalling by kallikrein-related peptidases KLK8 and KLK14, *Biol. Chem.* 383, 421–427, 2012.

68. Rajapakse, S., Ogiwara, K., Takano, N., et al., Biochemical characterization of human kallikrein 8 and its possible involvement in the degradation of extracellular matrix proteins, *FEBS Lett.* 579, 6879–6884, 2005.

69. Attwood, B.K., Bourgognon, J.M, Patel, S., et al., Neuropsin cleaves EphB2 in the amygdala to control anxieity, *Nature* 473, 372–375, 2011.

70. Yousef, G.M., Scorilas, A., Nakamura, T., et al., The prognostic value of the human kallikrein gene 9 (KLK9) in breast cancer, *Breast Cancer Res. Treat.* 78, 149–158, 2003.

71. Memari, N., Grass, L., Nakamura, T., et al., Human tissue kallikrein 9: Production of recombinant proteins and specific antibodies, *Biol. Chem.* 387, 733–740, 2006.

72. Tan, O.L., Whitbread, A.K., Clements, J.A., and Dong, Y., Kallikrein-related peptidase (KLK) family mRNA variants and protein isoforms in hormone-related cancers: Do they have a function, *Biol. Chem.* 387, 697–705, 2006.

73. Yousef, G.M. and Diamandis, E.P., The expanded human kallikrein gene family: Locus characterization and molecular cloning of a new member, KLK-L3 (KLK9), *Genomics* 65, 184–194, 2000.

74. Yousef, G.M., Kyrakopoulou, L.G., Scorillas, A., et al., Quantitative expression of the human kallikrein gene 9 (KLK9) in ovarian cancer: A new independent and favorable prognostic marker, *Cancer Res.* 61, 7811–7818, 2001.

75. Yoon, H., Balber, S.I., Debela, M., et al., A completed KLK activome profile: Investigation of activation profiles of KLK9, 10, and 15, *Biol. Chem.* 390, 373–377, 2009.

76. Liu, X.-L., Wazer, D.E., Watanabe, K., and Band, V., Identification of a novel serine protease-like gene, the expression of which is down-regulated during breast cancer progression, *Cancer Res.* 56, 3371–3379, 1996.

77. Goyal, J., Smith, K.M., and Cowan, J.M., The role for NES1 serine protease as a novel tumor suppressor, *Cancer Res.* 58, 4782–4786, 1998.

78. Luo, L., Herbrick, J.A., Scherer, S.W., et al., Structural characterization and mapping of the normal epithelial cell-specific 1 gene, *Biochem. Biophys. Res. Commun.* 247, 580–586, 1998.

79. Sauter, E.R., Linnger, J., Maglara, A., et al., Association of kallikrein in nipple aspirate fluid with breast cancer risk, *Int. J. Cancer* 108, 588–591, 2004.

80. Talleri, M., Alexopoulou, D.K., Scorilas, A., et al., Expression analysis and clinical evaluation of kallikrein-related peptidase (KLKL10) in colorectal cancer, *Tumour Biol.* 32, 737–744, 2011.

81. Koh, S.C., Razvi, K., Chan, Y.H., et al., The association with age, human tissue kallikreins 6 and 10 and hemostatic markers for survival outcome from epithelial ovarian cancer, *Arch. Gynecol. Obstet.* 284, 183–190, 2011.

82. Darling, M.R., Hashem, N.N., Zhang, I., et al., Kallikrein-related peptidase 10 expression in salivary gland tissue and tumours, *Int. J. Biol. Markers* 27:e38i-e388, 2012.

83. Petraki, C., Youssef, Y.M., Dubinski, W., et al., Evaluation and prognostic significance of human tissue kallikrein-related peptidase 10 (KLK10) in colorectal cancer, *Tumour Biol.* 33, 1209–1214, 2012.

84. Yoshida, S., Taniguchi, M., Suemoto, T., et al., cDNA cloning and expression of a novel serine protease, TLSP, *Biochim. Biophys. Acta* 1399, 335–228, 1998.

85. Mitsui, S., Yamada, T., Okui, A., et al., A novel isoform of a kallikrein-like protease, TLSP/hippostasin, (PRSS20), is expressed in the human brain and prostate, *Biochem. Biophys. Res. Commun.* 272, 205–211, 2000.

86. Mitsui, S., Okui, A., Kominami, K., et al., cDNA cloning and tissue-specific splicing variants of mouse hippostasin/TLSP (PRSS20), *Biochim. Biophys. Acta* 1494, 206–210, 2000.

87. Scorilas, A. and Gregorakis, A.K., mRNA expression analysis of human kallikrein 11 (KLK11) may be useful in the discrimination of benign prostatic hyperplasia from prostate cancer after needle prostate biopsy, *Biol. Chem.* 387, 789–793, 2006.

88. Sano, A., Sangai, T., Maeda, H., et al., Kallikrein 11 expressed in human breast cancer cells releases insulin-like growth factor through degradation of IGFBP-3, *Int. J. Oncol.* 30, 1493–1498, 2007.

89. Yousef, G.M., Luo, L.Y., and Diamandis, E.P., Identification of novel human kallikrein-like genes on chromosome 19q13.3-q13.4, *Anticancer Res.* 19, 2843–2852, 1999.

90. Yousef, G.M., Magklara, A., and Diamandis, E.P., KLK12 is a novel serine protease and a new member of the human kallikrein gene family -differential expression in breast cancer, *Genomics* 69, 331–341, 2000.

91. Gan, L., Lee, I., Smith, R., et al., Sequencing and expression analysis of the serine protease gene cluster located in chromosome 19q13 region, *Gene* 257, 119–130, 2000.

92. Komatsu, N., Takata, M., Otsuki, N., et al., Expression and localization of tissue kallikrein mRNAs in human epidermis and appedages, *J. Invest. Dermatol.* 121, 542–549, 2003.

93. Memari, N., Jiang, W., Diamandis, E.P., and Luo, L.Y., Enzymatic properties of human kallikrein-related peptidase 12 (KLK12), *Biol. Chem.* 388, 427–435, 2007.

94. Guillon-Munos, A., Oikonomopoulou, K., Michel, N., et al., Kallikrein-related peptidase 12 hydrolyzes matricellular proteins of the CCN family and modifies interactions of CCN1 and CCN5 with growth factors, *J. Biol. Chem.* 286, 25505–25518, 2011.

95. Kryza, T., Achard, C., Parent, C., et al., Angiogenesis stimulated by human kallikrein-related peptidase 12 acting via a platelet-derived growth factor B-dependent paracrine pathway, *FASEB J.* 28, 740–751, 2014.

96. Kryza, T., Lalmanach, G., Lavergne, M., et al., Pro-angiogenic effect of human kallikrein-related peptidase 12 (KLK12) in lung endothelial cells does not depend on kinin-mediated activation of B2 receptor, *Biol. Chem.* 394, 385–391, 2013.

97. Yousef, G.M., Chang, A., and Diamandis, E.P., Identification and characterization of KLK-L4, a new kallikrein-like gene that appears to be down-regulated in breast cancer tissues, *J. Biol. Chem.* 275, 11891–11898, 2000.

98. Chang, A., Yousef, G.M., Jung, K., et al., Identification and molecular characterization of five novel kallikrein gene 13 (KLK13, KLK-L4) splice variants: Differential expression in the human testis and testicular cancer, *Anticancer Res.* 21, 3147–3152, 2001.

99. Petraki, C.D., Karavana, V.N., and Diamandis, E.P., Human kallikrein 13 expression in normal tissues: An immunohistochemical study, *J. Histochem. Cytochem.* 51, 493–501, 2003.

100. Kapadia, C., Chang, A., Sotiropoulou, G., et al., Human kallikrein 13: Production and purification of recombinant protein and monoclonal and polyclonal antibodies, and development of a sensitive and specific immunofluorometric assay, *Clin. Chem.* 49, 77–86, 2003.

101. Andrade, D., Assis, D.M., Santos, J.A., et al., Substrate specificity of kallikrein-related peptidase 13 activated by salts or glycosaminoglycans and a search for natural substrate candidates, *Biochimie* 93, 1701–1709, 2011.

102. Kapadia, C., Ghosh, M.C., Grass, L., and Diamandis, E.P., Human kallikrein 13 involvement in extracellular matrix degradation, *Biochem. Biophys. Res. Commun.* 323, 1084–1090, 2004.

103. Kapadia, C., Yousef, G.M., Mellati, A.A., et al., Complex formation between human kallikrein 13 and serum protease inhibitors, *Clin. Chim. Acta* 339, 157–167, 2004.

104. Luo, L.-Y. and Jiang, W., Inhibition profiles of human tissue kallikreins by serine protease inhibitors, *Biol. Chem.* 387, 813–816, 2006.

105. Yousef, G.M., Magklara, A., Chang, A., et al., Cloning of a new member of the kallikrein gene family, KLK14, which is down-regulated in different malignancies, *Cancer Res.* 61, 3425–3431, 2001.

106. Eissa, A. and Diamandis, E.P., Kallikrein-related peptidase 14, in *Handbook of Proteolytic Enzymes*, eds. N.D. Rawlings and G. Salvesen, Vol. 3., Chapter 618, pp. 2809–2813, Elsevier/Academic Press, Amsterdam, Netherlands, 2013.

107. Rajapakse, S. and Takahashi, T., Expression and enzymatic characterization of recombinant human kallkrein 14, *Zoolog. Sci.* 24, 774–780, 2007.

108. Stefansson, K., Brattsand, M., Ny, A., et al., Kallikrein-related peptidase 14 may be a major contributor to trypsin-like proteolytic activity in human stratum corneum, *Biol. Chem.* 387, 761–768, 2006.

109. Gratis, V., Lorion, C., Virca, G.D., et al., Kallikrein-related peptidase 14 acts on proteinase-activated receptor 2 to induce signaling pathway in colon cancer cells, *Am. J. Pathol.* 179, 2625–2636, 2011.

110. de Veer, S.J., Swedberg, J.E., Parker, E.A., and Harris, J.M., Non-combinatorial library screening reveals subsite cooperativity and identifies new high-efficiency substrates for kallikrein-related peptidase 14, *Biol. Chem.* 393, 331–341, 2012.

111. Emami, N. and Diamandis, E.P., Human kallikrein-related peptidase 14 (KLK14) is a new activator component of the KLK proteolytic cascade. Possible functions in seminal plasma and skin, *J. Biol. Chem.* 283, 3031–3041, 2008.

112. Brattsand, M., Stefansson, K., Lundh, C., et al., A proteolytic cascade of kallikreins in the stratum corneum, *J. Invest. Dermatol.* 124, 198–203, 2005.

113. Emami, N. and Diamandis, E.P., Potential role of multiple members of the kallikrein-related peptidase family of serine proteases in activated latent TFFβ1 in semen, *Biol. Chem.* 391, 85–95, 2010.

114. Oikonomopoulou, K., DeAngelis, R.A., Chen, H., et al., Induction of complement C1a receptors responses by kallikrein-related peptidase 14, *J. Immunol.* 191, 3858–3866, 2013.

115. Takayama, T.K., Carter, C.A., and Deng, T., Activation of prostate-specific antigen precursor (pro-PSA) by prostin, a novel serine protease identified by degenerate PCR, *Biochemstry* 40, 1679–1687, 2001.

116. Shaw, J.L., Grass, L., Sotiropoulou, G., and Diamandis, E.P., Development of an immunofluorometric assay for human kallikrein 15 (KLK15) and identification of KLK15 in tissues and biological fluids, *Clin. Biochem.* 40, 104–110, 2007.

117. Batra, J. and Clements, J., Kallikrein-related peptidase 15 (prostinogen), in *Handbook of Proteolytic Enzymes,* 3rd edn., eds. N.D. Rawlings and G. Salvensen, Vol. 3, Chapter 619, pp. 2814–2817, Academic Press/Elsevier, Amsterdam, Netherlands, 2013.

118. Yousef, G.M., Scorilas, A., Jung, K., et al., Molecular cloning of the human *Kallkrein 15* gene (*KLK15*). Up-regulation in prostate cancer, *J. Biol. Chem.* 276, 53–61, 2001.

119. Ervin, L.B., Vasquez, J.R., and Craik, C.S., Substrate specificity of trypsin investigated by using a genetic selection, *Proc. Natl. Acad. Sci. USA* 87, 6659–6663, 1990.

120. Fink, E., Bhoola, K.D., Snyman, C., Neth, P., and Figueroa, C.D., *Biol. Chem.* 388, 957–963, 2007.

121. Cerf, M.E. and Raidoo, D.M., Immunolocalization on plasma kallikrein in human brain, *Metab. Brain Dis.* 15, 315–323, 2000.

122. Adamopoulos, P.G., Kontos, C.K., Papgeorgiou, S.G., Pappa, V., and Scorilas, A., *KLKB1* mRNA overexpression: A novel molecular biomarker for the diagnosis of chronic lymphocytic leukemia, *Clin. Biochem.* 48, 849–854, 2015.

123. Schmaier, A.H. and McCrae, K.R., The plasma kallikrein-kinin system: Its evolution from contact activation, *J. Thromb. Haemost.* 5, 2323–2329, 2007.
124. Ichinose, A., Fujikawa, K., and Suyama, T., The activation of pro-urokinase by plasma kallikrein and its inactivation by thrombin, *J. Biol. Chem.* 261, 3486–3489, 1986.
125. Nishimura, H., Kakizaki, T., Muta, T., et al., cDNA and deduced amino acid sequence of human PK-120, a plasma kallikrein-sensitive glycoprotein, *FEBS Lett.* 357, 207–211, 1995.
126. Liu, J., Gao, B.B., and Feener, E.P., Proteomic identification of novel plasma kallikrein substrates in the astrocyte secretome, *Transl. Stroke Res.* 1, 276–286, 2010.

occurred in hepatocytes, with secretion into the blood stream followed by extravasation to the interstitial space. Yamamoto and coworkers[7] used immunochemical techniques to demonstrate the presence of HMWK in the dermal interstitial space. Analysis of an extract from skin with an ELISA assay suggested that the concentration of HMWK was 23% that of the plasma concentration. HMWK is a relatively large single-chain protein with a mass of approximately 120 kDa, and has difficulty passing from the vascular bed into the interstitial space. Since we could find no data to support basolateral secretion, restricted extravasation might explain the lower concentration of HMWK in the interstitial space. These studies were suggestive of the presence of KLK-B1 in the interstitial space but definitive data were missing. While hepatocytes are the primary site of synthesis of KLK-B1, Fink and coworkers[8] have reported the presence of prekallikrein mRNA in other tissues, including kidney, ovary, parotid gland, skin, prostate, and breast.

Lewis and Wawretschek[9] observed that low levels of kallikrein activity were present in lymph and plasma (kallikrein activity was measured by the formation of kinin measured with rat uterus contraction assay).[10,11] Kallikrein activity was

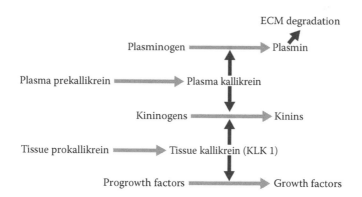

FIGURE 6.1 Activation and actions of plasma and tissue kallikreins. Shown here are the canonical mechanisms for the activation of plasma prekallikrein and tissue prokallikrein and suggested substrates within the interstitial space. The point here is that these two enzymes occur in their precursor or zymogen forms, which require activation for full expression of activity. This requirement for activation provides one of the more significant control mechanisms. Plasma prekallikrein is activated by factor XIIa in plasma, while a physiological activator of tissue prokallikrein remains to be identified.

enhanced in either fluid by treatment with glass or acid. The increase in activity seen with glass is consistent with the presence of prekallikrein, HMWK, and blood coagulation factor XII in lymph (see Chapter 8 for more discussion of contact activation in lymph).[12] Garbe and Vogt[13] had previously reported bradykinin formation in acid-treated plasma, providing support for the presence of kallikrein activity in lymph; earlier work by Vogt[14] showed that kininogenase I was activated in plasma by acid or acetone-activated kininogen I (LMWK) to produce kinins, and this would suggest that kininogenase I is KLK-1. Kininogenase II is activated by glass and produces kinins from kininogen II. Kininogen II is HMWK, suggesting that kininogenase II is KLK-B1. Early work by Jacobsen[15] showed low levels or the absence of kallikrein in either dog or rabbit lymph, though he did show substantial amounts of kininogen. This does not preclude the function of KLK-B1 or KLK-1 at the local level in the interstitial space, as there are several protein protease inhibitors (Chapter 9) that would provide *in situ* inhibition of either KLK-B1 or KLK-1. C1-inhibitor (C1-INH) is an inhibitor of a number plasma proteases, including factor XIIa and KLK-B1.[16] C1-IHN has been suggested to be a major inhibitor of KLK-B1 and has been demonstrated to be present in cellular secretions and interstitial fluid.[17]

Prekallikrein can be converted to KLK-B1 in blood and presumably in the interstitial space by the action of blood coagulation factor XIIa.[18] This activation reaction can be amplified, as factor XII may also be activated by KLK-B1 in a positive-feedback reaction. Recent work by Kusumam and coworkers[19] has shown that the complex of prekallikrein and HMWK can produce KLK-B1 in a reaction augmented by the presence of heat shock protein 90. It is suggested that the active site of kallikrein is generated from prekallikrein in the complex with HMWK. This observation is significant, as it shows that the zymogen form of an enzyme can possess activity without processing by limited proteolysis. This reaction could be of considerable importance in the interstitial space in tumors. While heat shock protein 90 is considered to function primarily as an intracellular chaperone, secreted heat shock protein has been suggested to be crucial in prostate tumor development.[20] The activity of the complex of HMWK and prekallikrein is inhibited by C1-INH (serpin G1). Ravindran and coworkers[21] have shown that type IV collagen, which is found in the basement membrane[22] (Table 2.1), affects the activity of KLK-B1. The rate of reaction of kallikrein with C1-INH is decreased in the presence of type IV collagen. However, the interpretation of this result is complicated by the observation that both KLK-B1 and C1-INH are absorbed into type IV collagen. KLK-B1 also activates matrix metalloproteinase (MMP)-1[23] and may have a role in tissue remodeling. Durham and coworkers[24] reported that prekallikrein bound to the heparin-binding domain of insulin-like growth factor binding protein (IGFBP)-3, forming a co-binary complex that in turn could bind to insulin-like growth factor (IGF)-1, forming a ternary complex. The prekallikrein in the ternary complex could be activated by factor XIIa to form kallikrein. The kallikrein thus formed could degrade IGFBP-3 with the release of IGF-1. The association of prekallikrein with IGFBP-3 provides a mechanism for the localization of a protease to preferentially degrade IGFBP-3. Proteolysis of IGFBPs has been suggested as a mechanism for controlling the levels of IGF.[25] The association of prekallikrein with IGF has also been demonstrated by other investigators.[26]

Schousboe and Nystrom[27] reported that HMWK bound to laminin (Table 2.1) in the basement membrane, where it can be digested with KLK-B1, promoting an inflammatory response and influencing the process of angiogenesis.

6.3   TISSUE KALLIKREIN AND KALLIKREIN-RELATED PEPTIDASES

KLK-1 is a member of the KLK family, which is composed of 15 proteins.[2,3,28–30] It is reasonable to assume that these proteases function primarily within the interstitial space; however, there is little evidence to support the presence of active enzymes. It is likely that these proteases function in a local environment and are regulated by the presence of protease inhibitors (Chapter 9).

Proud and coworkers[31] reported the presence of immunoreactive KLK-1 in rat renal lymph; however, it was not possible to demonstrate the presence of active enzymes. These investigators also showed the presence of kininogen, based on the formation of kinin on treatment with rat urinary kallikrein as well as the presence of rennin and angiotensin I. Rahman and coworkers[32] showed that KLK-1 in synovial fluid is modulated by various inhibitors. A consideration of these results suggests that there is little active kallikrein in lymph.[6] Low levels of active KLK-1 in lymph have also been reported by other workers.[33,34] Maier and coworkers[35] suggest that parotitis results from the leakage of KLK-1 into the interstitial space, with the subsequent generation of kinin (kallidin) from kininogen. Under normal conditions, KLK-1 is not found in substantial amounts in the interstitial space of salivary glands.[36] There are several other studies that support the presence of KLK-1 in the interstitial space. Using immunochemical techniques, Ramsaroop and coworkers[37] showed major luminal distribution of KLK in kidney transplants, but there was some basolateral localization. These investigators suggest that acute rejection results in more distribution of KLK-1 into the interstitial space. Another study[38] showed that there was a marked increase in the destitution of KLK-1 and kallistatin in the interstitial space of the intestine in subjects with inflammatory bowel disease. The release of KLK-1 into the intestine interstitial space as a result of inflammation has been observed by another worker.[39] Immunoreactive KLK-1 (urinary kallikrein) has been measured in human blood serum (approximately 3.8 ng/mL);[40] this does not represent free KLK-1 but rather KLK-1 in a complex, such as would have been formed with α_2-macroglobulin.

There has been an increase in the number of studies describing cascade systems of zymogens and active proteases,[41,42] ever since these were described in the process of blood coagulation.[43,44] These *waterfall* or *cascade* systems provide a mechanism for the signal amplification critical for the formation of fibrin clots in the process of hemostasis. These systems also provide a mechanism for the regulation of a biological response. Cascade systems have been either suggested or demonstrated for several families of proteinases found in the interstitial space. Interactions for the fibrinolytic system are described in Chapter 5, MMPs in Chapter 7, and coagulation proteases in Chapter 8. As the various members of the KLK family are synthesized as precursor or zymogen forms (Figure 6.1), it is not unreasonable to suggest that the various KLKs and KLK-B1 could participate in regulatory cascades (Figure 6.2).[45–47] It is also possible that enzymes such as plasmin or thrombin will participate with

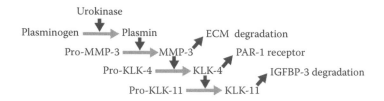

FIGURE 6.2   A regulatory cascade of kallikrein peptidases in the interstitial space. Shown here is a proteolytic cascade involving different proteases that could operate within in the interstitial space. While the individual proenzyme–enzyme conversions have been documented, the cascade reaction presented here has yet to be demonstrated.

members of the KLK family in such regulatory processes.[46] It is suggested that the various KLKs have diverse functions in the extracellular space, including the processing of growth factors, cleavage of extracellular matrix (ECM) proteins, and activation of other proteases, and are involved in tumorogenesis.[48] With the exception of KLK-4,[49] the KLKs function as secretory factors and/or in the extracellular space. Classic KLK-1 (KLK-L1) is partially activated during the secretory process. Saliva contains both enzymatically active kallikrein and prokallikrein;[50] the prokallikrein can be activated by the addition of trypsin. This study also validated the amidolytic assay for KLK-1. A variety of enzymes activate prokallikrein, including trypsin, thermolysin, and clostripain, but a physiological activator has not been identified.[51] The failure to detect significant active KLK-1 in the various biological fluids is likely a consequence of a reaction with various inhibitors, including α_2-macroglobulin and α_1-antitrypsin.[52] Kallistatin has been described as a specific serpin inhibitor of KLK-1[53] and has been found in synovial fluid.[54] We could not find data on the concentration of kallistatin in interstitial fluid or lymph. However, it is not unreasonable to suggest that it would be present in interstitial fluid as it is a single-chain protein with a molecular weight of 54 kDa.[55]

KLK-1 activity has been found in lymph[17,18] and could be derived from interstitial fluid or another source, such as synovial fluid,[56–58] where it may be derived from neutrophils.[57–59] KLK-1 could be derived from other sources such as cardiac tissue,[60] other vascular tissue,[61,62] stromal endothelial cells,[63] or vascular endothelial cells.[64] KLK-1 mediates proinflammatory pathways and the activation of protease-activated receptors (PARs) in proximal tubular epithelial cells.[65] KLK-1 is also suggested to have an important role in vascular development via kinin interaction with the B1 and B2 receptors, increasing the expression of vascular endothelial growth factor (VEGF).[66,67] Bledsoe and coworkers[116] showed that the infusion of KLK-1 could reverse gentamicin-induced renal injury. Specifically, the infusion of KLK-1 prevented apoptosis and reduced fibrosis. The use of bradykinin antagonists suggested the involvement of the B2 bradykinin receptor on renal proximal tubular cells in the effect observed with KLK-1. While KLK-1 expression is highest in the kidney, pancreas, and salivary glands, it is also expressed in circulating proangiogenic cells.[68] Proangiogenic cells are mononuclear cells derived from bone marrow that function in vascular repair and neovascularization.[69,70] The effect of KLK-1 on vascular development may well be dependent on the tissue. Fukuhara and coworkers[71] reported that the subcutaneous administration of KLK-1 inhibited choroidal neovascularization in a murine model. These workers showed that the subcutaneous administration of KLK-1 resulted in the cleavage of VEGF in the retinal pigmented epithelium (REP)–choroid complex, inhibiting angiogenesis. Nakamura and coworkers[72] had earlier reported that subcutaneous KLK-1 could cleave VEGF-165 in the C-terminal region, inhibiting its ability to promote angiogenesis. In subsequent work, Masuda and coworkers[73] reported that subcutaneous KLK-1 could prevent retinal ischemic damage in a murine model, possibly by preventing the activation of nitric oxide synthesis. In subsequent work, Masuda and coworkers[74] reviewed the role of the kallikrein system in the retina. KLK-B1, which directly forms bradykinin, stimulated vascular permeability and intraocular hemorrhage, while KLK-1, which forms kallidin (lysylbradykinin, which can be converted to bradykinin by an aminopeptidase), normalized retinal vascular permeability and inhibited retinal neovascularization and ischemic damage.

KLK-1 can also directly influence cell behavior. Biyashev and coworkers[75] reported the direct activation of bradykinin B2 receptors in transfected Chinese hamster ovary (CHO) cells with KLK-1. There are several examples of KLK-1 and other kallikrein-related proteases acting on PARs[76–79] as well as interacting with epidermal growth factor receptors (EGFRs).[80–82] KLK-1 has been suggested to be involved in the processing of pro-EGF to mature EGF,[83,84] but such processing is tissue specific[85] and may involve enzymes other than or in addition to kallikrein.[85–87] It is important to note that it is reasonable that there would be degeneracy in the processing of EGF.[88] There are some data suggesting the activation of a type IV collagenase/gelatinase/MMP-9[89] by KLK-1.[90–92]

KLK-2 and KLK-3 (prostate-specific antigen [PSA]) are products of the prostate and have been used for prostate cancer screening.[93,94] Immunoreactive PSA is also found in breast tumors,[95,96] with low immunoreactivity in other tissues. Both KLK-2 and KLK-3 have been isolated from seminal plasma.[97–99]

KLKs 4–15 (Table 6.1) are, in general, widely distributed and have been identified by analysis of a specific gene region and subsequently expressed by recombinant DNA technology. There are a few examples where KLKs other than 1–3 were evaluated by immunohistochemistry[100–111] and immunological assay of tissue extracts.[100] KLK-2 (hK2) has kininogenase activity,[112,113] while PSA has little[114] or no kininogenase activity.[113] Both KLK-2 and PSA are considered primary secretory products of the prostate and, as with other KLKs, there are products derived by alternative splicing.[115] These enzymes are thought to participate in the function of seminal plasma, but it is not clear as to whether there is a function in the interstitial space. Both PSA and KLK-2 are found in the circulation and used as biomarkers for prostate health.[116] We could find no evidence for the presence of either PSA or KLK-2 in lymph or interstitial fluid. It should be noted that KLK-1 is a glandular secretion, while PSA and KLK-2 are secreted with seminal plasma.

Dorn and coworkers[100] were able to show a prognostic value for KLK-7 antigen levels in a tissue extract, but not by immunohistochemical analysis. Bandiera and coworkers[108] measured serum levels of KLK-5 in normal subjects and individuals with ovarian cancer with an ELISA assay, using recombinant KLK-5 as a standard. Bandiera and coworkers[108] also showed that the expression of KLK-5 in patients with benign masses, borderline tumors, or ovarian cancer was associated with the development of IgG and IgM antibodies to KLK-5. There are no studies where the proposed activity of a given KLK is measured *in situ* by enzyme histochemistry. Petraki and coworkers,[117] using immunohistocytochemistry, established that KLKs 5–7 and 10–14 were found in the cytoplasm of glandular epithelial cells and in cellular secretions. There is wide tissue distribution of these KLKs. Regardless of tissue distribution, it is remarkably difficult to find laboratory studies describing the function of KLKs in the interstitial space.

The strongest evidence for the extracellular function of KLKs appears to be in tumor stromal cells. KLK-12 has been suggested to promote angiogenesis. Guillon-Munos and coworkers[118] treated MDA-MB-231 cells in cell culture with KLK-12, resulting in the cleavage of several members of the CCN protein family. These investigators suggest that the cleavage of CCN-1 results in the shedding of this protein from the cell surface. Cleavage of CCN-1 is associated with the release of VEGF, which promotes angiogenesis. KLK-12 also releases BMP-2, TGF-β1, and FGF-2 from the CCN surface protein complex. Kryza and coworkers[119] showed that the promotion of angiogenesis in lung endothelial cells did not depend on kinin generation. More recently, Kryza and coworkers[120] showed that KLK-12 converted platelet-derived growth factor B (PDGF-B) bound to the ECM into a soluble form. Soluble PDGF-B and VEGF-A induce endothelial tube formation, thus providing an end mechanism for the proangiogenic action of KLK-12.

Wei and coworkers[121] reported that KLK-1 (immunohistochemical) in left ventricular interstitial fluid was increased in a rodent model of chronic volume overload. In addition, mast cells were increased and interstitial collagen was decreased. Treatment with aprotinin, an inhibitor of KLK-1, prevented the decrease in collagen. These investigators also showed that mRNA for KLK-1 and KLK-10 was increased in chronic volume overload. These investigators evaluated kallikrein expression in cultured cardiomyocytes and fibroblasts (cultured on laminin-coated Flexcell® plates) and found an increase in the expression of mRNA for KLK-1 and KLK-10. KLK-10 is an epithelial cell–specific enzyme found in a variety of tissues.[122]

The degradation of collagen IV by KLK-8 has been reported by Rajapakse and coworkers.[123] Rajapakse and Takahashi[124] have also reported the degradation of collagen IV by KLK-14. KLK-8 and KLK-14 also degrade other ECM proteins, including fibronectin. Schanstra and coworkers[125] have shown that bradykinin activates the B2 receptor in renal tissue, which is associated with an increase in plasminogen activator and MMP-2 activities, which reduce tubular fibrosis by an increase in ECM degradation, including a loss of collagen IV and fibronectin.

6.3.1 MISCELLANEOUS OBSERVATIONS ON KALLIKREINS AND OTHER KININ-FORMING ENZYMES IN INTERSTITIAL SPACE

Various KLKs including KLK-1 are suggested to be important in tumor development and metastasis.[126,127] Endothelial cells are a source of KLK-1,[128,129] and there is one report of the direct interaction of KLK-1 with endothelial B1 receptor.[130] There are processes other than the actions of KLK-B1 or KLK-1 by which kinins can be formed from kininogen in the interstitial space. Kinin activity can be released from

HMWK by proteases derived from neutrophils[131] and by a cysteine proteinase from *Trypanosoma cruzi*.[132] PSA (KLK-3) has been reported to release a kinin-like material from a glycoprotein in semen.[133] A number of snake venoms have also been reported to have kininogenase activity.[134–137] Snake venoms are known to exert toxic responses in the extravascular space.[138–141]

6.3.2 HYALURONAN AND TISSUE KALLIKREIN

There is evidence to suggest KLK-1 activity can be mediated by interaction with hyaluronan. Fontreza and coworkers[142] showed that KLK-1 was physically bound to hyaluronan in primary cultures of submucosal gland cells. First, KLK-1 obtained from the conditioned media of the submucosal gland cells was heterogeneous on native gel electrophoresis; the heterogeneity was eliminated by digestion with hyaluronidase. Second, digestion of conditioned media from the submucosal gland cell culture with hyaluronidase resulted in a greater than eightyfold increase in KLK-1 enzyme activity (peptide nitroanilide substrate). Subsequent work by Forteza and coworkers[143] showed that KLK-1 was bound to hyaluronan on the apical surface of airway epithelium, and was thus protected from ciliary clearance. KLK-1 bound to the apical surface is inactive, while lactoperoxidase, which is also bound, retains catalytic activity. Casalino-Matsuda and coworkers[144] later showed that fragmentation of hyaluronan with reactive oxygen species (xanthine/xanthine oxidase) resulted in the release of KLK-1 in cultures of submucosal gland cells. The KLK-1 then processed pro-EGF bound to the submucosal cell surface, resulting in submucosal gland hypertrophy, hyperplasia, and mucous hypersecretion. Casalino-Matsuda and coworkers[145] followed their earlier study[144] with a similar study using cultures of human bronchial epithelial cells grown at an air–liquid interface. The generation of reactive oxygen species (xanthine/xanthine oxidase) results in activation of EGF receptors on goblet cells, resulting in metaplasia and mucous hypersecretion. These investigators suggested that fragmentation of hyaluronan by reactive oxygen species releases KLK-1 with the subsequent processing of EGF. In later work, Yu and coworkers[146] suggested that, in addition to the KLK-1–EGF pathway, the hyaluronan fragments generated by reactive oxygen species induce an interaction between EGF receptors and CD44, resulting in increased expression of mucin 5AC. These investigators suggest an interaction between KLK-1 and hyaluronan in the airway. No such interaction has been demonstrated in the interstitial space, but we are unaware of any study on the interaction of hyaluronan and a KLK. In fact, we could find few, if any, studies on the interaction of hyaluronan with other proteases. It is noted that a hyaluronan-binding protease in plasma has been reported to release kinin activity from HMWK or LMWK,[147] and thus is similar to KLK-1. While there are no specific studies on the presence of this enzyme in the interstitial space, there are some studies that suggest that it would be active outside the vascular bed.[148–151]

6.4 KININS

Kinins are products of the limited proteolysis of kininogens by either KLK-B1 or KLK-1. Bradykinin is produced by KLK-B1 acting on HMWK, while lysylbradykinin (kallidin) is produced by KLK-1 from either HMWK or LMWK. Lysylbradykinin can be converted to bradykinin through the action of an aminopeptidase. Both bradykinin and lysylbradykinin can be converted to active derivatives by the action of an enzyme such as carboxypeptidase M.[152] Both bradykinin and kallidin are subject to rapid degradation by various proteases.[153] Bradykinin can be degraded by carboxypeptidase M (kininase I)[152,154] and angiotensin-converting enzyme (ACE; kininase II);[155] kallidin is also degraded by ACE[156–158] and, as with bradykinin, proteolysis is associated with the loss of agonist activity.

Bradykinin is produced in the vascular space by the interaction of KLK-B1 with HMWK and binds to specific receptors on endothelial cells,[159–162] resulting in vasodilation[163,164] and increased vascular permeability,[165,155] which can result in edema.[167,168] The deficiency of C1-INH results in hereditary angioedema due to increased activity of KLK-B1.[169–171] The effect of bradykinin on vasodilation is mediated, in part, by nitric oxide (originally described as endothelium-derived relaxing factor [EDRF]).[163,172] Bradykinin and related peptides, such as kallidin, exert their physiological effect by interacting with specific G-coupled receptors.[173–176] Bradykinin is found in the vascular space and kallidin in urine.[177]

Degradation of either bradykinin or kallidin with carboxypeptidase M results in a derivative that no longer binds to B2 receptors but does bind to the B1 kinin receptor. Carboxypeptidase M is found as a membrane-associated protein in a number of different cell types.[178–181] It has been suggested that there is functional interaction between carboxypeptidase M and B1 receptors on endothelial cells,[182,183] enhancing nitric oxide output.[184] Carboxypeptidase M is found in tumors and has been suggested as a therapeutic target.[179,185,186]

Dendorfer and coworkers[187] studied the degradation of bradykinin in the intravascular space and the interstitial space. Aminopeptidase P (APP) and ACE are found on the luminal endothelial surface, while neutral endopeptidase (NEP) is membrane bound within the interstitial space of the heart. Dendorfer and coworkers[187] suggest that ACE and APP form a "metabolic barrier," preventing bradykinin from passing from the intravascular space into the extravascular space. This is consistent with earlier work by Adamski and Graga[188] on the role of ACE in the regulation of bradykinin in the vascular space. ACE is bound to the luminal vascular surface, so while there is some degradation of bradykinin in plasma, most of the enzyme reaction occurs on the endothelial cell surface.[189] The degradation of bradykinin in plasma is relatively slow (i.e., hours)[153] while the degradation in the circulation is fast (i.e., seconds).[190,191] Neutral endopeptidase functions within the interstitial space to degrade bradykinin. Neutral endopeptidase also functions in the interstitial space to degrade kallidin (lysylbradykinin).[192] Kallidin forms from kininogens through the action of KLK-1 and is likely the major kinin in the interstitial space. Bradykinin can be formed from kallidin by the action of an aminopeptidase.[193] KLK-B1 is generally considered to form bradykinin from HMWK in the vascular space; KLK-1 forms kallidin from either HMWK or LMWK in the interstitial space. Both KLK-2 and KLK-3 have been suggested to have low kininogenase activity. It is noted that most of the *in vitro* studies have been performed in the presence of components of interstitial fluid, such as hyaluronan. The work with kinins in the intravascular space has focused on their effect on vasodilation and vascular permeability. Kinins within the interstitial space have a broader range of potential activity. Yu and coworkers[194] have reported that bradykinin increases VEGF expression and angiogenesis in prostate cancer. Takano and coworkers[195] have suggested that B2 bradykinin receptor has a cell surface and nuclear location. The bradykinin B2 receptor forms a heterodimer with lamin C, promoting its nuclear localization and enabling the role of bradykinin in cell signaling. B2 kinin receptors are widely distributed, but B1 receptors appear to be inducible, in the sense that they are upregulated during inflammation and are involved with pain.[196] A recent observation suggests the involvement of the B1 receptor in skin with the itch response (alloknesis).[197] KLK-8 is found in skin and degrades HMWK, but kinin formation has not been reported.[123]

Bradykinin causes ATP release from human subcutaneous fibroblasts through intracellular calcium ion mobilization in a process involving B2 receptors and P2Y12 receptors.[198] This is suggested to be involved in chronic musculoskeletal pain, secondary to connective tissue remodeling. Bradykinin also influences the differentiation of human fibroblasts[199] and induces the expression of α-smooth muscle actin in mesenchymal stem cells.[200]

There is little definitive information on the formation and actions of kinins in the interstitial space. Both HMWK and LMWK are present, and the presence of both KLK-B1 and KLK-1 is also likely. It appears that KLK-1 is the predominant kininogenase in the interstitial space, suggesting in turn that kallidin is the predominant kinin. It is most likely that kallidin is converted to bradykinin through the action of kininase I activity.[201] There are also B2 and B1 kinin receptors in epithelial cells[202–204] and fibroblasts.[205–207]

REFERENCES

1. Schachter, M., Kallikreins (kininogenases): A group of serine proteases with bioregulatory actions, *Pharmcol. Rev.* 31, 1–17, 1979.
2. Pathak, M., Wong, S.S., Dreveny, I., and Emsley, J., Structure of plasma and tissue kallikreins, *Thromb. Haemost.* 110, 423–433, 2013.
3. Yousef, G.M. and Diamandis, E.P., The new human tissue kallikrein gene family: Structure, function, and association to disease, *Endocr. Rev.* 22, 184–204, 2001.
4. Björkqvist, J., Jämsä, A., and Renné, T., Plasma kallikrein: The bradykinin-producing enzyme, *Thromb. Haemost.* 110, 399–407, 2013.
5. Saito, H. and Ratnoff, O.D., Interactions among Hageman factor (HG, Factor XII), plasma thromboplastin antecedent (PTA, Factor XI), plasma prekallikrein (PK, Fletcher factor) and high molecular weight kininogen (HMW-K, Fitzgerald factor) in blood coagulation, *Adv. Exp. Med. Biol.* 120B, 61–70, 1979.
6. Tsuruta, J., Yamamoto, T., and Kambara, T., Immunohistochemical studies on synthesis and distribution of Hageman factor and kininogen, *Adv. Exp. Med. Biol.* 198B, 63–70, 1986.
7. Yamamoto, T., Tsuruta, J., and Kambara, T., Interstitial-tissue localization of high-molecular-weight kininogen in guinea-pig skin, *Biochim. Biophys. Acta* 916, 332–342, 1987.
8. Fink, E., Bhoola, K.D., Snyman, C., et al., Cellular expression of plasma prekallikrein in human tissues, *Biol. Chem.* 388, 957–963, 2007.
9. Lewis, G.P. and Wawretschek, W.A., Effect of thermal injury on the kinin system in rabbit high limb lymph, *Br. J. Pharmacol.* 43, 127–139, 1971.

10. Orce, G.G., Carretero, O.A., Scicli, G., and Scicli, A.G., Kinins contribute to the contractile effects of rat glandular kallikrein on the isolated rat uterus, *J. Pharmacol. Exp. Ther.* 249, 470–475, 1989.

11. Meini, S., Cucchi, P., Catalani, C., et al., Pharmacological characterization of the bradykinin B2 receptor antagonist MEN16132 in rat *in vitro* bioassays, *Eur. J. Pharmacol.* 615, 10–16, 2009.

12. Schmaier, A.H., The contact activation and kallikrein/kinin systems: Pathophysiologic and physiologic activities, *J. Thromb. Haemost.* 14(1), 28–39, 2016.

13. Garbe, G. and Vogt, W., Zur Natur der in menschlichem Plasma durch Pancreakallikrein, Glaskontakt unter Säurebehandlung gebildeten Kinine, *Naunyn-Schmiedebergs Arch. Pharmak. u. exp. Path.* 256, 119–126, 1967.

14. Vogt, W., An active kallikrein–α_2-macroglobulin complex generated by treatment of human plasma with acetone, *Adv. Exp. Med. Biol.* 70, 281–284, 1976.

15. Jacobsen, S., Observations on the content of kininogen, kallikrein and kinase in lymph from hind limbs of dogs and rabbits, *Br. J. Pharmacol. Chemother.* 27, 213–221, 1966.

16. Davis, A.E., III, Mejia, P., and Lu, F., Biological activities of C1 inhibitor, *Mol. Immunol.* 45, 4057–4063, 2008.

17. Zvonic, S., Lefevre, M., Kilroy, G., et al., Secretome of primary cultures of human adipose-derived stem cells: Modulation of serpins by adipogenesis, *Mol. Cell. Proteomics* 6, 18–28, 2007.

18. Miyoshi, S. and Shinoda, S., Activation mechanism of human Hageman factor–plasma kallikrein–kinin system by *Vibrio vulnificus* metalloprotease, *FEBS Lett.* 308, 315–319, 1992.

19. Kusumam, J., Tholanikunnel, B.G., Bygum, A., et al., Factor XII–independent activation of the bradykinin-forming cascade: Implications the pathogenesis of hereditary angioedema types I and II, *J. Allergy Clin. Immunol.* 132, 470–475, 2013.

20. Bohonowyck, J.E., Hance, M.W., Nolan, K.D., et al., Extracellular Hsp90 mediates an NF-κB dependent stromal program: Implications for the prostate tumor microenvironment, *Prostate* 74, 395–407, 2014.

21. Ravindran, S., Shapira, M., and Preston, P.A., Modulation of C1-inhibitor and plasma kallikrein activities by type IV collagen, *Int. J. Biomater.* 2012, 212417, 2012.

22. Kühn, K., Basement membrane (type IV) collagen, *Matrix Biol.* 14, 439–445, 1995.

23. Saunders, W.B., Bayless, K.J., and Davis, G.E., MMP-1 activation by serine proteases and MMP-10 induces human capillary tubular network collapse and regression in 3D collagen matrices, *J. Cell. Sci.* 118, 2325–2340, 2005.

24. Durham, S.K., Suwanichikui, A., Hayes, J.D., et al., The heparin binding domain of insulin-like growth factor binding protein (IGFBP)-3 increases the susceptibility of IGFBP-3 to proteolysis, *Hormone Metabol. Res.* 31, 216–225, 1999.

25. Burns, R.C. and Fowlkes, J.L., Insulin-like growth factor binding protein proteolysis, *Trends Endocrinol. Metab.* 14, 176–181, 2003.

26. Oesterreicher, S., Blum, W.F., Schmidt, B., Braulke, T., and Kühler, B., Interaction of insulin-like growth factor II (IGF-II) with multiple plasma proteins: High affinity binding of plasminogen to IFG-II and IGF-binding protein, *J. Biol. Chem.* 280, 9994–10000, 2005.

27. Schousboe, I. and Nystrøm, B., High molecular weight kininogen binds to laminin: Characterization and kinetic analysis, *FEBS J.* 276, 5228–5238, 2009.

28. Harvey, T.J., Hooper, J.D., Myers, S.A., et al., Tissue-specific expression patterns and fine mapping of the human kallikrein (KLK) locus on proximal 19q13.4, *J. Biol. Chem.* 275, 37397–37406, 2000.

29. Lundwall, A., Clauss, A., and Olsson, A.Y., Evolution of kallikrein-related peptidases in mammals and identification of a genetic locus encoding potential regulatory inhibitors, *Biol. Chem.* 387, 243–249, 2006.

30. Lundwall, A., Band, V., Blaber, M., et al., A comprehensive nomenclature for serine proteases with homology to tissue kallikreins, *Biol. Chem.* 387, 637–641, 2006.

31. Proud, D., Nakamura, S., Carone, F.A., et al., Kallikrein–kinin and renin–angiotensin systems in rat renal lymph, *Kidney Int.* 24, 880–885, 1984.

32. Rahman, M.M., Worthy, K., Elson, C.J., et al., Inhibitor regulation of tissue kallikrein activity in the synovial fluid of patients with rheumatoid arthritis, *Br. J. Rheumatol.* 33, 215–223, 1994.

32. Girolami, J.P., Pecher, C., Bascanda, J.L., et al., Direct radioimmunoassay of active and inactive human glandular kallikrein: Some physiological and pathological variabilities, *J. Immunoassay* 10, 221–236, 1989.

34. Clement, C.C. and Santambrogio, L., The lymph self-antigen repertoire, *Front. Immunol.* 4, 424, 2013.

35. Maier, H., Adler, D., Menstell, S., and Lenarz, T., Glandular kallikrein in chronic recurrent parotitis, *Laryngol. Rhinol. Otol.* (Stuttg.) 63, 633–635, 1984.

36. Simson, J.A. and Chao, J., Subcellular distribution of tissue kallikrein and Na, K-ATPase α-subunit in rat parotid striated duct cells, *Cell Tissue Res.* 275, 407–417, 1994.

37. Ramsaroop, R., Naicker, S., Naicker, T., Naidoo, S., and Bhoola, K.D., Tissue kallikrein in transplant kidney, *Immunopharmacology* 36(2–3), 255–261, 1997.

38. Devani, M., Vecchi, M., Ferrero, S., et al., Kallikrein–kinin system in inflammatory bowel diseases: Intestinal involvement and correlation with the degree of tissue inflammation, *Dig. Liver Dis.* 37, 665–673, 2005.

39. Stadnicki, A., Intestinal tissue kallikrein–kinin system in inflammatory bowel disease, *Inflamm. Bowel Dis.* 17, 645–654, 2011.

40. Shimamoto, K., Mayfield, R.K., Margolius, H.S., et al., Immunoreactive tissue kallikrein in human serum, *J. Lab. Clin. Med.* 103, 731–738, 1984.

41. Mannelo, F., Tonti, G.A., Bagnara, G.P., and Papa, S., Role and function of matrix metalloproteinases in the differentiation and biological characterization of mesenchymal stem cells, *Stem Cells.* 24, 475–481, 2006.

42. Affara, N.I., Andreu, P., and Coussens, L.M., Delineating protease functions during cancer development, *Methods Mol. Biol.* 539, 1–32, 2009.

43. Davie, E.W. and Ratnoff, O.D., Waterfall sequence for intrinsic blood clotting, *Science* 145, 1310–1312, 1964.

44. MacFarlane, R.G., An enzyme cascade in the blood clotting mechanism, and its function as a biochemical amplifier, *Nature* 202, 498–499. 1964.

45. Yoon, H., Laxmikanthan, G., Lee, J., et al., Activation profiles and regulatory cascades of the human kallikrein-related peptidases, *J. Biol. Chem.* 282, 31852–31864, 2007.

46. Yoon, H., Blaber, S.I., Evans, D.M., et al., Activation profiles of human kallikrein-related peptidases by proteases of the thrombostasis axis, *Protein Sci.* 17, 1998–2007, 2008.

47. Yoon, H., Blaber, S.I., Debela, M., et al., A completed KLK activome profile: Investigation of activation profiles of KLK9, 10, and 15, *Biol. Chem.* 390, 373–377, 2009.

48. Dong, Y., Loessner, D., Irving-Rodgers, H., et al., Metastasis of ovarian cancer is mediated by kallikrein related peptidases, *Clin. Exp. Metastasis* 31, 135–147, 2014.

49. Korkmaz, K.S., Korkmaz, C.G., Pretlow, T.G., and Saatchioglu, F., Distinctly different gene structure of KLK4/KLK-L1/prostase/ARM1 compared with other members of the kallikrein family: Intracellular localization, alternative cDNA forms, and regulation by multiple hormones, *DNA Cell Biol.* 20, 435–445, 2001.

50. Jenzano, J.W., Coffey, J.C., Heizer, W.D., et al., The assay of glandular kallikrein and prekallikrein in human mixed saliva, *Arch. Oral Biol.* 33, 641–644, 1988.

51. Mauer, S. and Kemme, M., Magnetic beads capture assay for the study of zymogen activation, *Anal. Biochem.* 305, 284–287, 2002.
52. Rhaman, M.M., Worthy, K., Elson, C.J., et al., Inhibitor regulation of tissue kallikrein activity in the synovial fluid of patients with rheumatoid arthritis, *Br. J. Rheumatol.* 33, 215–223, 1994.
53. Chao, J., Chai, K.X., and Chao, L., Tissue kallikrein inhibitors in mammals, *Immunopharmacology* 32, 67–92, 1996.
54. Wang, C.R., Chen, S.Y., Shiau, A.L., et al., Upregulation of kallistatin expression in rheumatoid joints, *J. Rheumatol.* 34, 2171–2176, 2007.
55. Wang, M.Y., Day, J., Chao, L., and Chao, J., Human kallistatin, a new tissue kallikrein–binding protein: Purification and characterization, *Adv. Exp. Med. Biol.* 247B, 1–8, 1989.
56. Volpe-Júnior, N., Donadi, E.A., Carvalho, I.F., and Reis, M.L., Augmented plasma and tissue kallikrein like activity in synovial fluid of patients with inflammatory articular diseases, *Inflamm. Res.* 45, 198–202, 1996.
57. Williams, R.J., Henderson, L.M, Naidoo, Y., et al., Immunocytochemical analysis of tissue kallikrein and the kinin moiety in rheumatoid synovial fluid neutrophils, *Br. J. Rheumatol.* 36, 420–425, 1997.
58. Cassim, B., Shaw, O.M., Mazur, M., et al., Kallikreins, kininogens and kinin receptors on synovial fluid neutrophils: Role in kinin generation in rheumatoid arthritis, *Rheumatology (Oxford)* 48, 490–496, 2009.
59. Wu, H.F., Venezie, R.D., Cohen, W.M., et al., Identification of tissue kallikrein messenger RNA in human neutrophils, *Agents Actions* 38, 27–31, 1993.
60. Nolly, H., Carbini, L.A., Scicli, G., et al., A local kallikrein/kinin system is present in rat hearts, *Hypertension* 23, 919–923, 1994.
61. Madeddu, P., Gherli, T., Bacciu, P.P., et al., A kallikrein-like enzyme in human vascular tissues, *Am. J. Hypertens.* 6, 344–348, 1993.
62. Wolf, W.C., Harley, R.A., Sluce, D., et al., Localization and expression of tissue kallikrein and kallistatin in human blood vessels, *J. Histochem. Cytochem.* 47, 221–228, 1999.
63. Wu, H.F., Xu, L.H., Jenzano, J.W., et al., Expression of tissue kallikrein in normal and SV40-transfected human endometrial stromal cells, *Pathobiology* 61, 123–127, 1993.
64. Yayama, K., Kunimatsu, N., Teranishi, Y., et al., Tissue kallikrein is synthesized and secreted by human vascular endothelial cells, *Biochim. Biophys. Acta* 1593, 231–238, 2003.
65. Yiu, W.H., Wong, D.W., Chan, L.Y., et al., Tissue kallikrein mediates pro-inflammatory pathways and activation of protease-activated receptor-4 in proximal tubular epithelial cells, *PLoS One* 9(2), e88894, 2014.
66. Bader, M., Kallikrein–kinin system in neovascularization, *Arteriocler. Thromb. Vasc. Biol.* 29, 617–619, 2009.
67. Stone, O.A., Riches, C., Emanuel, C., et al., Critical role of tissue kallikrein in vessel formation and maturation: Implications for therapeutic revascularization, *Arterioscler. Thromb. Vasc. Biol.* 29, 657–664, 2009.
68. Spinetti, G., Fortunato, O., Cordella, D., et al., Tissue kallikrein is essential for the invasive capacity of circulating proangiogenic cells, *Circ. Res.* 108, 284–293, 2011.
69. Dimmeler, S., Regulation of bone marrow–derived vascular progenitor cell mobilization and maintenance, *Arterioscler. Thromb. Vasc. Biol.* 30, 1088–1093, 2010.
70. Honold, J., Fischer-Rasokat, U., Lehman, R., et al., G-CSF stimulation and coronary reinfusion of mobilized circulating mononuclear proangiogenic cells in patients with chronic ischemic heart disease: Five-year results of the TOPCARE-G-CSP trial, *Cell Transplant.* 21, 2325–2337, 2012.

71. Fukuhara, J., Noda, K., Murata, M., et al., Tissue kallikrein attenuates choroidal neovascularization via cleavage of vascular endothelial growth factor, *Invest. Opthalmol. Vis. Sci.* 54, 274–279, 2013.

72. Nakamura, S., Morimoto, N., Tsuruma, K., et al., Tissue kallikrein inhibits retinal neovascularization via the cleavage of vascular endothelial growth factor-165, *Arterioscler. Thromb. Vasc. Biol.* 31, 1041–1048, 2011.

73. Masuda, T., Shimazawa, M., Ishizuka, F., et al., Tissue kallikrein (kallidinogenase) protects against retinal ischemic damage in mice, *Eur. J. Pharmacol.* 5, 74–82, 2014.

74. Masuda, T., Shimazawa, M., and Hara, H., The kallikrein system in retinal damage/protection, *Eur. J. Pharmacol.* 749, 161–163, 2015.

75. Biyashev, D., Tan, F., Chen, Z., et al., Kallikrein activates bradykinin B2 receptors in absence of kininogen, *Am. J. Physiol. Heart Circ. Physiol.* 290, H1244–H1250, 2006.

76. Gao, L., Smith, R.S., Chen, L.M., et al., Tissue kallikrein promotes prostate cancer cell migration and invasion via a protease-activated receptor-1-dependent signaling pathway, *Biol. Chem.* 391, 803–812, 2010.

77. Rothmeier, A.S. and Ruf, W., Protease-activated receptor 2 signaling in inflammation, *Semin. Immunopathol.* 34, 133–149, 2012.

78. Chung, H., Hamza, M., Oikonomopoulou, K., et al., Kallikrein-related peptidase signaling in colon carcinoma cells: Targeting proteinase-activated receptors, *Biol. Chem.* 393, 413–420, 2012.

79. Ramachandran, R., Eissa, A., Mihara, K., et al., Proteinase-activated receptors (PARs): Differential signalling by kallikrein-related peptidases KLK8 and KLK14, *Biol. Chem.* 393, 421–427, 2012.

80. Gao, L., Chao, L., and Chao, J., A novel signaling pathway of tissue kallikrein in promoting keratinocyte migration: Activation of proteinase-activated receptor 1 and epidermal growth factor receptor, *Exp. Cell Res.* 316, 376–389, 2010.

81. Lu, Z., Cui, M., Zhao, H., et al., Tissue kallikrein mediates neurite outgrowth through epidermal growth factor receptor and flotillin-2 pathway *in vitro*, *Cell Signal.* 26, 220–232, 2014.

82. Lu, Z., Yang, Q., Cui, M., et al., Tissue kallikrein induces SH-SY5Y cell proliferation via epidermal growth factor receptor and extracellular signal-regulated kinase 1/2 pathway, *Biochem. Biophys. Res. Commun.*, 446(1), 25–29, 2014.

83. Jørgensen, P.E., Nexø, E., and Poulsen, S.S., The membrane fraction of homogenized rat kidney contains an enzyme that releases epidermal growth factor from the kidney membranes, *Biochim. Biophys. Acta* 1074, 284–288, 1991.

84. Jørgensen, P.E., Nexø, E., Poulsen, S.S., et al., Processing of epidermal growth factor in the rat submandibular gland by kallikrein-like enzymes, *Growth Factors* 11, 113–123, 1994.

85. Rousselet, E., Benjannet, S., Marcinkiewicz, E., et al., Proprotein convertase PC7 enhances the activation of the EGF receptor pathway through processing of the EGF precursor, *J. Biol. Chem.* 286, 9185–9195, 2011.

86. Le Gall, S.M., Meneton, P., Mauduit, P., and Dreux, C., The sequential cleavage of membrane anchored pro-EGF requires a membrane serine protease other than kallikrein in rat kidney, *Regul. Pept.* 122, 119–129, 2004.

87. Horiuchi, K., Le Gall, S., Schulte, M., et al., Substrate selectivity of epidermal growth factor–receptor ligand sheddases and their regulation by phorbol esters and calcium influx, *Mol. Biol. Cell* 18, 176–188, 2007.

88. Edelman, G.M. and Gally, J.A., Degeneracy and complexity in biological systems, *Proc. Natl. Acad. Sci. USA* 98, 13763–13768, 2001.

89. Tryggvason, K., Huhtala, P., Höyhtya, M., et al., 70 K type IV collagenase (gelatinase), *Matrix Suppl.* 1, 45–50, 1992.

90. Desrivières. S., Lu., H., Peyri, N., et al., Activation of the 92 kDa type IV collagenase by tissue kallikrein, *J. Cell Physiol.* 157, 587–593, 1993.

91. Menashi, S., Fridman, R., Desrivières, S., et al., Regulation of 92-kDa gelatinase B activity in the extracellular matrix by tissue kallikrein, *Ann. N.Y. Acad. Sci.* 732, 466–468, 1994.

92. Corthorn, J., Rey, S., Chacón, C., and Valdés, G., Spatio-temporal expression of MMP-9 and tissue kallikrein in uteroplacental units of the pregnant guinea-pig (*Cavia procelluls*), *Reprod. Biol. Endocrinol.* 5(27), 2007.

93. Lövgren, J., Piironen, T., Overmo, C., et al., Production of recombinant PSA and HK2 and analysis of their immunologic cross-reactivity, *Biochem. Biophys. Res. Commun.* 213, 888–895, 1995.

94. Voigt, J.D., Zappala, S.M., Vaughn, E.D., and Wein, A.J., The kallikrein panel for prostate cancer screening: Its economic impact, *Prostate* 74, 250–259, 2014.

95. Yu, H., Diamandis, E.P., and Sutherland, D.J., Immunoreactive prostate-specific antigen levels in female and male breast tumors and its association with steroid hormone receptors and patient age, *Clin. Biochem.* 27, 75–79, 1994.

96. Alanan, K.A., Kuopio, T., Koskinen, P.J., and Nevalainen, T.J., Immunohistochemical labelling for prostate-specific antigen in non-prostatic tissues, *Pathol. Res. Pract.* 192, 233–237, 1996.

97. Frenette, G., Deperthes, D., Tremblay, R.R., et al., Purification of enzymatically active kallikrein hK2 from human seminal plasma, *Biochim. Biophys. Acta* 1334, 109–115, 1997.

98. Lilja, H., A kallikrein-like serine protease in prostatic fluid cleaves the predominant seminal vesicle protein, *J. Clin. Invest.* 76, 1899–1903, 1985.

99. Sensabaugh, G.F. and Blake, E.T., Seminal plasma protein p30: Simplified purification and evidence for identify with prostate specific antigen, *J. Urol.* 144, 1523–1526, 1990.

100. Dorn, J., Gkazepis, A., Kotzsch, M., et al., Clinical value of protein expression of kallikrein-related peptidase 7 (KLK7) in ovarian cancer, *Biol. Chem.* 395, 95–107, 2014.

101. Wen, Y.G., Wang, Q., Zhou, C.Z., et al., Identification and validation of kallikrein-related peptidase 11 as a novel prognostic marker of gastric cancer based on immunohistochemistry, *J. Surg. Oncol.* 104, 516–524, 2011.

102. Seiz, L., Kotzsch, M., Grebenchtchikov, N.I., et al., Polyclonal antibodies against kallikrein-related peptidase 4 (KLK4): Immunohistochemical assessment of KLK4 expression in healthy tissues and prostate cancer, *Biol. Chem.* 391, 391–401, 2010.

103. Zhao, H., Dong, Y., Quan, J., et al., Correlation of the expression of human kallikrein-related peptidases 4 and 7 with the prognosis in oral squamous cell carcinoma, *Head Neck* 33, 566–572, 2011.

104. Petraki, C., Youssef, Y.M., Dubinski, W., et al., Evaluation and prognostic significance of human tissue kallikrein–related peptidase 10 (KLK10) in colorectal cancer, *Tumour Biol.* 33, 1209–1214, 2012.

105. Darling, M.R., Hashem, N.N., Zhang, I., et al., Kallikrein-related peptidase 10 expression in salivary gland tissues and tumours, *Int. J. Biol. Markers* 27, e381–388, 2012.

106. Seiz, L., Dorn, J., Kotzsch, M., et al., Stromal cell–associated expression of kallikrein-related peptidase 6 (KLK6) indicates poor prognosis of ovarian cancer patients, *Biol. Chem.* 393, 391–401, 2012.

107. Gabril, M., White, N.M., Moussa, M., et al., Immunohistochemical analysis of kallikrein-related peptidase in the normal kidney and renal tumors: Potential clinical implications, *Biol. Chem.* 391, 403–409, 2010.

108. Bandiera, E., Zanotti, L., Bignotti, E., et al., Human kallikrein 5: An interesting novel biomarker in ovarian cancer patients that elicits humoral response, *Int. J. Gynecol. Cancer* 19, 1015–1021, 2009.

109. Emami, N., Scorilas, A., Soosaipillai, A., et al., Association between kallikrein-related peptidases (KLKs) and macroscopic indicators of semen analysis: Their relation to sperm motility, *Biol. Chem.* 390, 921–929, 2009.

110. Chee, J., Singh, J., Naran, A., et al., Novel expression of kallikreins, kallikrein-related peptidases and kinin receptors in human pleural mesothelioma, *Biol. Chem.* 388, 1235–1242, 2007.

111. Memari, N., Diamandis, E.P., Earle, T., et al., Human kallikrein-related peptidase 12: Antibody generation and immunohistochemical localization in prostatic tissues, *Prostate* 67, 1465–1474, 2007.

112. Charlesworth, M.C., Young, C.Y.F., Miller, V.M., and Tindall, D.J., Kininogenase activity of prostate-derived human glandular kallikrein (hK2) purified from seminal fluid, *J. Andrology* 20, 220–229, 1999.

113. Deperthes, D., Marceau, F., Frenette, G., et al., Human kallikrein hK2 has low kininogenase activity while prostate-specific antigen (hK3) has none, *Biochim. Biophys. Acta* 1343, 102–106, 1997.

114. Andrade, D., Assis, D.M., Lima, A.R., et al., Substrate specificity and inhibition of human kallikrein-related peptidase 3 (KLK3 or PSA) activated with sodium citrate and glycosaminoglycans, *Arch. Biochem. Biophys.* 498, 74–82, 2010.

115. David, A., Mabjeesh, N., Azar, I., et al., Unusual alternative splicing within the human kallikrein genes KLK2 and KLK3 gives rise to novel prostate-specific proteins, *J. Biol. Chem.* 277, 18084–18090, 2002.

116. Sävblom, C., Halldén, C., Cronin, A.M., et al., Genetic variation in KLK2 and KLLK3 is associated with concentrations of hK2 and PSA in serum and seminal plasma in young men, *Clin. Chem.* 60, 490–499, 2014.

117. Petraki, C.D., Papanastasou, P.A., Karavana, V.N., et al., Cellular distribution of human tissue kallikreins: Immunochemical localization, *Biol. Chem.* 387, 653–663, 2006.

118. Guillon-Munos, A., Oikonomopoulou, K., Michel, N., et al., Kallikrein-related peptidase 12 hydrolyzes matricellular proteins of the CCN family and modifies interactions of CCN1 and CNN5 with growth factors, *J. Biol. Chem.* 286, 25505–25518, 2011.

119. Kryza, T., Lalmanach, G., Lavergne, M., et al., Pro-angiogenic effects of human kallikrein-related peptidase 12 (KLK12) in lung endothelial cells does not depend on kinin-mediated activation of B2 receptor, *Biol. Chem.* 394, 3385–391, 2013.

120. Kryza, T., Achard, C., Parent, C., et al., Angiogenesis stimulated by human kallikrein-related peptidase 12 acting via platelet-derived growth factor B-dependent paracrine pathway, *FASEB J.* 28, 740–751, 2014.

121. Wei, C.-C., Chen, Y., Powell, L.C., et al., Cardiac kallikrein-kinin system is upregulated in chronic volume overload and mediates an inflammatory collagen loss, *PLoS One* 7, e40110, 2012.

122. Shaw, J.L. and Diamandis, E.P., Distribution of 15 human kallikreins in tissues and biological fluids, *Clin. Chem.* 53, 1423–1432, 2007.

123. Rajapakse, S., Ogiwara, K., Takano, N., et al., Biochemical characterization of human kallikrein 8 and its possible involvement in the degradation of extracellular matrix protein, *FEBS Lett.* 579, 6879–6884, 2005.

124. Rajapakse, S. and Takahashi, T., Expression and enzymatic characterization of recombinant human kallikrein 14, *Zoolog. Sci.* 24, 774–780, 2007.

125. Schanstra, J.P., Neau, E., Drogoz, P., et al., *In vivo* bradykinin B2 receptor activation reduces renal fibrosis, *J. Clin. Invest.* 110, 371–279, 2002.

126. Clements, J.A., Willemsen, N.M., Myers, S.A., and Dong, Y., The tissue kallikrein family of serine proteases: Functional roles in human disease and potential as clinical biomarkers, *Crit. Rev. Clin. Lab. Sci.* 41, 265–312, 2004.

127. Mavridis, K., Avgeris, M., and Scorilas, A., Targeting kallikrein-related peptidases in prostate cancer, *Expert Opin. Ther. Targets* 18, 365–383, 2014.

128. Graf, K., Gräfe, M., Auch-Schwelk, W., et al., Tissue kallikrein activity and kinin release in human endothelial cells, *Eur. J. Clin. Chem. Clin. Biochem.* 32, 495–500, 1994.

129. Dedio, J., Wiemer, G., Rütten, H., et al., Tissue kallikrein is expressed *de novo* in endothelial cells and mediates relaxation of human umbilical veins, *Biol. Chem.* 382, 1483–1490, 2001.

130. Hecquet, C., Tan, F., Marcic, B.M., et al., Human bradykinin B(2) receptors is activated by kallikrein and other serine proteases, *Mol. Pharmacol.* 58, 828–836, 2000.

131. Kahn, R., Hellmark, T., Leeb-Lundberg, L.M., et al., Neutrophil-derived proteinase 3 induces kallikrein-independent release of a novel vasoactive kinin, *J. Immunol.* 182, 7906–7915, 2009.

132. Del Nery, E., Juliano, M.A., Lima, A.P., et al., Kininogenase activity by the major cysteinyl proteinase (cruzipain) from *Trypanosoma cruzi*, *J. Biol. Chem.* 272, 25713–25718, 1997.

133. Fichtner, J., Graves, H.C., Thatcher, K., et al., Prostate specific antigen releases a kinin-like substance on proteolysis of seminal vesicle fluid that stimulates smooth muscle contraction, *J. Urol.* 155, 738–742, 1996.

134. Yauki, Y., Oguchi, T., and Takahashi, H., Purification of a kininogenase (kininogenase-2) from the venom of *Agkistrodon caliginosus* (Kankoku-Mamushi), *Toxicon* 29, 73–84, 1991.

135. Hung, C.C. and Chiou, S.H., Fibrinogenolytic proteases isolated from the snake venom of Taiwan habu: Serine proteases with kallikrein-like and angiotensin-degrading activities, *Biochem. Biophys. Res. Commun.* 281, 1012–1018, 2001.

136. Felicori, L.F., Souza, C.T., Velarde, D.T., et al., Kallikrein-like proteinase from bushmaster snake venom, *Protein Expr. Purif.* 30, 32–42, 2003.

137. Weinberg, M.L., Felicori, L.F., Bello, C.A., et al., Biochemical properties of a bushmaster snake venom serine proteinase (LV-Ka), and its kinin releasing activity evaluated in rat mesenteric arterial rings, *J. Pharmacol. Sci.* 96, 333–342, 2004.

138. Baramova, E.N., Shannon, J.D., Bjarnason, J.B., and Fox, J.W., Degradation of extracellular matrix proteins by hemorrhagic metalloproteinases, *Arch. Biochem. Biophys.* 275, 63–71, 1989.

139. Soe, S., Win, M.M., Htwe, T.T., et al., Renal histopathology following Russell's viper (*Vipera russelli*) bite, *Southeast. Asian. J. Trop. Med.* 24, 193–197, 1993.

140. Gutiérez, J.M., León, G., and Lomonte, B., Pharmacokinetic-pharmacodynamic relationships of immunoglobulin therapy for envenomation, *Clin. Pharmacokinet.* 42, 721–741, 2003.

141. Francisco, G., Zara, F.J., Maria, D.A., and Cruz-Neto, A.P., Toxin jarahagin in low doses induces interstitial edema and increases the metabolic rate and red blood cells in mice, *Toxicon* 48, 1060–1067, 2006.

142. Forteza, R., Lauredo, I., Abraham, W.M., and Conner, G.E., Bronchial tissue kallikrein activity is guided by hyaluronic acid binding, *Am. J. Respir. Cell Mol. Biol.* 21, 666–674, 1999.

143. Forteza, R., Lieb, T., Aoki, T., et al., Hyaluronan serves a novel role in airway mucosal host defense, *FASEB J.* 15, 2179–2186, 2001.

144. Casalino-Matsuda, S.M., Monzon, M.E., Conner, G.E., et al., Role of hyaluronan and reactive oxygen species in tissue kallikrein–mediated epidermal growth factor activation in human airways, *J. Biol. Chem.* 279, 21606–21615, 2004.

145. Casilino-Matsuda, S.M., Monzón, M.E., and Forteza, R.M., Epidermal growth factor receptor activation by epidermal growth factor mediates oxidant-induced goblet cell metaplasia in human airway epithelium. *Am. J. Respir. Cell. Mol. Biol.* 34, 581–591, 2006.

146. Yu, H., Li, Q., Zhou, X., et al., Role of hyaluronan and CD44 in reactive oxygen species–induced mucin hypersecretion, *Mol. Cell. Biochem.* 352, 65–75, 2011.

147. Etscheid, M., Beer, N., Fink, E., et al., The hyaluronan-binding serine protease from human plasma cleaves HMW and LWM kininogen and releases bradykinin, *Biol. Chem.* 383, 1633–1643, 2002.

148. Etscheid, M., Beer, N., Kress, J.A., et al., Inhibition of bFGF/EGF-dependent cell proliferation by the hyaluronan-binding protease from human plasma, *Eur. J. Cell Biol.* 82, 597–604, 2004.

149. Nakazawa, F., Kannemeier, C., Shibamiya, A., et al., Extracellular RNA is a natural cofactor for the (auto-)activation of Factor VII-activating protease (FSAP), *Biochem. J.* 385, 831–838, 2005.

150. Etscheid, M., Beer, N., and Dodt, J., The hyaluronan-binding protease upregulates ERK1/2 and PI3K/Akt signalling pathways in fibroblasts and stimulates cell proliferation and migration, *Cell. Signal.* 17, 1486–1494, 2005.

151. Borkham-Kamphorst, E., Zimmerman, H.W., Gassler, N., et al., Factor VII activating protease (FSAP) exerts anti-inflammatory and anti-fibrotic effects in liver fibrosis in mice and men, *J. Hepatol.* 58, 104–111, 2013.

152. Skidgel, R.A., McGwire, G.B., and Li, X.Y., Membrane anchoring and release of carboxypeptidase M: Implications for extracellular hydrolysis of peptide hormones, *Immunopharmacology* 32, 48–52, 1996.

153. Mirgorodskaya, O.A. and Shevehenko, A.A., Bradykinin degradation pathways in human blood plasma, *FEBS Lett.* 307, 263–266, 1992.

154. Skidgel, R.A., Davis, R.M., and Tan, R., Human carboxypeptidase M. Purification and characterization of a membrane-bound carboxypeptidase that cleaves peptide hormones, *J. Biol. Chem.* 264, 2236–2241, 1989.

155. Dorer, F., Ryan, J.W., and Stewart, J.M., Hydrolysis of bradykinin and its higher homologues by angiotensin-converting enzyme, *Biochem. J.* 141, 915–917, 1974.

156. Sheikh, I.A. and Kaplan, A.P., Studies of the digestion of bradykinin, lys-bradykinin, and des-Arg9-bradykinin by angiotensin converting enzyme, *Biochem. Pharmacol.* 35, 1951–1956, 1986.

157. Sheikh, I.A. and Kaplan, A.P., Mechanism of digestion of bradykinin and lysylbradykinin (kallidin) in human serum: Role of carboxypeptidase, angiotensin-converting enzyme and determination of final degradation products, *Biochem. Pharmacol.* 38, 993–1000, 1989.

158. Wolfrum, S., Dendorfer, A., and Dominiak, P., Identification of kallidin degrading enzymes in the isolated perfused rat heart, *Jpn. J. Pharmacol.* 79, 117–120, 1999.

159. Sheng, Z., Yao, Y., Li, Y., et al., Bradykinin preconditioning improves therapeutic potential of human endothelial progenitor cells in infarcted myocardium, *PLoS One* 8(12), e81505, 2013.

160. Ghebrehiwet, B., Ji, Y., Valentino, A., et al., Soluble gC1qR is an autocrine signal that induces B1R expression on endothelial cells, *J. Immunol.* 192, 377–384, 2014.

161. Veronez, C.L., Nascimento, F.D., Melo, K.R., et al., The involvement of proteoglycans in the human plasma prekallikrein interaction with the cell surface, *PLoS One* 9(3), e91280, 2014.

162. Kajdácsi, E., Jani, P.K., Csuka, D., et al., Endothelial cell activation during edematous attacks of hereditary angioedema types I and II, *J. Allergy Clin. Immunol.* 133(6), 1686–1691, 2014.

163. Marshall, J.M. and Kontos, H.A., Endothelium-derived relaxing factors: A perspective from *in vivo* data, *Hypertension* 16, 371–386, 1990.

164. Kasuba, E., Bailey, J., Allsup, D., and Cawkwell, L., The kinin–kallikrein system: Physiological roles, pathophysiology and its relationship to cancer biomarkers, *Biomarkers* 18, 279–296, 2013.

165. Bossi, F., Peerschke, E.I., Ghebrehiwet, B., and Tedesco, F., Cross-talk between the complement and the kinin system in vascular permeability, *Immunol. Lett.* 140, 7–13, 2011.

166. Phipps, J.A., Clermont, A.C., Sinha, S., et al., Plasma kallikrein mediates angiotensin II type 1 receptor–stimulated retinal permeability, *Hypertension* 53, 175–181, 2009.

167. Rocha, E., Silva, M., and Antonio, A., Release of bradykinin and the mechanism of production of "thermic edema (45 degrees C)" in the rat's paw, *Med. Exp. Int. J. Exp. Med.* 3, 371–382, 1960.

168. Wahl, M., Whalley, E.T., Unterberg, A., et al., Vasomotor and permeability effects of bradykinin in the cerebral microcirculation, *Immunopharmacology* 33, 257–263, 1996.

169. Bork, K. and Davis-Lorton, M., Overview of hereditary angioedema caused by C1-inhibitor deficiency: Assessment and clinical management, *Eur. Ann. Allergy Clin. Immunol.* 45, 7–16, 2013.

170. Suffritti, C., Zanichelli, A., Maggioni, L., et al., High-molecular-weight kininogen cleavage correlates with disease states in the bradykinin mediated angioedema due to hereditary c1-inhibitor deficiency, *Clin. Exp. Allergy* 44(12), 1503–1514, 2014.

171. Defendi, F., Charignon, D., Ghannam, A., et al., Enzymatic assays for the diagnosis of bradykinin-dependent angioedema, *PLoS One* 8(8), e70140, 2013.

172. Romero, J.C, Lahera, V., Salom, M.G., and Biondi, M.L., Role of the endothelium-dependent relaxing factor nitric oxide on renal function, *J. Am. Soc. Nephrol.* 2, 1371–1387, 1992.

173. Petho, G. and Reeh, P.W., Sensory and signaling mechanisms of bradykinin, eicosanoids, platelet-activating factor, and nitric oxide in peripheral nociceptors, *Physiol. Rev.* 92, 1699–1775, 2012.

174. Steranka, L.R., Farmer, S.G., and Burch, R.M., Antagonists of B2 bradykinin receptors, *FASEB J.* 3, 2019–2025, 1989.

175. Marceau, F., Sabourin, T., Houle, S., et al., Kinin receptors: Functional aspects, *Int. Immunopharmacology* 2, 1729–1739, 2002.

176. Alla, S.A., Buschko, J., Quitterer, U., et al., Structural features of the human bradykinin B2 receptor probed by agonists, antagonists, and anti-idiotypic antibodies, *J. Biol. Chem.* 268, 17277–17285, 1993.

177. Campbell, D.J., The kallikrein–kinin system in humans, *Clin. Exp. Pharmacol. Physiol.* 28, 1060–1065, 2001.

178. Skidgel, R.A., Johnson, A.R., and Erdös, E.G., Hydrolysis of opioid hexapeptides by carboxypeptidase N: Presence of carboxypeptidase in cell membranes, *Biochem. Pharmacol.* 33, 3471–3478, 1984.

179. Denis, C.J., Van Acker, N., De Schepper, S., et al., Mapping of carboxypeptidase m in normal human kidney and renal cell carcinoma: Expression in tumor-associated neovasculature and macrophages, *J. Histochem. Cytochem.* 61, 218–235, 2013.

180. Schremmer-Danniger, E., Nägler, D.K., Miska, K., et al., Kinin receptors in stimulated and characterized decidua tissue-derived cells, *Int. Immunopharmacol.* 7, 103–112, 2007.

181. Wang, C.H., Lee, Y.S., Lin, S.J., et al., Surface markers for heterogeneous peripheral blood-derived smooth muscle progenitor cells, *Arterioscler. Thromb. Vasc. Biol.* 32, 1875–1883, 2012.

182. Zhang, X., Tan, F., Zhang, Y., and Skidgel, R.A., Carboxypeptidase M and kinin B1 receptors interact to facilitate efficient b1 signaling from B2 agonists, *J. Biol. Chem.* 283, 7994–8004, 2008.

183. Zhang, X., Tan, F., and Skidgel, R.A., Carboxypeptidase M is a positive allosteric modulator of the kinin B1 receptor, *J. Biol. Chem.* 288, 33226–33240, 2013.

184. Zhang, X., Tan, F., Brovkovych, V., et al., Carboxypeptidase M augments kinin B1 receptor signaling by conformational crosstalk and enhances endothelial nitric oxide output, *Biol. Chem.* 394, 335–345, 2013.

185. Denis, C.J., Deiteren, K., Hendriks, D., et al., Carboxypeptidase M in apoptosis, adipogenesis and cancer, *Clin. Chim. Acta* 415, 306–316, 2013.

186. Denis, C.J. and Lambeir, A.M., The potential of carboxypeptidase M as a therapeutic target in cancer, *Expert Opin. Ther. Targets* 17, 265–279, 2013.

187. Dendorfer, A., Wolfram, S., Wellhöner, P., et al., Intravascular and interstitial degradation of bradykinin in isolated perfused rat heart, *Brit. J. Pharmacol.* 122, 1179–1187, 1997.

188. Adamski, S.W. and Grega, G.J., Contribution of kininase II to the waning of vascular actions of bradykinin, *Am. J. Physiol.* 254, H1042–H1050, 1988.

189. Bénéteau-Burnat, B. and Baudin, B., Angiotensin-converting enzyme: Clinical applications and laboratory investigations on serum and other biological fluids, *Crit. Rev. Clin. Lab. Sci.* 28, 337–356, 1991.

190. Ferreira, S.H. and Vane, J.R., Half-lives of peptides and amines in the circulation, *Nature* 215, 1237–1240, 1967.

191. Pojda, S.M. and Vane, J.R., Inhibitory effects of aprotinin on kallikrein and kininases in dog's blood, *Brit. J. Pharmacol.* 42, 558–568, 1971.

192. Rosenbaum, C., Cardoza, C., and Lesser, M., Degradation of lysylbradykinin by endopeptidase 24.11 and endopeptidase 24.15, *Peptides* 16, 523–525, 1995.

193. Campbell, D.J., Towards understanding the kallikrein–kinin system: Insights from measurements of kinin peptides, *Braz. J. Med. Biol. Res.* 33, 665–677, 2000.

194. Yu, H.S., Wang, S.W., Chang, A.C., et al., Bradykinin promotes vascular endothelial growth factor expression and increases angiogenesis in human prostate cancer cells, *Biochem. Pharmacol.* 87, 243–253, 2014.

195. Takano, M., Kanoh, A., Amako, K., et al., Nuclear localization of bradykinin B_2 receptors reflects binding to the nuclear envelope protein lamin C, *Eur. J. Pharmacol.* 723, 507–514, 2014.

196. Calixto, J.B., Medieros, R., Fernandes, E.S., et al., Kinin B_1 receptors: Key G-protein-coupled receptors and their role in inflammatory and painful processes, *Brit. J. Pharmacol.* 143, 803–818, 2004.

197. Feng, J., Chen, Y., Xiong, J., et al., The kinin B1 receptor mediates alloknesis in a murine model of inflammation, *Neurosci. Lett.* 560, 31–35, 2014.

198. Pinheiro, A.R., Paramos-de-Carvalho, K., Certal, M., et al., Bradykinin-induced Ca^{2+} signaling in human subcutaneous fibroblasts involves ATP release via hemichannels leading to P2Y12 receptors activation, *Cell Commun. Signal.* 11(70), 2013.

199. Vancheri, C., Gili, E., Failla, M., et al., Bradykinin differentiates human lung fibroblasts to a myofibroblast phenotype via the B2 receptor, *J. Allergy Clin. Immunol.* 116, 1242–1246, 2005.

200. Kim, Y.M., Jeoon, E.S., Kim, M.R., et al., Bradykinin-induced expression of α-smooth muscle actin in human mesenchymal stem cells, *Cell. Signal.* 20, 1882–1889, 2008.

201. Sangsree, S., Borvkovych, V., Minshall, R.D., and Skidgel, R.A., Kininase I-type carboxypeptidases enhance nitric oxide production in endothelial cells by generating bradykinin B1 receptor antagonists, *Am. J. Physiol. Heart Circ. Physiol.* 284, H1959–1968, 2003.

202. Chen, B.C., Yu, C.C., Lei, H.C., et al., Bradykinin B2 receptor mediates NF-κB activation and cyclooxygenase-2 expression via the Ras/Raf-1/ERK pathway in human airway epithelial cells, *J. Immunol.* 173, 5219–5228, 2004.

203. Greco, S., Muscella, A., Elia, M.G., et al., Mitogenic signalling by B2 bradykinin receptor in epithelial breast cells, *J. Cell Physiol.* 201, 84–96, 2004.

204. Ricciardolo, F.L., Sorbello, V., Benedetto, S., et al., Bradykinin- and lipopolysaccharide-induced bradykinin B2 receptor expression, interleukin 8 release and "nitrosative stress" in bronchial epithelial cells BEAS-2B: Role for neutrophils, *Eur. J. Pharmacol.* 694, 30–38, 2012.

205. Vancheri, C., Gili, E., Failla, M., et al., Bradykinin differentiates human lung fibroblasts to a myofibroblast phenotype via the B2 receptor, *J. Allergy Clin. Immunol.* 116, 1242–1248, 2005.

206. Catalán, M., Smolic, C., Contreras, A., et al., Differential regulation of collagen secretion by kinin receptors in cardiac fibroblast and myofibroblast, *Toxicol. Appl. Pharmacol.* 261, 300–308, 2012.

207. Souza, P.P., Brechter, A.B., Reis, R.I., et al., IL-4 and IL-13 inhibit IL-1β and TNF-α induced kinin B1 and B2 receptors through a STAT6-dependent mechanism, *Br. J. Pharmacol.* 169, 400–412, 2013.

7 Matrix Metalloproteinases in the Interstitial Space

7.1 MATRIX METALLOPROTEINASES

Matrix metalloproteinases (MMPs) are a family of proteases that function in the extravascular space (see Appendix). The MMP system is an important component of the interstitial system of degradation of the extracellular matrix (ECM) during normal tissue remodeling or during metastatic disease.[1–5] MMPs have broad specificity, with many having similar sites of cleavage,[6] and can be considered both digestive proteases and regulatory proteases as well as being evaluated as biomarkers. It can be argued that, for some MMPs, their most significant role is in the degradation of collagen, as demonstrated by the roles of MMP-1 and MMP-3 as effectors of TNF-α action on the skin.[7] Here, MMP-3 can be considered a regulatory protease for its role in stimulating MMP-1 activity[8] (Table 7.1). It should be noted that MMP-1 digestion of collagen enables the subsequent digestion of collagen by MMP-9.[9] The ability of other proteases such as plasmin and thrombin to activate MMPs results in a carefully regulated environment for phenomena such as tumor progress, tissue remodeling, and wound healing.[10] Exposure to cigarette smoke not only induces the production of MMP-1 but also promotes the activation of pro-MMP-1.[11] This observation is noted to indicate the complexity of factors that govern MMP functional expression, including redox systems.[12–14] The suggestion that oxidants in cigarette smoke may be responsible for the activation of pro-MMP-1 has to be considered speculation in the absence of other data.

MMPs are also known as *matrixins* and are numbered MMP-1 to MMP-28, with various members missing as they were discovered to be identical to a previously defined member. For example, MMP-6[15] was found to be identical to MMP-3.[16] Woessner presented a full discussion of the "missing" MMPs in 2001.[17] The Appendix also contains the "trivial" names for the various MMPs with their number designation. There does not appear to be rigorous adherence to the numbering system, as papers do appear with only the trivial name. Thus, a literature search should include multiple names and multiple databases. While much interest in MMPs has focused on the degradation of the ECM and, in particular, collagen, MMPs also influence cell behavior[18] either directly through, for example, PAR receptors[19] or through CD44.[20,21]

MMPs can also be found in the vascular space,[22,23] in synovial fluid,[24–26] and in cerebrospinal fluid.[27,28] The great majority of these studies are performed in disease states and it is not unusual to be unable to find MMP expression in normal tissues. The source of MMPs in the vascular space is not clear. There is no evidence to support the presence of MMPs in lymph; however, the majority of these studies are based on activity measurements and may not measure MMPs bound to inhibitors.

TABLE 7.1
Activation of Pro-MMPs by Proteases

MMP[a]	Furin[b]	Trp[a]	Plm[a]	IIa[a]	CHT[a]	FXa[a]	MMP-3[a]	MMP-10[a]	MMP-13[a]	MMP-14[a]	PKA[a]	Tryptase	Tgn-2[a]
1		+	+				+	+					+
2	+	+	+	+			+			+			
3		+	+		+						+	+	
7		+	+				+						
8							+			+			+
9		+	+		+		+		+		+		
10		+	+		+								
11	+												
12		+	+										
13		+	+							+			+
14	+												
15	+												
16	+												
17	+												
18													
19		+											
20										+			
21													
22													
23													
24													
25													
26													
27													
28													

Note: As reported in the peer-reviewed literature, only positive results are reported.

[a] Matrix metalloproteinase (MMP).

[b] Furin is one of several proprotein convertases, which are a family of proteolytic enzymes involved in the processing of proteins either for secretion or expression on the cell surface. In most cases, a specific proprotein convertase is not identified. (From Seidah, N.G., et al., *J. Biol. Chem.* 288, 21473–21481, 2013.)

It is likely that the expression of MMPs is both temporally and spatially controlled. In other words, the "normal" synthesis and secretion of a specific MMP likely occurs in a discrete tissue site over a defined period in a highly controlled process.[29–33] Regardless, the presence of selected MMPs in the circulation is increased in the presence of tumors and there is interest in the use of MMPs as biomarkers.[34–38] The factors promoting the secretion of MMPs into the synovium[24–26] and cerebrovascular space[27,28] are likely the same as those functioning in the interstitial space.

MMP-9, some characteristics of which can be found in the Appendix, may be the most highly cited member of the MMP family. There is much interest in the use of MMP-9 as a biomarker, but its use is complicated by an increase in a variety of inflammatory states.[39–43] There is also the issue of spatial and temporal expression of MMP-9, together with fact that it has a normal function in tissue remodeling. Further complication is provided by the association of MMP-9 with neutrophil gelatinase–associated lipocalin (NGAL), an acute phase reactant, to form a complex with enhanced MMP-9 activity and enhanced stability.[44] Halade and coworkers[40] describe MMP-9 as a proximal biomarker for cardiac remodeling and a distal biomarker for inflammation. These investigators[40] define a proximal biomarker as one showing a close relationship to a biological process, while a distal biomarker is less strongly related to a specific process. As a proximal biomarker, it is argued that MMP-9 is directly involved in the process of tissue remodeling, while as a distal marker it is a less specific biomarker of the inflammatory response. Christensen and coworkers[41] made a similar observation of MMP-9 in primary hyperthyroidism. MMP-9 levels were elevated prior to parathyroidectomy, as were other biomarkers of inflammation such as S100A4 and sCD14; while the levels of S100A4 and sCD14 decreased following surgery, the level of MMP-9 remained elevated, reflecting its role in tissue remodeling. Chang and coworkers[42] reviewed the role of MMP-9 in intracerebral hemorrhage and suggested, as with the above studies,[40,41] that MMP-9 has temporally variable functions, detrimental in the acute phase through tissue destruction but therapeutic in tissue remodeling, including angiogenesis.

The fact that MMPs function in the interstitial space is usually ignored, and the effect of a major interstitial constituent such as hyaluronan (Chapter 3) on MMPs is poorly understood. There is a considerable body of work on the effect of hyaluronan on the expression of MMPs. Much of this work has been performed in a synovium model, reflecting the use of hyaluronan in osteoarthritis.[45] Santangelo and coworkers[46] have shown that hyaluronic acid can block the increased expression of MMP-3 in lipopolysaccharide (LPS)-challenged synovial fibroblasts, with no difference between high- and low-molecular-weight synovial fibroblasts. Nie and Cai[47] presented data suggesting that hyaluronan enhanced MMP-9 expression in a rat sciatic nerve model. Julovi and coworkers[48] reported that hyaluronan inhibited the IL-1β-induced expression of MMP-13 in chondrocytes obtained from either osteoarthritic or rheumatoid arthritic patients.

7.2 ACTIVATION OF MATRIX METALLOPROTEINASES

The majority of MMPs are secreted into the interstitial space as proenzymes that require activation (Appendix; Table 7.1). As can be seen, the enzymes shown to be involved in the activation of MMPs are diverse. With several exceptions, the structure of a typical MMP consists of a proenzyme domain, a catalytic domain, and a hemopexin domain (Figure 7.1). The zymogen form of the MMP is maintained by a bond between the sulfhydryl group of a cysteine residue in the prodomain and a catalytic zinc atom at the enzyme active site. The prodomain can be removed by proteolysis either by an exogenous enzyme such as plasmin or by autolysis, secondary to disruption of the bond between the thiol group of cysteine and the zinc atom.

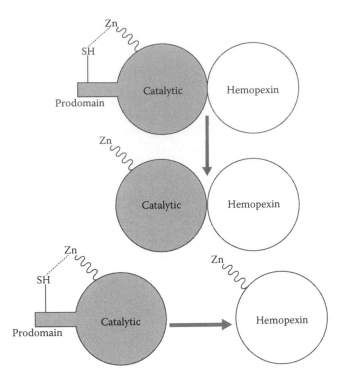

FIGURE 7.1 Canonical structure of MMPs. The majority of MMPs consist of a hemopexin domain, which contributes to the specificity of MMPs, and a catalytic domain, which contains the enzyme active site, as shown at the top. Activation occurs by disruption of a bond between a cysteine residue and zinc atom at the active site, freeing the zinc to participate in catalysis. Several MMPs (e.g., MMP-7, MMP-26) do not contain a hemopexin subunit.

Modification of the cysteine in pro-MMPs with a mercury-containing compound such as 4-aminophenylmercuric acid (APMA) also results in activation. Of more physiological interest is the activation of MMPs by hypochlorite or peroxynitrite, both of which can result from oxidative stress. Hypochlorite can oxidize cysteine to cysteine sulfinic acid, which peroxynitrite can nitrosylate to a cysteine residue, resulting in S-nitrosocysteine. Figure 7.2 presents the activation of pro-MMP-2 by reactive nitrogen species.[49] Jacob-Ferreira and Schultz[49] review the intracellular activation of MMP-2 by peroxynitrite in cardiac tissue and the subsequent degradation of intracellular proteins such as troponin. This is an example of the intracellular activity of MMP-2. MMP-2 is unique among MMPs in that there is both intracellular and extracellular distribution of the enzyme (see Appendix). Also shown in Figure 7.2 is the regulation of MMP-2 by phosphorylation.[50] Phosphorylation appears to decrease activity, and dephosphorylation as treatment with alkaline phosphatase increases activity. These investigators also suggest that the degree of phosphorylation can influence the reaction of peroxynitrite with MMP-2. These investigators also observed that S-nitrosocysteine can react with reduced glutathione to form an S-glutathione derivative of MMP-2. Hydrogen sulfide (H_2S) has been demonstrated to block oxidative activation of pro-MMP-2 in cardiac tissue.[51] Mishra and

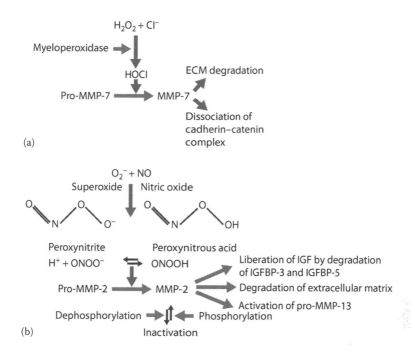

FIGURE 7.2 Activation of matrix metalloproteinases by oxidative stress. In panel A, oxidation of the cysteine residue frees the zinc atom to participate in catalysis. In the example shown, pro-MMP-7 is activated to MMP-7, resulting in disruption of the E-cadherin–β-catenin complex, enhancing the dissociation of cells and the change to a more invasive species. (From Davies, G., et al., *Clin. Cancer Res.* 7, 3289–3297, 2001; Alfackry, H., et al., *Innate Immun.* 22, 85–99, 2016.) Oxidation of the cysteine residue frees the zinc atom to participate in catalysis. In panel B, activation occurs via nitrosylation of the cysteine residue, freeing the zinc atom to participate in catalysis. (From Gu, Z., et al., *Science* 297, 1186–1190, 2002.) Also shown in panel B is the regulation of MMP-2 by phosphorylation. (From Sariahmetoglu, M., et al., *FASEB J.* 21, 2486–2495, 2007.)

coworkers[51] also observed a reduction in the level of MMP-9 activity with H_2S. Other investigators[52] had previously observed a reduction in MMP-2 and MMP-9 activity with hydrogen sulfide in hyperhomocysteinemia-associated renal failure. Hydrogen sulfide is known to reduce cysteine sulfinic acid to cysteine, which would result in the restoration of the zinc–sulfhydryl bridge and an inactive enzyme. Hypochlorite (Figure 7.2) activates pro-MMP-7[53] and subsequently inactivates MMP-7 through the formation of a unique tryptophan–glycine adduct.[54] Albumin modified with advanced oxidation end products increased the expression of MMP-3 in fibroblast-like synocytes[55] while buthionine sulfoximine, a modulator of oxidative stress, increased expression of MMP-3 n intestinal subepithelial fibroblasts.[56] Pro-MMP-2 is also subject to oxidative activation.[57] The activation of pro-MMP-2 as well as the active MMP-2 are inhibited by a catechin derived from green tea.[58] Resveratrol, an antioxidant in red wine, decreases the expression of pro-MMP-2[59] and inhibits the active enzyme.[60,61] MMP-9 is also inhibited by resveratrol.[60,61] N-acetylcysteine reduces pro-MMP-2 secretion from intestinal subepithelial myofibroblasts and the level of active MMP-2.[62] The effect of N-acetylcysteine is thought to be mediated through an increase in the ratio of reduced glutathione to oxidized glutathione. Jacob-Ferreira and coworkers[63] showed that peroxynitrite in the presence of glutathione resulted in the activation of MMP-2. It is unclear if this is exclusively an intracellular event or whether it could occur in the interstitial space. There are, however, mechanisms for the generation of peroxynitrite in the interstitial space.[64] The nitration of pro-MMP-2 by peroxynitrite resulting in the development of collagenase activity was reported by Rajagopalan and coworkers[65] in 1996; activation was also observed with hydrogen peroxide, suggesting modification of the cysteine residue in the prodomain. Sorsa and coworkers[66] suggested that oxidative activation of MMPs is important for bone and tissue destruction in inflammatory diseases. The oxidative activation of MMPs was blocked with analogs of tetracycline. Ottonello and coworkers[67] suggested the formation of reactive oxygen species with the myeloperoxidase system activated MMPs and inactivated α_1-proteinase inhibitor, contributing to tissue destruction. Intracellular activity of MMP-2 is also influenced by phosphorylation.[68] Phosphorylation (protein kinase C) decreases activity, while dephosphorylation (alkaline phosphatase) increased activity (fluorogenic peptide substrate). It is difficult to assess the importance of oxidation in the "normal" function of MMPs in the interstitial space. Control of activity by phosphorylation or nitrosylation may be associated with normal function, but this appears to be associated with a single MMP (MMP-2) and most likely is an intracellular event.

7.3 MEMBRANE-TYPE MATRIX METALLOPROTEINASES

Membrane-type matrix metalloproteinases (MT-MMPs) are covalently associated with cell membrane either by a transmembrane segment terminating with a cytoplasmic domain (Figure 7.3) or a glycosylphosphatidylinositol (GPI) linkage (Figure 7.4; see Appendix). MMPs bound by a transmembrane segment attached to a cytoplasmic domain have the ability to initiate an intracellular signaling pathway;[69,70] those with a GPI linkage do not have this capability.

Activation of the various MT-MMPs can be accomplished during intracellular transport by the action of furin, a proprotein convertase. MMP-27 appears to be retained as a zymogen in endoplasmic reticulum.[71,72] Autoactivation is proposed for several MMPs, including MMP-26, which is expressed in both placenta and tumor cells. MMP-26 expression during fetal development is likely to be temporally controlled and it is suggested to be involved in trophoblast invasion.[73] The involvement of MMP-26 in tumor development is more complex in that it has been suggested to correlate with positive outcomes in colorectal[74] and breast cancer.[75] It has been suggested[76] that internal retention of the activated MMP-26 in breast tumors is associated with a positive outcome; MMP-26 is one of two MMPs that has been suggested to be associated with antitumor activity. A direct role for secreted MMP-26 in the invasive process observed with colorectal cancer[77] is difficult to assess, as MMP-26 can activate pro-MMP-9, which would in turn lead to the fragmentation of fibronectin.[78,79]

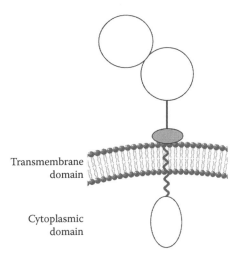

FIGURE 7.3 MT-MMP with a cytoplasmic tail. Several MT-MMPs are bound to the cell via atransmembrane segment connected to a cytoplasmic tail. The presence of a cytoplasmic tail permits signaling by MT-MMPs by mechanisms unrelated to proteolytic function. (From Sina, A., et al., *J. Cell Commun. Signal.* 4, 31–38, 2010.) MMP-14 (MT1-MMP), MMP-15 (MT2-MMP), MMP-16 (MT3-MMP), and MMP-24 (MT4-MMP) are bound by a transmembrane segment connected to a cytoplasmic tail.

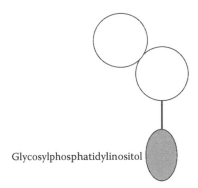

FIGURE 7.4 MT-MMP with a GPI tail. These MMPs lack a cytoplasmic domain and thus lack intracellular signaling capability. This group includes MMP-17 (MT4-MMP) and MMP-25 (MT6-MMP).

7.4 MATRIX METALLOPROTEINASES AND REGULATORY PROTEOLYSIS

The activation of pro-MMPs by limited proteolysis is likely of more importance in the current work as there is interaction between MMPs and with other proteases in the interstitial space (Table 7.1). Blaber and coworkers[80] have proposed such interactions between kallikrein-like peptidases (KLKs) and coagulation proteases.

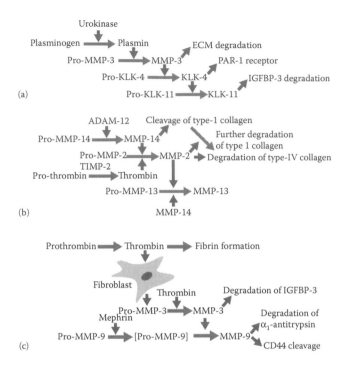

FIGURE 7.5 Some examples of MMP cascades that could occur in the interstitial space. Shown are some potential regulatory cascades involving MMPs that also involve proteases from different classes, including fibrinolytic, coagulation, and kallikrein. These cascades have not been documented with data but the assumptions are reasonable considering the information available for individual enzymes.

Beaufort and coworkers[81] reported that pro-KLK-11 can be activated by KLK-4, KLK-5, KLK-6, and KLK-8, and pro-KLK-4 can be activated by MMP-3 (See Figure 7.5). As shown in Figure 7.5, there is a cascade activation system for the production of MMP-3, KLK-4, and KLK-11, starting with urokinase. Also shown is a more complex cascade initiated by ADAM-12,[82] resulting in the formation of MMP-2 and MMP-13. MMP-2 and MMP-14 associated with TIMP-2 and CD44 have been described as a minidegradome.[83] The interaction of MMP-14 and CD44 may be involved in tumor cell migration.[84] Kung and coworkers[84] reported that hyaluronan oligosaccharides enhanced the expression of MMP-14, resulting in CD44 cleavage and tumor cell migration. There are studies supporting the cleavage of CD44 by MMP-14 in promoting cell motility.[85] CD44 is important for the MMP-14-dependent activation of pro-MMP-9.[86,87] An earlier study by Kajita and coworkers[88] showed that MMP-14 cleaved CD44, releasing a fragment into the medium with the stimulation of cell motility. MMP-9 also cleaves CD44, resulting in cell motility[89] or apoptosis.[90] MMP-9 specifically cleaves osteopontin, an ECM protein with diverse activities,[91] into fragments with biological activity. Takafuji and coworkers[92] showed that fragmentation of osteopontin with MMP-9 produced an important peptide for tumor cell invasion in hepatocellular carcinoma, while Tan and coworkers[93] suggested that the MMP-9 cleavage of osteopontin contributed to renal fibrosis. As discussed in Section 6.3, thrombin is suggested to have an important role in interstitial fibrosis by other mechanisms.[94]

Such cascade systems are seen in other processes, such as blood coagulation, and may or may not be associated with signal amplification.[95] We simply do not have enough information on the solution chemistry of the various MMPs to validate the presence of amplification processes. There is one possible exception: MMP-14 (MT1-MMP) and MMP-2 (gelatinase A) interact to activate pro-MMP-13[96] and the coordinate action of MMP-14 and MMP-2 on collagen. However, it is far more likely that the interplay of the various proteases in the interstitial space has more to do with regulation than amplification. It is abundantly clear that there are a number of proteases in the interstitial space with the ability to activate various pro-MMPs (Table 7.1), with the potential for regulation.

Roderfeld and coworkers[97] have described regeneration from liver fibrosis as a four-step process, one of which is the remodeling of the ECM by the coordinate action of several MMPs. One of the factors in the development of liver fibrosis is the activation of hepatic stellate cells, resulting in an altered phenotype, the hepatic myofibroblast, and the replacement of collagen IV with the fibrillar collagens I and III.[98] Hemmann and coworkers[99] organized a systematic review of the role of MMPs and TIMPs in liver fibrosis. The one major point is that much of the information on MMP function has been based on studies in murine model systems. Roderfeld and coworkers[97] note that the information obtained from animal systems is not readily transferrable to human systems. A further point raised by Hemmann and coworkers[99] is the poor quality of many of the studies. Regardless, it is clear that MMPs and TIMPs have a key role in the normal maintenance of the ECM and are likely important in any antifibrotic therapy.

A striking example of the functional nonequivalence of orthologous systems is provided by a recent study by Fleetwood and coworkers[100] on the role of urokinase plasminogen activator as a major factor in the macrophage degradation of the ECM. These investigators demonstrate that urokinase plasminogen activator bound to its receptor on the macrophage surface activates plasminogen to plasmin, which in the mouse system activates MMP-9, which then degrades the ECM. This conclusion is based on the ability of GM6001, an inhibitor of MMPs, which inhibited the murine system in the degradation of a 3D Matrigel® barrier but had no effect on a human system. These results suggest the involvement of another protease in the human system. These results have great importance in the development of inhibitors of MMPs; such inhibitors are of interest in the treatment of various tumors.[101]

7.5 MATRIX METALLOPROTEINASES AS BIOPHARMACEUTICALS

While most of the interest in MMPs has been focused on the inhibition of these enzymes, there has been some interest in their therapeutic use. Bedair and coworkers[102] used a mouse model to show that the injection of MMP-1 could enhance muscle healing by reducing fibrosis and increasing the number of myofibrils. The results were obtained after a relatively short exposure. These investigators suggest that the success reflected the use of a mixture of active enzymes and zymogen. The injection of

MMP-1 into normal muscle did not result in a negative effect on the muscle or the ECM. Subsequent work from this group[103] showed that MMP-1 enhanced myoblast migration and differentiation. Zheng and coworkers[104] showed that MMP-1 had no deleterious effect on murine bone marrow-derived mesenchymal stem cells but did promote *in vitro* myogenic differentiation of bone marrow-derived mesenchymal stem cells as assessed by increases in myoD and desmin. Mu and coworkers[105] showed that MMP-1 enhanced soft tissue regeneration. We could find no further published work on biopharmaceutical applications of MMP-1. The work cited is confined to rodent systems and might not be useful in human systems. There has been a report[106] on the use of directed mutagenesis in the catalytic domain of human MMP-1, which regulates activity by varying calcium concentration. The goal of this work was the development of a form of MMP-1 that would be useful in fibrotic disease. There is one report[107] on the acceleration of wound healing with MMP-3 in a rat model of tooth pulp injury.

While the application of MMP-1 to muscle may be useful, there are potential hazards in the use of MMPs for the resolution of fibrotic disease. McKleroy and coworkers[108] describe pulmonary fibrosis as resulting from an imbalance of collagen synthesis and collagen degradation. These investigators note the risks of protease-based therapeutics and suggest that inhibiting collagen cross-linking may be a more viable option. Cross-linked collagen is more resistant to degradation by MMPs and other proteases in the interstitial space.[109–112] However, the approach to blocking collagen cross-linking must take into account that cross-linkage can occur by the canonical route mediated through lysyl oxidase or via the action of tissue trans-glutaminase.[111] Olsen and coworkers[113] have reported the development of two novel inhibitors of tissue transglutaminase 2 for the treatment of pulmonary fibrosis. The potential value of thrombin inhibition in the prevention of fibrotic disease is discussed in Section 6.4.1.

7.6 DEVELOPMENT OF INHIBITORS OF MATRIX METALLOPROTEINASES FOR THERAPEUTIC USE

MMPs are implicated in a number of disease processes, including aneurysm development, tumor metastasis, chronic obstructive pulmonary disease, and periodontal disease. As a result, there is considerable interest in the development of specific inhibitors for use as therapeutics, such as those developed for HIV proteases[114,115] and coagulation proteases.[116] It is, however, difficult to develop a unique inhibitor for each of the several MMPs given their considerable similarity in specificity as well as the complexity in the binding of substrates. As a note of caution in the development of MMP inhibitors, MMPs have been suggested to have pleiotropic functions. Deryugina and Quigley[117] observed that antiangiogenic therapeutic approaches using MMP inhibitors can promote metastasis. MMPs have a variety of substrates in the interstitial space.[6,118]

7.6.1 Substrate Specificity of Matrix Metalloproteinases

The most useful approach to the development of drugs that are inhibitors to proteases (and other enzymes) is to identify the structural determinants in a substrate protein that are critical for recognition by the protease. This information can then be used to identify a target that can be developed into a lead compound, which can subsequently be used to develop a drug.[119] Target proteases such as thrombin tend to recognize sequences preceding the amino acid, contributing the carboxyl group to the scissile peptide bond. In the case of thrombin, the amino acid contributing the carboxyl group is arginine, leading to the development of inhibitors such as dabigatran etexilate. Plasmin (Chapter 5) has a specificity toward peptide bonds in which the carboxyl group is contributed by lysine, resulting in the use of primary amines such as ε-aminocaproic acid as inhibitors. MMPs present a larger challenge for the development of inhibitors, as MMPs recognize both the carboxyl-terminal and amino-terminal amino acid sequences surrounding the scissile peptide bond. To use the nomenclature developed by Schechter and Berger,[120] both P and P' residues in the protein substrate are recognized by S and S' sites (Figure 7.6) on the protease. As such, specific protease substrates, such as the peptide nitroanilides, are not very useful for defining MMP specificity. Fluorescence resonance energy transfer (FRET) peptide[121–123] substrates (Figure 7.7) have been more useful.[124,125] FRET peptide substrates can be used to study both intracellular and extracellular proteases.[126] The similarity between the various MMPs in specificity of peptide bond cleavage[127] as well as the importance of various exosite interactions[128,129] presents a challenge. However, similar issues exist in blood coagulation proteases and specific inhibitors have been developed for thrombin and factor Xa. One such inhibitor is dabigatran etexilate,[130] which is recognized by thrombin as a substrate, forming a stable acyl-enzyme intermediate that undergoes very slow deacylation. Unlike thrombin, which is a serine protease, or caspases, which are cysteine-aspartic proteases, MMPs do not have functional groups at the enzyme active site that are available for chemical modification. This issue has been addressed by the use of photoaffinity probes for the detection of active MMPs[131] that are not dependent on the presence of a functional group at the enzyme active site. The attachment of a reporter function such as radioactivity enables the detection of active MMPs in tissues and fluids. Finally,

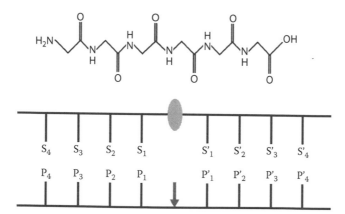

FIGURE 7.6 Substrate determinants of protease specificity. This model is based on the original work of Schechter and Berger (*Biochem. Biophys. Res. Commun.* 27, 157–162, 1967). S_n indicates binding sites on the protease for sites P_n on the peptide/protein substrate.

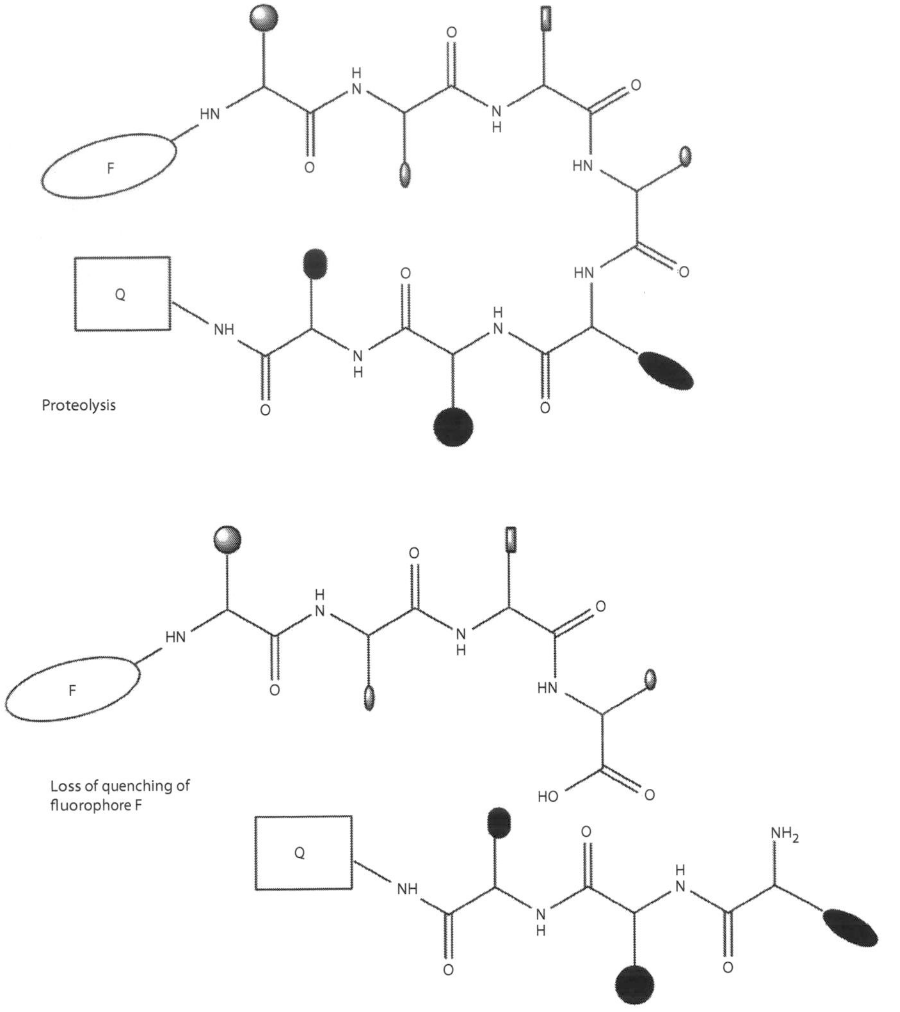

FIGURE 7.7 Hydrolysis of a FRET substrate. Shown is a model for a FRET substrate for a peptidase/protease. These substrates have the advantage of recognizing both P and P' sites in the substrate. (From Kojima, K., et al., *J. Biol. Chem.* 276, 2115–2121, 2001.) The assay is based on the increase in fluorescence when the acceptor (quencher) is removed from the donor.

another issue with the development of drugs to inhibit MMPs is the spatial and temporal expression of active MMPs (Section 7.7), which would suggest that timing is critical for therapeutic intervention.

While the development of MMP inhibitors has presented considerable challenges, there is continued interest because of the putative role that MMPs play in the metastatic process of tumors.[132–134] Phosphinic acid peptides,[135] for example, are transition state analogs that are stable and can recognize both P and P' positions, thus potentially taking advantage of data obtained with FRET systems. Phage display has also been used to identify potential peptide inhibitors.[136] Other peptides have been identified from natural sources that decrease MMP expression.[137,138] A peptide inhibitor labeled with Technetium (^{99m}Tc)[139] or Gallium (^{68}Ga)[140] has been developed for *in vivo* visualization of MMPs.

7.6.2   TISSUE INHIBITORS OF METALLOPROTEINASES

The tissue inhibitors of metalloproteinases (TIMPs) are four "specific" inhibitors of MMPs.[141–144] These inhibitors also inhibit other metalloproteinases such ADAM and ADAMTS (Chapter 4).

TIMP-1 is a poor inhibitor of several MMPs, while TIMP-2, TIMP-3, and TIMP-4 are potent inhibitors of all MMPs. While these proteins do inhibit MMPs, they are suggested to be pleiotropic[143] (as with some SERPINs described in Chapter 9), and the expression of the various activities is dependent on tissue location and time.[142–145] Moore and Crocker[146] have recently reviewed the pleiotropic activities of TIMPs. TIMP-1 reportedly is involved in a variety of central nervous system functions, including plasticity and oligodendrocyte differentiation. Baker and coworkers[143] reviewed the various activities of TIMPs, including the many pleiotropic effects. There is one report of the modification of TIMP-2 to obtain a more specific inhibitor of MMP-2.[147] Higashi and coworkers[147] prepared a fusion protein of a decapeptide and TIMP-2, which was a potent inhibitor of MMP-2 ($K_i \approx 0.6$ pmol); the inhibitory activity against other MMPs was μmol or greater.

7.6.3   CHELATION OF ZINC IONS AND INHIBITION
OF MATRIX METALLOPROTEINASES

The work suggesting that MMPs are zinc metalloenzymes dates back at least to 1970, with the work of Seifter and coworkers[148] showing that the inhibition of a collagenase from *Clostridium histolyticum* by cysteine and 2,3-dimercaptopropanol (BAL) involved the chelation of a zinc ion at the enzyme active site. Seltzer and coworkers[149] subsequently demonstrated that mammalian collagenases are zinc metalloenzymes. These early observations have led to the development of a number of inhibitors based their ability to chelate zinc ions.[150–156] Since all MMPs have zinc at their active sites, it has been necessary to build specificity into the inhibitors to enable selective modification of a single MMP. Jin and coworkers[155] have developed a series of inhibitors based on 3-mercaptopyrrolidine. Varying the P and P' sides (Figure 7.6), they were able to obtain considerable but not absolute specificity for several MMPs. These investigators also observe that while hydroxamic acid derivatives were useful in the early development of inhibitors for MMPs, the avidity of the hydroxamic acid for zinc precluded building P and P' specificity into the inhibitors based on this chemistry. Mori and coworkers[156] took advantage of the availability of crystal structures for MMPs in docking experiments to optimize arylsulfonamide derivatives and, as with Jin and coworkers,[155] were able to obtain enhanced specificity but not absolute specificity.

There is an interesting story about zinc in MMPs related to the inhibition of collagenase by tetracycline. Golub and coworkers[157] had observed increased collagen destruction in gingiva in patients with diabetes. They hypothesized that the overgrowth of gram-negative bacteria released endotoxin, which increased collagenase production in the gingival crevice. In studies with minocycline, a derivative of tetracycline, a decrease in collagen destruction was observed, but the effect was due to the inhibition of collagenase by minocycline. Subsequent work from this group[158] showed that tetracycline also inhibited collagenase activity and supported a mechanism of action for tetracycline in periodontal disease that combined antibacterial action and collagenase inhibition. Golub and coworkers[159] subsequently showed that a chemically modified derivative of tetracycline without antibacterial activity did inhibit tissue collagenase activity and is consistent with the effect of tetracycline being based on the ability to chelate zinc. Work continues to develop tetracycline derivatives with enhanced specificity for the inhibition of MMPs.[160]

7.7 COMPARTMENTALIZATION AND REGULATION OF MATRIX METALLOPROTEINASES

Tocchi and Parks[161] present an excellent case for the compartmentalization of MMP activity. Their argument is based, in part, on the interaction of MMPs with components of the ECM such as glycosaminoglycans; the importance of such interactions has previously been suggested by other workers.[162] Compartmentalization as a regulatory mechanism for the control of MMPs has been discussed by a number of investigators.[163–167] Ahmed and coworkers[166] remind us that the effect of compartmentalization on enzyme activity may be lost in the study of tissue homogenates. Temporal control of MMP expression[97,167–170] can also be a confounding factor for therapeutic intervention. It is likely that promoter polymorphism is important in the aberrant expression of MMPs.[171] It is also possible that environmental factors influence specific MMP gene expression.[172,173] There is potential for siRNA therapeutics in the inhibition of aberrant MMP activity.[174]

It is clear that MMPs have an important role in a variety of normal biological processes as well as pathologies such as inflammation and tumor metastasis. We have attempted to describe some of the properties of the various MMPs and factors that regulate their activity in the interstitial space. The spatial and temporal expressions of the various MMPs create challenges for the study of the *in vivo* function of these proteases. It is anticipated that advances in spectroscopy[175–177] will provide more information on the action of MMPs and other proteases in the skin, which is active tissue for such enzymes. Spectroscopy combined with the use of labeled inhibitors that can form covalent bonds with MMPs[131] will be useful, as well as inhibitors that can form noncovalent bonds.[139,140]

REFERENCES

1. Nagase, H. and Woessner, J.F., Jr., Matrix metalloproteinases, *J. Biol. Chem.* 274, 21491–21494, 1999.
2. Woessner, J.F., Jr., MMPs and TIMPs: An historical perspective, *Mol. Biotechnol.* 22, 33–49, 2002.
3. Spinale, F.G., Koval, C.N., Deschamps, A.M., et al., Dynamic changes in matrix metalloproteinase activity within the human myocardial interstitium during myocardial arrest and reperfusion, *Circulation* 118 (Suppl 14), S16–S23, 2008.

4. Lerchenberger, M., Uhl, B., Stark, K., et al., Matrix metalloproteinases modulate ameboid-like migration of neutrophils through inflamed interstitial tissue, *Blood* 122, 770–780, 2013.

5. Rawlings, N.D. and Barrett, A.J., Introduction: Metallopeptidases and their clans, in *Handbook of Proteolytic Enzymes*, 3rd edn., eds. N.D. Rawlings and G. Salvesen, Chapter 77, pp. 325–370, Elsevier, Amsterdam, Netherland, 2013.

6. Overall, C.M., Molecular determinants of metalloproteinase substrate specificity: Matrix metalloproteinase substrate binding domains, modules, and exosites, *Mol. Biotechnol.* 22, 51–86, 2002.

7. Ågren, M.S., Schnabel, R., Christensen, L.H., and Mirastschijski, U., Tumor necrosis factor-α-accelerated degradation of type I collagen in human skin is associated with elevated matrix metalloproteinase (MMP)-1 and MMP-3 *ex vivo*, *Eur. J. Cell Biol.* 94, 12–21, 2015.

8. Suzuki, K., Enghlid, J.J., Morodormi, T., Salvesen, G., and Nagase, H., Mechanisms of activation of tissue procollagenase by matrix metalloproteinase 3 (stromelysin), *Biochemistry* 29, 10261–10270, 1990.

9. Christiansen, V.J., Jackson, K.W., Lee, K.N., and McKee, P.A., Effect of fibroblast activation protein and α_2-antiplasmin cleaving enzyme on collagen types I, III, and IV, *Arch. Biochem. Biophys.* 457, 177–186, 2007.

10. Wilkins-Port, C.E., Higgins, S.P., Higgins, C.E., Kobori-Hotchkiss, I., and Higgins, P.J., Complex regulation of the pericellular proteolytic microenvironment during tumor progression and wound repair: Functional interactions between the serine protease and matrix metalloproteinase cascade, *Biochem. Res. Int.* 2012, 454368, 2012.

11. Kim, H., Liu, X., Kobyama, T., et al., Cigarette smoke stimulates MMP-1 production by human lung fibroblasts through the ERK1/2 pathway, *COPD* 1, 13–23, 2004.

12. Tyagi, S.C., Kumar, S., and Borders, S., Reduction-oxidation(redox) state regulation of extracellular matrix metalloproteinases and tissue inhibitors in cardiac normal and transformed fibroblasts, *J. Cell. Biochem.* 61, 139–151, 1996.

13. Nelson, S., Subbaram, S., Conner, K.M., et al., Redox-dependent matrix metalloproteinase-1 expression is regulated by JNK through Ets and AP-1 promoter motifs, *J. Biol. Chem.* 281, 14100–14110, 2006.

14. Koch, S., Volkmar, C.M., Kolb-Bachofen, V., et al., A new redox-dependent mechanism of MMP-1 activity control comprising reduced low-molecular weight thiols and oxidizing radicals, *J. Mol. Med.* 87, 261–272, 2009.

15. Azzo, W. and Woessner, J.F., Jr., Purification and characterization of an acid metalloproteinase from human articular cartilage, *J. Biol. Chem.* 261, 5434–5441, 1986.

16. Wilhelm, S.M., Shao, Z.H., Housley, T.J., et al., Matrix metalloproteinase-3 (stromelysin-1). Identification as the cartilage acid metalloprotease and effect of pH on catalytic properties and calcium affinity. *J. Biol. Chem.* 268, 21906–21913, 1993.

17. Woessner, J.F., Jr., MMPs and TIMPs: An historical perspective, in *Matrix Metalloproteinase Protocols*, ed. I. Clark, Chapter 1, pp. 1–23, Humana Press, Totowa, NJ, 2001.

18. Sternlicht, M.D. and Werb, Z., How matrix metalloproteinases regulate cell behavior, *Annu. Rev. Cell Dev. Biol.* 17, 463–536, 2001.

19. Jaffré, F., Friedman, A.E., Hu, Z., et al., β-Adrenergic receptor stimulation transactivates protease-activated receptor 1 via matrix metalloproteinase 13 in cardiac cells, *Circulation* 125, 2993–3003, 2012.

20. Yu, Q. and Stamenkovic, I., Localization of matrix metalloproteinase 9 to the cell surface provides a mechanism for CD44-mediated tumor invasion, *Genes Dev.* 13, 35–48, 1999.

21. Chetty, C., Vananmala, S.K., Gondi, C.S., et al., MMP-9 induces CD44 cleavage and CD44 mediated cell migration in glioblastoma xenograft cells, *Cell. Signal.* 24, 549–559, 2012.

22. Zucker, S., Hymowitz, M., Conner, C., et al., Measurement of matrix metalloproteinase and tissue inhibitors of metalloproteinases in blood and tissues: Clinical and experimental applications, *Ann. N.Y. Acad. Sci.* 870, 212–227, 1999.

23. Martin, G., Asensi, V., and Montes, A.H., Role of plasma matrix-metalloproteases (MMPs) and their polymorphisms (SNPs) in sepsis development and outcome in ICU patients, *Sci. Rep.* 4, 5002, 2014.

24. Huang, Y.C., Chiang, C.Y., Li, C.H., et al., Quantification of tumor necrosis factor-α and matrix metalloproteinase-3 in synovial fluid by a fiber-optic particle plasmon resonance sensor, *Analyst* 138, 4599–4606, 2013.

25. Niarakis, A., Giannopoulou, E., Ravaszoula, P., et al., Detection of a latent soluble form of membrane type 1 matrix metalloprotease bound with tissue inhibitor of matrix metalloproteinases-2 in periprosthetic tissues and fluids from loose arthroplasty endoprothesis, *FEBS J.* 280, 6541–6555, 2013.

26. Koskinen, A., Vuolteenaho, K., Moilanen, T., et al., Resistin as a factor in osteoarthritis: Synovial fluid resistin concentrations correlate positively with interleukin 6 and matrix metalloproteinases MMP-1 and MMP-3, *Scand. J. Rheumatol.* 43, 249–253, 2014.

27. Halliday, M.R., Pomara, N., Sagare, A.P., et al., Relationship between cyclophilin levels and matrix metalloproteinase 9 activity in the cerebrospinal fluid of cognitively normal apolipoprotein e4 carriers and blood barrier breakdown, *JAMA Neurol.* 70, 1198–1200, 2013.

28. Roberts, D.J., Jenne, C.N., Leger, C., et al., Association between the cerebral inflammatory and matrix metalloproteinase responses after severe traumatic brain injury in humans, *J. Neurotrauma* 30, 1727–1736, 2013.

29. Correale, J. and Bassani Molinas, M.L., Temporal variations of adhesion molecules and matrix metalloproteinases in the course of MS, *J. Neuroimmunol.* 140, 198–209, 2003.

30. Lichtinghagen, R., Bahr, M.J., Wehmeier, M., et al., Expression and coordinated regulation of matrix metalloproteinases in chronic hepatitis C and hepatitis C virus-induced liver cirrhosis, *Clin. Sci. (Lond.)* 105, 373–382, 2003.

31. Garg, P., Ravi, A., Patel, N.R., et al., Matrix metalloproteinase-9 regulates MUC-2 expression through its effect on goblet cell differentiation, *Gastroenterology* 132, 1877–1889, 2007.

32. Ghajar, C.M., George, S.C., and Putnam, A.J., Matrix metalloproteinase control of capillary morphogenesis, *Crit. Rev. Eurkaryot. Gene Expr.* 18, 251–278, 2007.

33. Hurley, J.R., Balaji, S., and Narmoneva, D.A., Complex temporal regulation of capillary morphogenesis by fibroblasts, *Am. J. Physiol. Cell Physiol.* 299, C444–C453, 2010.

34. Prince, H.E., Biomarkers for diagnosing and monitoring autoimmune diseases, *Biomarkers* 10(Suppl 1), S44–S49, 2005.

35. Nanda, D.P., Sil, H., Moulik, S., et al., Matrix metalloproteinase-9 as a potential tumor marker in breast cancer, *J. Environ. Toxicol. Oncol.* 32, 115–129, 2013.

36. Thorsen, S.B., Christensen, S.L., Würtz, S.O., et al., Plasma levels of the MMP-9: TIMP-1 complex as prognostic biomarker in breast cancer: A retrospective study, *BMC Cancer* 13, 598, 2013.

37. Sessa, C., Lorusso, P., Tolcher, A., et al., Phase I safety, pharmacokinetic and pharmacodynamic evaluation of the vascular disrupting agent ombrabulin (AVE8062) in patients with advanced solid tumors, *Clin. Cancer Res.* 19, 4832–4842, 2013.

38. Braicu, E.I., Gasimli, K., Richter, R., et al., Role of serum VEGFA, TIMP2, MMP2, and MMP9 in monitoring the response to adjuvant radiochemotherapy in patients with primary cervical cancer: Results of a companion protocol of the randomized NOGGO-AGO phase III clinical trial, *Anticancer Res.* 34, 385–391, 2014.

39. Holmey, T., Løken-Amsrud, K.I., Bakke, S.J., et al., Inflammation markers in multiple sclerosis: CXCL16 reflects and may predict disease activity, *PLoS One* 8(9), e75021, 2013.

40. Halade, G.V., Jin, Y.E., and Lindsey, M.L., Matrix metalloproteinase (MMP-9): A proximal biomarker for cardiac remodeling and a distal biomarker for inflammation, *Pharmacol. Ther.* 139, 32–40, 2013.

41. Christensen, M.H., Fenne, I.S., Nordbø, Y., et al., Novel biomarkers in primary hypothyroidism, *Eur. J. Endocrinol.* 173, 9–17, 2015.

42. Chang, J.J., Emanuel, B.A., Mack, W.J., Tsivgoulis, G., and Alexandrov, A.V., Matrix metalloproteinase-9: Dual role and temporal profile in intracerebral hemorrhage, *J. Stroke Cerebrovasc. Dis.* 23, 2498–2505, 2014.

43. Wang, M., Zhang, Q., Zhao, X., Dong, G., and Li, C., Diagnostic and prognostic value of neutrophil gelatinase–associated lipocalin, matrix metalloproteinease-9, and tissue inhibitor of matrix metalloproteinase-1 for sepsis in the emergency department: An observational study, *Crit. Care* 18(6), 634, 2014.

44. Helanova, K., Spinar, J., and Parenica, J., Diagnostic and prognostic utility of neutrophil gelatinase–associated lipocalin (NGAL) in patients with cardiovascular disease: A review, *Kidney Blood Press. Res.* 39, 623–629, 2014.

45. Trigkilidas, D. and Anand, A., The effectiveness of hyaluronic acid intra-articular injections in managing osteoarthritic knee pain, *Ann. R. Coll. Surg. Engl.* 95, 545–551, 2013.

46. Santangelo, K.S., Johnson, A.L., Ruppert, A.S., and Bertone, A.L., Effects of hyaluronan treatment on lipopolysaccharide-challenged fibroblast-like synovial cells, *Arthritis Res. Ther.* 9(1), R1, 2007.

47. Nie, Y. and Cia, G., Upregulation of matrix metalloproteinase-9 dependent on hyaluronan synthesis after sciatic nerve injury, *Neurosci. Lett.* 444, 259–263, 2008.

48. Julovi, S.M., Ito, H., Nishitani, K., et al., Hyaluronan inhibits matrix metalloproteinase-13 in human arthritic chondrocytes via CD44 and P38, *J. Orthoped. Res.* 29, 256 264, 2011.

49. Jacob-Ferreira, A.L. and Schulz, R., Activation of intracellular matrix metalloproteinase-2 by reactive oxygen–nitrogen species: Consequences and therapeutic strategies in the heart, *Arch. Biochem. Biophys.* 540, 82–93, 2013.

50. Jacob-Ferreira, A.L., Kondo, M.Y., Baral, P.K., et al., Phosphorylation status of 72 kDa MMP-2 determines its structure and activity in response to peroxynitrite, *PLoS One* 8(8), e71794, 2013.

51. Mishra, P.K., Tyagi, N., Sen, U., et al., H₂S ameliorates oxidative and proteolytic stresses and protects the heart against remodeling in chronic heart failure, *Am. J. Physiol. Heart Circ. Physiol.* 298, H451–456, 2010.

52. Sen, U., Basu, P., Abe, O.A., et al., Hydrogen sulfide ameliorates hyperhomocysteinemia-associated chronic renal failure, *Am. J. Physiol. Renal Physiol.* 297, F410–419, 2009.

53. Fu, X., Kassim, S.Y., Parks, W.C., and Heinecke, J.W., Hypochlorous acid oxygenates the cysteine switch domain of pro-matrilysin (MMP-7): A mechanism for matrix metalloproteinase activation and atherosclerosis plaque rupture by myeloperoxidase, *J. Biol. Chem.* 276, 41279–41287, 2001.

54. Fu, X., Kao, J.L., Bergt, C., et al., Oxidative cross-linking of tryptophan to glycine restrains matrix metalloproteinase activity: Specific structural motifs control protein oxidation, *J. Biol. Chem.* 279, 6209–6212, 2004.

55. Zheng, S., Zhong, Z.M., Qin, S., et al., Advanced oxidation protein products induce inflammatory response in fibroblast-like synoviocytes through NADPH oxidase-dependent activation of NF-κB, *Cell Physiol. Biochem.* 32, 972–985, 2013.

56. Fontani, F., Marcucci, T., Picariello, L., et al., Redox regulation of MMP-3/TIMP-1 ratio in intestinal myofibroblasts: Effect of N-acetylcysteine and curcumin, *Exp. Cell Res.* 323, 77–86, 2014.

57. Ranganathan, A.C., Nelson, K.K., Rodriguez, A.M., et al., Manganese superoxide dismutase signals matrix metalloproteinase expression via H_2O_2-dependent ERK1/2 activation, *J. Biol. Chem.* 276, 14264–14270, 2001.

58. Maeda, K., Kuzuya, M., Cheng, X.W., et al., Green tea catechins inhibit the cultured smooth muscle cell invasion through the basement barrier, *Atherosclerosis* 166, 23–30, 2003.

59. Lee, S.J. and Kim, M.M., Resveratrol with antioxidant activity inhibits matrix metalloproteinase via modulation of STRT1 in human fibrosarcoma cells, *Life Sci.* 88, 465–472, 2011.

60. Gweon, E.J. and Kim, S.J., Resveratrol attenuates matrix metalloproteinase-9 and -2 regulated differentiation of HTB94 chondrosarcoma cells through the p38 kinase and JNK pathways, *Oncol. Rep.* 32, 71–78, 2014.

61. Lin, Y.C., Chen, L.H., Varadharajan, T., et al., Resveratrol inhibits glucose-induced migration of vascular smooth muscle cells mediated by focal adhesion kinase, *Mol. Nutr. Food Res.* 58, 1389–1401, 2014.

62. Tyagi, S.C., Kumar G.S., and Borders, S., Reduction-oxidation (Redox) state regulation of extracellular matrix metalloproteinase and tissue inhibitors in cardiac normal and transformed fibroblast cells, *J. Cell. Biochem.* 61, 139–151, 1996.

63. Jacob-Ferreira, A.L., Kondo, M.Y., Baral, P.K., et al., Phosphorylation status of 72 kDa MMP-2 determines its structure and activity in response to peroxynitrite, *PLoS One* 8(8), e71794, 2013.

64. Ding, J.W., Dickie, J., O'Brodovich, H., et al., Inhibition of amiloride-sensitive sodium channel activity in distal lung epithelial cells by nitric oxide, *Am. J. Physiol.* 274, L378–L387, 1998.

65. Rajagopalan, S., Meng, X.P., Ramasamy, S., et al., Reactive oxygen species produced by macrophage-derived foam cells regulate the activity of vascular matrix metalloproteinases *in vitro*: Implications for atherosclerotic plaque stability, *J. Clin. Invest.* 98, 2572–2679, 1996.

66. Sorsa, T., Ramamurthy, N.S., Vernillo, A.T., et al., Functional sites of chemically modified tetracyclines: Inhibition of the oxidative activation of human neutrophil and chicken osteoclast pro-matrix metalloproteinases, *J. Rheumatol.* 25, 975–982, 1998.

67. Ottonello, L., Dapino, P., and Sallegri, F., Inactivation of alpha-1-proteinase inhibitor by neutrophil metalloproteinases: Crucial role of the myeloperoxidase system and effects of the anti-inflammatory drug nimesulide, *Respiration* 60, 32–37, 1993.

68. Sariahmetoglu, M., Crawford, B.D., Leon, H., et al., Regulation of matrix metalloproteinase-2 (MMP-2) activity by phosphorylation, *FASEB J.* 21, 2486–2495, 2007.

69. Sina, A., Prouix-Bonneau, S., Roy, A., et al., The lectin concanavalin-A signals MT1-MMP catalytic independent induction of COX-2 through an IKKγ/NF-κB-dependent pathway, *J. Cell Commun. Signal.* 4, 31–38, 2010.

70. Valacca, C., Tassone, E., and Mignatti, P., TIMP-2 interaction with MT1-MMP activates the AKT pathway and protects tumor cells from apoptosis, *PLoS One* 10(9), e136797, 2015.

71. Cominelli, A., Halbout, M., N'Kull, F., et al., A unique C-terminal domain allows retention of matrix metalloproteinase-27 in the endoplasmic reticulum, *Traffic* 15, 401–417, 2014.

72. Cominelli, A., Gaide Chevronnay, H.P., Lemoine, P., et al., Matrix metalloproteinase-27 is expressed in CD163+/CD206+ M2 macrophages in cycling human endometrium and in superficial endometriotic lesions, *Mol. Hum. Reprod.* 20, 767–775, 2014.

73. Liu, J., Cao, B., Li, Y.X., et al., GnRNI and II up-regulate MMP-26 expression through the JNK pathway in human cytotrophoblasts, *Reprod. Biol. Endocrinol.* 8(5), 2010.

74. Hu, Q., Yan, C., Xu, C., et al., Matrilysin-2 expression in colorectal cancer is associated with overall survival of patients, *Tumour Biol.* 35, 3569–3574, 2014.

75. Savinov, A.Y., Remacle, A.G., and Golubkov, V.S., Matrix metalloproteinase 26 proteolysis of the NH$_2$-terminal domain of the estrogen receptor β correlates with the survival of breast cancer patients, *Cancer Res.* 66, 2716–2724, 2006.

76. Strongin, A.Y., Mislocalization and unconventional functions of cellular MMPs in cancer, *Cancer Metastasis Rev.* 25, 87–98, 2006.

77. Gutschalk, C.M., Yanamadra, A.K., Linde, N., et al., GM-CSF enhances tumor invasion by elevated MMP-2, -9, and -26 expression, *Cancer Med.* 2, 117–129, 2013.

78. Zhao, Y.G., Xiao, A.Z., Newcomer, R.G., et al., Activation of pro-gelatinase B by endometase/matrilysin-2 promotes invasion of human prostate cancer cells, *J. Biol. Chem.* 278, 15056–15064, 2003.

79. Yamamoto, H., Vinitketkumnuen, A., Adachi, Y., et al., Association of matrilysin-2 (MMP-26) expression with tumor progression and activation of MMP-9 in esophageal squamous cell carcinoma, *Carcinogenesis* 25, 2353–2360, 2004.

80. Blaber, M., Yoon, H., Juliano, M.A., et al., Functional intersection of the kallikrein-related peptidases (KLKs) and thrombostasis axis, *Biol. Chem.* 391, 311–320, 2010.

81. Beaufort, N., Plaza, K., Utzschneider, D., et al., Interdependence of kallikrein-related peptidases in proteolytic networks, *Biol. Chem.* 391, 581–587, 2010.

82. Albrechtsen, R., Kveiborg, M., Stautz, D., et al., ADAM12 redistributes and activates MMP-14, resulting in gelatin degradation, reduced apoptosis and increased tumor growth, *J. Cell Sci.* 126, 4707–4720, 2013.

83. Hornebeck, W. and Maquart, F.X., Proteolyzed matrix as a template for the regulation of tumor progression, *Biomed. Pharmacother.* 57, 223–230, 2003.

84. Kung, C.I., Chen, C.Y., Yang, C.C., et al., Enhanced membrane-type 1 matrix metalloproteinase expression by hyaluronan oligosaccharides in breast cancer cells facilitates CD44 cleavage and tumor cell migration, *Oncol. Rep.* 28, 1808–1814, 2012.

85. Marrero-Diaz, R., Bravo-Cordero, J.J., Megías, D., et al., Polarized MT1-MMP-CD44 interaction and CD44 cleavage during cell retraction reveal an essential role for MT1-MMP in CD44-mediated invasion, *Cell Motil. Cytoskeleton* 66, 48–61, 2009.

86. Samanna, V., Ma, T., Mak, T.W., et al., Actin polymerization modulates CD44 surface expression, MMP-9 activation, and osteoclast function, *J. Cell. Physiol.* 213, 710–720, 2007.

87. Chellaiah, M.A., and Ma, T., Membrane localization of membrane type 1 matrix metalloproteinase by CD44 regulates the activation of pro-matrix metalloproteinase 9 in osteoclasts, *Biomed. Res. Int.* 2013, 302–392, 2013.

88. Kajita, M, Itoh, Y., Chiba, T., et al., Membrane-type 1 matrix metalloproteinase cleaves CD44 and promotes cell migration, *J. Cell Biol.* 28, 893–904, 2001.

89. Chetty, C., Vanamala, S.K., Gondi, C.S., et al., MMP-9 induces CD44 cleavage and CD44 mediated cell migration in glioblastoma xenograft cells, *Cell Signal.* 24, 549–559, 2012.

90. Kim, Y.H. and Jung, J.C., Suppression of tunicamycin-induced CD44v6 ectodomain shedding and apoptosis is correlated with temporal expression patterns of active ADAM10, MMP-9 and MMP-13 proteins in Caki-2 renal carcinoma cells, *Oncol. Rep.* 28, 1869–1874, 2012.

91. Kahles, F., Findeisen, H.M., and Bruemmer, D., Osteopontin: A novel regulation at the cross roads of inflammation, obesity and diabetes, *Mol. Metab.* 3, 384–393, 2014.

92. Takafuji, V., Forgnes, M., Unsworth, E., et al., An osteopontin fragment is essential for tumor cell invasion in hepatocellular carcinoma, *Oncogene* 26, 6361–6371, 2007.

93. Tan, T.K., Zheng, G., Hsu, T.T., et al., Matrix metalloproteinase-9 of tubular and macrophage origin contributes to the pathogenesis of renal fibrosis via macrophage recruitment through osteopontin cleavage, *Lab. Invest.* 93, 434–449, 2013.

94. Atanelishvili, I., Liang, J., Akter, T., et al., Thrombin increases lung fibroblast survival while promoting alveolar epithelial cell apoptosis via the endoplasmic reticulum stress marker, CCAAT enhancer-binding homologous protein, *Am. J. Respir. Cell Mol. Biol.* 50, 893–902, 2014.

95. Neurath, H. and Walsh, K.A., Role of proteolytic enzymes in biological regulation, *Proc. Natl. Acad. Sci. USA* 73, 3825–3832, 1976.

96. Knäuper, V., Will, H., López-Otin, C., et al., Cellular mechanisms for human procollagenase-3 (MMP-13) activation: Evidence that MT1-MMP (MMP-14) and gelatinase A (MMP-2) are able to generate active enzyme, *J. Biol. Chem.* 271, 17124–17131, 1996.

97. Roderfeld, M., Herrmann, S., and Roeb, E., Mechanisms of fibrinolysis in chronic liver injury (with special emphasis on MMPs and TIMPs), *Z. Gastroenterol.* 45, 25–33, 2007.

98. Mallat, A. and Lotersztain, S., Cellular mechanisms of tissue fibrosis: 5. Novel insights into liver fibrosis, *Am. J. Physiol. Cell. Physiol.* 305, C789–C799, 2013.

99. Hemmann, S., Graf, J., Rodereld, M., and Roeb, E., Expression of MMPs and TIMPs in liver fibrosis: A systematic review with special emphasis on anti-fibrotic strategies, *J. Hepatol.* 46, 955–975, 2007.

100. Fleetwood, A.J., Achuthan, A., Schultz, H., et al., Urokinase plasminogen activator is a central regulator of macrophage three-dimensional invasion, matrix degradation, and adhesion, *J. Immunol.* 192, 3540–3547, 2014.

101. Dufour, A. and Overall, C.M., Missing the target: Matrix metalloproteinase antitargets in inflammation and cancer, *Trends Pharmcol. Sci.* 34, 233–242, 2013.

102. Bedair, H., Liu, T.T., Kaar, J.L., et al., Matrix metalloproteinase-1 therapy promotes muscle healing, *J. Appl. Physiol.* 102, 2338–2345, 2007.

103. Wang, W., Pan, H., Murray, R., et al., Matrix metalloproteinase-1 promotes muscle cell migration and differentiation, *Am. J. Pathol.* 175, 1905–1914, 2009.

104. Zheng, Z., Leng, Y., Zhou, C., et al., Effect of matrix metalloproteinase-1 on the myogenic differentiation of bone marrow–derived mesenchymal stem cells *in vitro*, *Biochem. Biophys. Res. Commun.* 428, 309–314, 2012.

105. Mu, X., Bellayr, I., Pan, H., et al., Regeneration of soft tissue is promoted by MMP1 treatment after digit amputation in mice, *PLoS One* 8(3), e59105, 2014.

106. Paladini, R.D., Wei, G., Kundu, A., et al., Mutations in the catalytic domain of human matrix metalloproteinase-1 (MMP-1) that allow for regulated activity through the use of Ca^{2+}, *J. Biol. Chem.* 288, 6629–6639, 2013.

107. Zheng, L., Amano, K., Ichara, K., et al., Matrix metalloproteinase-3 accelerates wound healing following dental pulp injury, *Am. J. Pathol.* 175, 1905–1914, 2009.

108. McKleroy, W., Lee, T.-H., and Atabai, K., Always clean up your mess: Targeting collagen degradation to treat tissue fibrosis, *Am. J. Physiol. Lung Cell. Mol. Physiol.* L709–L721, 2013.

109. Johnson, T.S., Skill, N.J., El Nahas, A.M., et al., Transglutaminase transcription and antigen translocation in experimental renal scarring, *J. Am. Soc. Nephrol.* 10, 2140–2151, 1999.

110. van der Slot-Verhoeven, A.J., van Durg, E.A., Attema, J., et al., The type of collagen cross-link determines the reversibility of experimental skin fibrosis, *Biochim. Biophys. Acta* 1740, 60–67, 2005.

111. Fisher, M., Jones, R.A., Huang, L., et al., Modulation of tissue transglutaminase in the tubular epithelial cells alters extracellular matrix levels: A potential mechanism of tissue scarring, *Matrix Biol.* 28, 20–31, 2009.

112. Nowotny, K. and Grune, T., Degradation of oxidized and glycoxidized collagen: Role of collagen cross-linking, *Arch. Biochem. Biophys.* 542, 56–64, 2014.
113. Olsen, K.C., Epa, A.P., Kulkarni, A.A., et al., Inhibition of transglutaminase 2, a novel target for pulmonary fibrosis by two small electrophilic molecules, *Am. J. Respir. Cell Biol.* 50, 737–747, 2014.
114. Blundell, T.L., Lapatto, R., Wilderspin, A.F., et al., The 3-D structure of HIV-1 protein-ase and the design of antiviral agents for the treatment of AIDS, *Trend Biochem. Sci.* 15, 425–430, 1990.
115. Debouk, C., The HIV-1 protease as a therapeutic target for AIDS, *AIDS Res. Hum. Retroviruses* 8, 153–164, 1992.
116. Mani, H. and Lindhoff-Last, E., New oral anticoagulants in patients with nonvalvular atrial fibrillation: A review of pharmacokinetics, safety, efficacy, quality of life, and cost effectiveness, *Drug Des. Devel. Ther.* 8, 789–798, 2014.
117. Deryugina, E.I. and Quigley, J.P., Pleiotropic roles of matrix metalloproteinases in tumor angiogenesis: Contrasting overlapping and compensatory functions, *Biochim. Biophys. Acta* 1803, 103–120, 2010.
118. Overall, C.M. and Dean, R.A., Degradomics: Systems biology of the protease web; Pleiotropic roles of MMPs in cancer, *Cancer Metastasis Rev.* 25, 69–75, 2006.
119. Lundblad, R.L., Drug design, in *Encyclopedia of Cell Biology*, Vol. 1, eds. R.A. Bradshaw and P. Stahl, pp. 135–140, Academic Press, Waltham, MA, 2016.
120. Schechter, I. and Berger, A., On the size of the active site in proteases, *Biochem. Biophys. Res. Commun.* 27, 157–162, 1967.
121. Matayoshi, E.D., Wang, G.T., Krafft, G.A., and Erickson, J., Novel fluorogenic sub-strates for assaying retroviral proteases by resonance energy transfer, *Science* 247, 954–958, 1990.
122. Taliani, M., Bianchi, E., Narjes, F., et al., A continuous assay of hepatitis C virus pro-tease based on resonance energy transfer depsipeptide substrates, *Anal. Biochem.* 240, 60–67, 1996.
123. Liu, Y., Kati, W., Chen, C.-M., et al., Use of a fluorescence plate reader form measur-ing kinetic parameters with inner filter effect correction, *Anal. Biochem.* 267, 331–335, 1999.
124. Raysberg, N., Monitoring matrix metalloproteinase activity using FRET peptide sub-strates and assay kits, *PharmaChem* 6, 442–444, 2007.
125. Fields, G.B., Using fluorogenic peptide substrates to assay matrix metalloproteinases, *Methods Mol. Biol.* 622, 393–433, 2010.
126. Meyer, B.S. and Rademann, J., Extra- and intracellular imaging of human matrix metalloprotease 11 (hMMP-11) with a cell-penetrating FRET substrate, *J. Biol. Chem.* 287, 37857–37867, 2012.
127. Murphy, G., Fell-Muir Lecture: Metalloproteinases; From demolition squad to master regulators, *Int. J. Exp. Pathol* 91, 303–313, 2010.
128. Fulcher, Y.G. and Van Doren, S.R., Remote exosites of the catalytic domain of matrix metalloproteinase-12 enhanced elastin degradation, *Biochemistry* 50, 9488–9499, 2011.
129. Manka, S.W., Carafoli, F., Visse, R., et al., Structural insights into triple-helical collagen cleavage by matrix metalloproteinase 1: Structural insights into triple-helical collagen cleavage by matrix metalloproteinase 1, *Proc. Natl. Acad. Sci. USA* 109, 12461–12466, 2012.
130. Hauel, N.H., Nar, H., Priepke, H., et al., Structure-based design of novel potent nonpep-tide thrombin inhibitors, *J. Med. Chem.* 45, 1757–1766, 2002.
131. Nury, C., Czarny, B., Cassar-Lajeunesse, E., et al., A pan photoaffinity probe for detect-ing active forms of matrix metalloproteinases, *ChemBioChem.* 14, 107–114, 2013.

132. Shay, G., Lynch, C.C., and Fingleton, B., Moving targets: Emerging roles for MMPs in cancer progression and metastasis, *Matrix Biol.* 44–46, 200–206, 2015.
133. Brown, G.T. and Murray, G.I., Current mechanistic insights into the roles of matrix metalloproteinases in tumour invasion and metastasis, *J. Pathol.* 237, 273–281, 2015.
134. Deryugina, E.I. and Quigley, J.P., Tumor angiogenesis: MMP-mediated induction of intravasation- and metastasis-sustaining neovasculature, *Matrix Biol.* 44–46, 94–112, 2015.
135. Dive, V., Georgiadis, D., Matziari, M., et al., Phosphinic peptides as zinc metalloproteinase inhibitors, *Cell. Mol. Life Sci.* 61, 2010–2019, 2004.
136. Ndinguri, M.W., Bhowmick, M., Tokmina-Roszyk, D., Robichaud, T.K., and Fields, G.B., Peptide-based selective inhibitors of matrix metalloproteinase-mediated activities, *Molecules* 17, 14230–14248, 2012.
137. Kim, D.-H., Han-Hyuk, K., Hyeon-Jeong, J., et al., CopA3 peptide prevents ultraviolet-induced inhibition of type-I procollagen and induction of matrix metalloproteinase-1 in human skin fibroblasts, *Molecules* 19, 6407–6414, 2014.
138. LIui, G., Ming, W., Jianteng, H., et al., CS5931, a novel polypeptide in *Ciona savignyi*, represses angiogenesis via inhibiting vascular endothelial growth factor (VEGF) and matrix metalloproteinases (MMPs), *Mar. Drugs* 12, 1530–1544, 2014.
139. Altiparmak, B., Burcu, L., Fatma, Y., and Citak, A., Design of radiolabeled gelatinase inhibitor peptide (^{99m}Tc-CLP) and evaluation in rats, *Appl. Radiat. Isot.* 89, 133–133, 2014.
140. Liu, O., Pan, D., Cheng, C., et al., Targeting of MMP2 activity in malignant tumors with a ^{68}Ga-labeled gelatinase inhibitor cyclic peptide, *Nuc. Med. Biol.* 42, 939–944, 2015.
141. Edwards, D.R., Beaudry, P.P., Laing, T.D., et al., The roles of tissue inhibitors of metalloproteinases in tissue remodeling and cell growth, *Int. J. Obes. Relat. Metab. Disord.* 20(Suppl 3), S9–S15, 1996.
142. Henriet, P., Blavier, L., and Declerk, Y.A., Tissue inhibitors of metalloproteinases (TIMP) in invasion and proliferation, *APMIS* 107, 111–119, 1999.
143. Baker, A.H., Edwards, D.R., and Murphey, G., Metalloproteinase inhibitors: Biological actions and therapeutic opportunities, *J. Cell. Sci.* 115, 3719–3727, 2002.
144. Jiang, Y., Goldberg, I.D., and Shi, Y.E., Complex roles of tissue inhibitors of metalloproteinases in cancer, *Oncogene* 21, 2245–2252, 2002.
145. Cruz-Munoz, W. and Khokha, R., The role of tissue inhibitors of metalloproteinases in tumorogenesis and metastasis, *Crit. Rev. Clin. Lab. Sci.* 45, 291–338, 2008.
146. Moore, C.S. and Crocker, S.J., An alternative perspective on the roles of TIMPs and MMPs in pathology, *Am. J. Pathol.* 180, 12–16, 2012.
147. Higashi, S., Hirose, T., Takeuchi, T., and Miyazaki, K., Molecular design of a highly selective and strong protein inhibitor against matrix metalloproteinase-2 (MMP-2), *J. Biol. Chem.* 288, 9066–9076, 2013.
148. Seifter, S., Takahashi, S., and Harper, E., Further demonstration that cysteine reacts with the metal component of collagenase, *Biochim. Biophys. Acta* 214, 559–561, 1970.
149. Seltzer, J.L., Jeffrey, J.J., and Eisen, A.Z., Evidence for mammalian collagenases as zinc ion metalloenzymes, *Biochim. Biophys. Acta* 485, 179–185, 1977.
150. Ferry, G., Boutin, J.A., Hennig, P., et al., A zinc chelator inhibiting gelatinases exerts potent *in vitro* anti-invasive effects, *Eur. J. Pharmacol.* 351, 225–233, 1998.
151. Jacobsen, F.E., Lewis, J.A., and Cohen, S.M., A new role for old ligands: Discerning chelators for zinc metalloproteinases, *J. Am. Chem. Soc.* 128, 3156–3157, 2006.
152. Serra, P., Bruczko, M., Zapico, J.M., et al., MMP-2 selectivity in hydroxamate-type inhibitors, *Curr. Med. Chem.* 19, 1036–1064, 2012.
153. De Savi, C., Waterson, D., Pape, A., et al., Hydantoin based inhibitors of MMP13: Discovery of AZD6605, *Bioorg. Med. Chem.* 23(16), 4706–4712, 2013.

154. Marques, S.M., Abate, C.C., Chaves, S., et al., New bifunctional metalloproteinase inhibitors: An integrated approach towards biological improvements and cancer therapy, *J. Inorg. Biochem.* 127, 188–202, 2013.
155. Jin, Y., Roycik, M.D., Bosco, D.B., et al., Matrix metalloproteinase inhibitors based on the 3-mercaptopyrrolidine core, *J. Med. Chem.* 56, 4357–4373, 2013.
156. Mori, M., Massaro, A., Calderone, V., et al., Discovery of a new class of potent MMP inhibitors by structure-based optimization of the arylsulfonamide scaffold, *ACS Med. Chem. Lett.* 4, 565–569, 2013.
157. Golub, L.M., Lee, H.M., Lehrer, G., et al., Minocycline reduces gingival collagenolytic activity during diabetes, *J. Perio. Res.* 18, 516–524, 1983.
158. Golub, L.M., Ramamurthy, N., McNamare, T.E., et al., Tetracycline inhibits tissue collagenase activity: A new mechanism in the treatment of periodontal disease, *J. Perio. Res.* 19, 651–655, 1984.
159. Golub, L.M., McNamara, T.F., D'Angelo, G., Greenwald, R.A., and Ramamurthy, N.S., A non-antibacterial chemically-modified tetracycline inhibits mammalian collagenase activity, *J. Dent. Res.* 66, 1310–1314, 1987.
160. Marcial, B.L., Sousa, S.F., Barbosa, I.L., Dos Santos, H.F., and Ramos, M.J., Chemically modified tetracyclines as inhibitors of MMP-2 matrix metalloproteinase: A molecular and structural study, *J. Phys. Chem.* 116, 13644–13654, 2012.
161. Tocchi, A. and Parks, W.C., Functional interactions between matrix metalloproteinases and glycosaminoglycans, *FEBS J.* 280, 2332–2341, 2013.
162. Hadler-Olsen, E., Fadries, B., Sylte, I., et al., Regulation of matrix metalloproteinase activity in health and disease, *FEBS J.* 278, 28–45, 2011.
163. Tomlinson, J., Barsky, S.H., Nelson, S., et al., Different patterns of angiogenesis in sarcomas and carcinomas, *Clin. Cancer Res.* 5, 3516–3522, 1999.
164. Phillips, P.G. and Birnby, L.M., Nitric oxide modulates caveolin-1 and matrix metalloproteinase-9 expression and distribution at the endothelial cell/tumor cell interface, *Am. J. Physiol. Lung Cell. Mol. Physiol.* 286, L1055–L1065, 2004.
165. Plantner, J.J. and Drew, T.A., Polarized distribution of metalloproteinases in the bovine interphotoreceptor matrix, *Expt. Eye Res.* 59, 577–585, 1994.
166. Ahmed, A.K., Haylor, J.L., El Nathas, A.M., and Johnson, T.S., Localization of matrix metalloproteinases and their inhibitors in experimental kidney scarring, *Kid. Int.* 71, 756–763, 2007.
167. Sato, H. and Takino, T., Coordinate action of membrane-type matrix metalloproteinase-1 (MT1-MMP) and MMP-2 enhances pericellular proteolysis and invasion, *Cancer Sci.* 101, 843–847, 2010.
168. Liaw, L. and Crawford, H.C., Functions of the extracellular matrix and matrix degrading proteases during tumor progression, *Braz. J. Med. Biol. Res.* 32, 805–812, 1999.
169. Gillard, J.A., Reed, M.W.R., Buttle, D., et al., Matrix metalloproteinase activity and immunohistochemical profile of matrix metalloproitnease-2 and -9 and tissue inhibitor of metalloproteinase-1 during human dermal wound healing, *Wound Rep. Reg.* 12, 295–304, 2004.
170. Wang, P., Zhu, F., and Konstantopoulos, K., The antagonistic actions of endogenous interleukin-1β and 15-deoxy-Δ12,14-prostaglandin J2 regulate the temporal synthesis of matrix metalloproteinase-9 in sheared chondrocytes, *J. Biol. Chem.* 287, 31877–31893, 2012.
171. Yan, C. and Boyd, D.D., Regulation of matrix metalloproteinase gene expression, *J. Cell. Physiol.* 211, 19–26. 2007.
172. Bartling, T., Subbaram, S., Clark, R., et al., Redox-sensitive gene-regulatory events controlling aberrant matrix metalloproteinase-1 expression, *Free Radic. Biol. Med.* 74, 99–107, 2014.

173. Sun, Y., Lin, Z., Ding, W.J., et al., Secondhand smoking and matrix metalloproteinase-12 and -9 gene expression in saphenous veins of women nonsmokers, *Ann. Thorac. Surg.*, 98, 556–562, 2014.

174. Akagi, R., Sasho, T., Saito, M., et al., Effective knock down of matrix metalloproteinase-13 by an intra-articular injection of small interfering RNA (siRNA) in a murine surgically-induced osteoarthritis model, *J. Orthop. Res.* 32, 1175–1180, 2014.

175. Andrew Chan, K.L., Zhang, G., Tomic-Canic, M., et al., A coordinated approach to cutaneous wound healing: Vibrational microscopy and molecular biology, *J. Cell. Mol. Med.* 12, 2145–2154, 2008.

176. Mohammed, D., Crowther, J.M., Matts, P.J., Hadgraft, J., and Lane, M.E., Influence of niacinamide containing formulations on the molecular and biophysical properties of the stratum corneum, *Int. J. Pharm.* 441, 192–201, 2013.

177. Bocklitz, T., Bräutigam, K., Urbanek, A., et al., Novel workflow for combining Raman spectroscopy and MALDI-MSI for tissue based studies, *Anal. Bioanal. Chem.* 407, 7865–7873, 2015.

APPENDIX: MATRIX METALLOPROTEINASES

Matrix Metalloproteinase (MMP)	Characteristics, Specificity, and Function
MMP-1 (interstitial collagenase; tissue collagenase)	MMP-1 was one of the first MMPs[1] and was purified from human skin fibroblasts.[2,3] Much of the work on MMP-1 was performed with the enzyme purified by the tissue culture[4] (purification from the tissue was difficult).[2] MMP-1 differs from many of the MMPs described later in that it was (1) identified in tissue by biological activity and (2) purified from tissue culture media; early work described MMP-1 as *tissue collagenase*. Most of the later MMPs were identified by PCR cloning and only the recombinant form has been evaluated. A generic structure for MMP-1 is shown in Figure 7.1. A mutant enzyme missing the C-terminal hemopexin domain is similar to the native purified enzymes in the hydrolysis of synthetic substrates but does not cleave collagen.[5] The hemopexin domain is thought to contribute to the specificity of MMP-1. MMP-1 degrades collagens I, II, III, VII, and X,[6,7] and IGFBP-3.[8] MMP-1 preferentially degrades collagen III. The rate of fibrillar collagen cleavage is slow; cleavage of collagen III in solution is more rapid.[9,10] Application of a mechanical load to the collagen substrate increases rate of cleavage.[11] MMP-1 is less active in the degradation of gelatin than collagen.[10] The cleavage of native collagen involves a conformational change in the substrate collagen induced by binding MMP-1.[12] MMP-1 is produced in a wide variety of tissues[13] and the expression of MMP-1 is increased in tumors and thought to be involved, with other MMPs, in the metastatic process.[14] MMP-1 is inhibited by α_2-macroglobulin[15] and TIMP-1.[16] α_1-Protease inhibitor is degraded by MMP-1,[17,18] yielding fragments[a,b] with proinflammatory activity with monocytes[19] and neutrophils.[20] MMP-1 has a therapeutic application for muscle healing by degrading fibrous tissue and releasing local growth factors.[21]

Matrix Metalloproteinase (MMP)	Characteristics, Specificity, and Function
MMP-2 (gelatinase A)	MMP-2[22] is produced in a variety of normal tissues as well as by various tumors. MMP-2 is also known as the *72 kDa gelatinase/type IV collagenase*.[22,23] MMP-2 is a separate gene product from the 92 kDa gelatinase (gelatinase b; MMP-9).[22] However, MMP-9 expression is frequently concomitant with MMP-2 expression.[24–28] A gelatinase is defined as a proteolytic enzyme that will work on gelatin (denatured collagen). In MMP-2, that means that it does not degrade collagens I–III but is highly specific for the degradation of collagen IV, a major component of the basement membrane.[29–31] The ability of MMP-2 to degrade collagen IV in the basement membrane is considered critical to the process of tumor metastasis.[32] Degradation of collagen IV in the ECM by MMP-2 (and/or MMP-9) exposes an important cryptic epitope for angiogenesis.[33,34] While TIMP-2 is a specific inhibitor of MMP-2,[31,35] TIMP-2 also functions a *cofactor* in the activation of pro-MMP-2 by MT1-MMP (MMP-14).[36] The association between MMP-2 and TIMP-2 and the resulting activation on the cell surface by MMP-14 is thought to represent a unique regulatory mechanism.[37] MMP-2 is unique in that there is intracellular and extracellular expression of the active enzyme.[38,39] It has been noted that MMP-27 is confined to an intracellular site. MMP-2 contains three tandem fibronectin domains, which are important in MMP-2 binding to collagen in the ECM.[40–42] Endogenous MMP-2 in fibroblasts is activated by culturing on collagen I.[43] MMP-2 cannot cleave native collagen I but can degrade collagen I fragments produced by MMP-14.[44] Angiostatin is produced by cleavage of plasminogen by MMP-2.[45,46] It is of interest that MMP-2 is inhibited by red wine, providing an explanation for the protective effect of red wine in coronary disease.[47,48] MMP-2 acting with MMP-14 activates pro-MMP-13.[49] Pro-MMP-2 can be activated by a number of proteases including thrombin.[50–52] The activation of pro-MMP-2 by thrombin has been suggested to require the participation of MMP-14[30] or the presence of heparan sulfate.[53] Other work[54] suggests the participation of activated protein C in processing pro-MMP-2 to an intermediate form, which is then activated by thrombin. There are earlier data to suggest that thrombin does not activate pro-MMP-2.[55] It does appear that the activation of pro-MMP-2 by thrombin is a complex process occurring on a cell surface. Genetic polymorphism of MMP-2 is associated with a number of disparate pathologies from ischemic stroke to cancer.[56–59]
MMP-3 (stromelysin 1)[b1]	MMP-3 is a stromal cell–derived MMP that degrades the ECM, hence the alternative designation as stromelysin 1.[60] MMP-3 was originally described as an enzyme that hydrolyzed proteoglycans and hence was referred to as *proteoglycanase*.[61–63] Approximately 20% of pro-MMP-3 is produced as a glycosylated form.[64] MMP-3 is also referred to as transin.[65] Pro-MMP-3 can be activated by thrombin,[66] cathepsin G,[67] neutrophil elastase,[67] KLK-B1,[64] trypsin,[64] plasmin,[64] and chymotrypsin.[64] MMP-3 activates KLK-4[68] as well as pro-MMP-9.[69] MMP-3 has broad pH dependence for both activity and reaction with inhibitors.[70] Digestion of fibronectin and gelatin was more extensive at pH 5.5, while the digestion of azocoll was more

(Continued)

Matrix Metalloproteinase (MMP)	Characteristics, Specificity, and Function
	extensive at pH 6.2.[71] MMP-3 digestion of collagen IX was performed at pH 7.4[72] or 7.5,[73] but it is not clear that this is optimum pH. MMP-3 has broad specificity in degrading collagens II, IX, X, and XI,[73] as well as proteoglycans, casein, fibronectin, laminin, collagen IV, and gelatin, but not collagen I.[74] MMP-3 also degrades IGFBP,[75] substance P,[76] fetuin,[77] plasminogen activator inhibitor 1 (PAI-1),[78] and plasminogen with the generation of angiostatin.[79] MMP-3 is inhibited by α_2-macroglobulin[75,80] and by TIMP.[60,81,82]
MMP-4 (procollagen peptidase)	MMP-4 activity is reported to be identical with that of MMP-3, with possible contributions from MMP-13.
MMP-5 (3/4 collagenase)	MMP-5 is reported to be identical to MMP-2.
MMP-6[c]	MMP-6 is reported to be identical to MMP-3.
MMP-7 (matrilysin)	MMP-7[83,84] is one of the better-known MMPs and is also known as *matrin,*[85] *uterine metalloproteinase* (UPP), *putative metalloproteinase I* (pump-1), or *punctuated metalloproteinase.* MMP-7 is unique among MMPs in that it is small; its zymogen form has a molecular mass of 28 kDa, the active enzyme approximately 20 kDa.[84,85] MMP-7 lacks the hemopexin domain that appears to confer specificity to other MMPs.[86,87] As with other MMPs, pro-MMP-7 is activated by mercurials,[85,88] trypsin,[88] and heat.[89] Pro-MMP-7 can be activated[90] and inactivated by hypochlorite.[91] Pro-MMP-7 can also be activated by reaction with an electrophilic derivative of nitro-oleic acid, a fatty acid.[92] MMP-7 degrades a broad range of proteins in the interstitium, including fibronectin, laminin, collagen IV, and gelatin.[85,93] MMP-7 degrades fetuin.[77] MMP-7 also regulates β-catenin function in epithelial cell growth via degradation of the adherens junction protein E-cadherin.[85] As with other MMPs, MMP-7 is inhibited by TIMP-1[57] and α_2-macroglobulin.[94]
MMP-8 (neutrophil collagenase)	MMP-8 is synthesized and secreted from neutrophils as a zymogen or latent form from neutrophil,[95] which can be activated via limited proteolysis[95] by several enzymes, including cathepsin G[96] or stromelysin (MMP-3).[97] Activation of MMP-8 by nitric oxide has also been reported.[98] Reversible activation of MMP-8 by hypochlorous acid (HOCl) has been reported.[99,100] MMP-8 degrades triple-helical collagens I, II, and III; it also degrades other proteins including fibronectin, fibrinogen, and cartilage aggrecan.[95] There has been considerable work on the mechanism of collagen cleavage by MMP-8. As with other MMPs, the latent form of MMP-8 can be activated with mercuric chloride.[99,101] There has been work on the role of the hemopexin domain of MMP-8 in recognizing the substrate collagen molecule.[102,103] MMP-8 degrades α_1-antitrypsin.[101,104] Degradation of α_1-antitrypsin permits enhanced expression of neutrophil elastase.[105] As with other MMPs, MMP-8 can be inhibited by doxycycline,[93,106] α_2-macroglobulin, and TIMPs.[107,108] MMP-8 bound to the neutrophil membrane is protected from inhibition by TIMP-1 or TIMP-2.[109] MMP-8 stability is also increased when bound to the neutrophil membrane.[109]

Matrix Metalloproteinase (MMP)	Characteristics, Specificity, and Function
MMP-9 (gelatinase B)	MMP-9 was first described as a *gelatin-specific protease* from human leucocytes (neutrophils) in 1974.[110] Later work[111] reported neutrophil gelatinase was secreted as a monomer (92 kDa), a dimer (220 kDa) that reduced to a monomer (92 kDa), and a 130 kDa species that could also be converted to a monomer (92 kDa). In addition to secretion by leukocytes, MMP-9 is produced in a variety of other tissues.[112] MMP-9 is also known as the 92 kDa/type IV collagenase and is a distinct gene product to MMP-2.[111] As with other MMPs, MMP-9 is activated as a zymogen (pro-MMP-9) and can be activated by reaction with organic mercurials, cathepsin G, trypsin, α-chymotrypsin, and MMP-3.[113] Pro-MMP-9 can also be partially activated by hypochlorite[113,114] and by a protease from German cockroach frass.[115] Pro-MMP-9 derived from neutrophils occurs as heterodimer with lipocaliin.[116] Pro-MMP-9 derived from a macrophage cell line (THP-1) covalently links chondroitin sulfate proteoglycan.[117] Disulfide bonds have been suggested to be involved in heterodimer/oligomer formation,[117] but other data suggest alternatives to disulfide bonds.[118] MMP-9 binds to CD44 and promotes cell migration.[119,120] CD44 is a receptor found on a number of hematopoietic and nonhematopoietic cells and is important for cell–cell and cell–matrix interactions.[121,122] MMP-9 can cleave collagen IV and collagen V, forming discrete fragments.[123] MMP-9 is able to specifically cleave soluble collagens I and III.[124] However, MMP-9 does not cleave native triple-helical collagen I.[125,126] MMP-1 cleavage of triple-helical collagen I facilitates subsequent degradation by MMP-9.[125] MMP-9 has also been suggested to be important for the generation of active IL-1β, being much more effective than either MMP-2 or MMP-3 in this process.[127] MMP-9 can degrade a number of other proteins in the interstitium,[122,128] and is inhibited by TIMPs[129] and α_2-macroglobulin.[130] MMP-9 can form angiostatin from plasminogen.[131,132] As observed with other MMPs, MMP-9 can degrade α_1-protease inhibitors;[104,133,134] the degraded α_1-protease inhibitor is proinflammatory.[135] α_1-antichymotrypsin attenuates MMP-9 activation in the skin during wound healing.[136,137] Increased expression of MMP-9 results in poor wound healing; a porcine matrix product used in the promotion of wound healing in periodontal disease, EMD®, contains α_1-antichymotrypsin.[138]
MMP-10 (stromelysin 2)	As with MMP-3, MMP-10 degrades various components of the ECM, including collagens III, IV, and V, and fibronectin.[139] MMP-3 and MMP-10 are not isozymes but do demonstrate approximately 80% homology based on analysis of cDNA sequences.[140,141] There are differences in the regulation of the expression of the two proteins.[141,142] MMP-10, together with other MMPs, is suggested to be important for angiogenesis.[143] MMP-10 is inhibited by TIMP-1 and TIMP-2 but with less avidity than that observed with MMP-3.[144,145]

(Continued)

Matrix Metalloproteinase (MMP)	Characteristics, Specificity, and Function
MMP-11 (stromelysin 3)	Native MMP-11[146] has restricted substrate specificity, with early studies showing only cleavage of α_1-antiprotease inhibitor.[147] Deletion of approximately 175 amino acids from the C-terminal (hemopexin domain) and substitution of proline for ala235 resulted in a mutant enzyme that can now degrade casein, laminin, and collagen IV.[148] More recent work with phage display suggests that there are unique substrates for MMP-11 in tumors that remain to be identified.[149] The degradation of IGFBP by MMP-11 has been reported, which would favor cellular proliferation.[150] The development of a novel FRET[d] substrate permitted the intracellular and extracellular localization of MMP-11 in tumor cells.[151] MMP-11 is found in tissues undergoing rapid remodeling, as observed in tumor growth and wound healing as well as embryonic development.[152–154] Furin activates the zymogen form of MMP-11.[153,155]
MMP-12 (macrophage elastase)[e]	MMP-12 is also known as *macrophage metalloelastase*.[156] Murine macrophage elastase was described in 1975,[157] while the human enzyme was not characterized until 1993.[158] The murine enzyme has a mass of 22 kDa.[157] Subsequent isolation and characterization of the cDNA for the human protein showed a proenzyme (pro-MMP-12) of 54 kDa, which is processed to a 45 kDa product with removal of an N-terminal region, resulting in an active enzyme containing a catalytic domain and a hemopexin domain.[158] The 45 kDa species is subject to autolysis, yielding a 22 kDa catalytic domain that can cleave a triple-helical fluorescent peptide derived from collagen V.[159] MMP-12 degradation of human α_1-protease inhibitor by murine MMP-12[157] has been observed and the degradation product has been suggested to have chemotactic activity.[160] There are no studies with human MMP-12, nor are there any other studies with the murine enzyme; there are a number of other studies on the activity of peptide fragments obtained from α_1-proteinase inhibitor.[a,b] MMP-12 is also efficient at generating angiostatin from plasminogen.[161] MMP-12 degrades a large number of ECM proteins including fibronectin, laminin, collagen IV, and α_1-protease inhibitor.[162] Oxidation of α_1-antiprotease inhibitor resulting in the formation of methionine sulfoxide at Met[358] changes the site of cleavage from Pro[357]–Met[358] to Phe[352]–Leu[353].[163] MMP-12 is less effective than neutrophil elastase in solubilizing elastin.[162] MMP-12 stimulates IL-9/CXCL8 release from alveolar epithelium by EGF receptor-mediated pathway.[164]
MMP-13 (collagenase III)	MMP-13 degrades collagen II more rapidly than either collagen I or III.[165] MMP-13 also has general protease activity degrading: for example, fibrinogen and fibronectin. MMP-13 was first described in breast tumor tissue and subsequently in chondrocytes.[166] α_1-acid glycoprotein inhibits MMP-3 collagenolytic activity as well as the binding of MMP-3 to collagen.[167] As with other metalloproteinases, MMP-13 occurs as a precursor that can be activated by a variety of agents, including MMP-10.[168] MMP-13-activated PAR-1 receptors at a noncanonical site resulted in cellular activation via a tethered ligand.[169] Thrombin promotes MMP-13 expression in chondrocytes.[170] As with other MMPs, MMP-13 is inhibited by TIMPs and α_2-macroglobulin.[171]

Matrix Metalloproteinase (MMP)	Characteristics, Specificity, and Function
MMP-14 (MT1-MMP)	MMP-14 is an integral membrane protein[172] that was discovered by cloning technology[173] focused on identifying the factor(s) responsible for the activation of pro-MMP-2 (progelatinase A). MT1-MMP is expressed as a proenzyme that is activated in at least a two-step process[174] involving furin, possibly in complex with Golgi-reassembly stacking protein.[175] MT1-MMP initiates the degradation of collagen I followed by the action of MMP-2.[176,177] TIMP-2, TIMP-3, and TIMP-4 have been shown to inhibit the MT1-MMP,[94] although the relationship of TIMP-2 and MT1-MMP is complex, as both stimulation and inhibition of MT1-MMP activity is reported with this TIMP.[177–180] TIMP-2 forms a complex with MT1-MMP and pro-MMP-2, leading to the formation of MMP-2 and efficient degradation of collagen.[181] MT1-MMP is not inhibited by TIMP-1.[182] MT1-MMP also acts as a sheddase in releasing extracellular matrix metalloproteinase inducer (EMMPRIN)[183–185] from tumor cells.[186] There is considerable interest in the role of MT1-MMP in cancer biology[86,187] as well as in the etiology of rheumatoid arthritis.[188] MMP-14 is synthesized in a latent or zymogen form that is activated by furin or other convertases.[189] The activation of pro-MMP-14 and the subsequent production of brain-specific angiogenesis inhibitor 1 (BAI-1) is viewed as a proteolytic cascade.[190,f]
MMP-15 (MT2-MMP)	MMP-15[191] was identified by PCR cloning of a human lung cDNA library.[192] MMP-15 shows extensive structural homology to MMP-14 and is bound by a transmembrane domain to the cell surface. MMP-15 activates pro-MMP-2 in a process not requiring the participation of TIMP-2.[193,194] As with MMP-14, MMP-15 is inhibited by TIMP-2, TIMP-3, and TIMP-4, but not by TIMP-1.[181,191] Despite the structural homology between MMP-14 and MMP-15, the two proteins show different expression profiles.[195–197]
MMP-16 (MT3-MMP)	MMP-16 was identified by PCR cloning of a cDNA library from human tissues.[198,199] MMP-16 is similar to MMP-14 and MMP-15 (and MMP-24) in that it is attached to the membrane though a stem from a catalytic domain to a transmembrane domain with a cytoplasmic tail (Figure 7.3).[200] While MMP-14 and MMP-15 are widely distributed, MMP-16 expression is restricted to brain, lung, heart, and placenta.[200] MMP-16, as with MMP-14 and MMP-15, is an activator of pro-MMP-2 in the presence of either TIMP-2 or TIMP-3; TIMP-3 is also a high-affinity inhibitor of MMP-16 ($K_i = 0.008$ nM).[201] Inhibition of MMP-16 is observed with TIMP-2 (0.17 nM) and TIMP-4 (0.34 nM). MMP-16 can degrade fibronectin and collagen II.[200] A soluble form of MMP-16 resulting from alternative splicing has been described and has been suggested to have a direct role in the degradation of the ECM in addition to the activation of pro-MMP-2.[202] A recombinant soluble form of MMP-16 lacking the transmembrane and cytoplasmic domains degraded collagen III but not collagen I.[203] The truncated MMP-16 also degraded cartilage proteoglycan, gelatin, fibronectin, vitronectin, laminin-1, α_1-proteinase inhibitor, and α_2-macroglobulin, yielding fragments identical to those obtained with a truncated MMP-14.

(Continued)

Matrix Metalloproteinase (MMP)	Characteristics, Specificity, and Function
MMP-17 (MT4-MMP)	MMP-17 was identified by PCR cloning of a human breast carcinoma cDNA library.[204,205] It was not possible to express the first cDNA isolate;[205] subsequent work[206] identified a novel transcript that could be expressed. Other work[207] showed that MMP-17 differed from the other MT-MMPs in that MMP-17, and MMP-25, are linked to the membrane via linkage to GPI (Figure 8.4).[208] The catalytic domain of MMP-17 (Figure 7.4) has been expressed as an inclusion body and purified after solubilization in 8 M urea and renaturation.[209] The MMP-17 catalytic domain degrades gelatin and was a poor activator of pro-MMP-2 (progelatinase A). The MMP-17 catalytic domain was inactive in the degradation of other ECM proteins such as collagen I, collagen IV, fibronectin, and laminin. It has been suggested that the absence of the hemopexin domain might influence the observed activities. Another study[210] on the MMP-17 catalytic domain obtained similar results, except it was not possible to show activation of pro-MMP-2. Both studies[209,210] showed that, differing from other MT-MMPs, the MMP-17 catalytic domain was inhibited by TIMP-1; inhibition was also observed with TIMP. The recombinant murine MMP-17 catalytic domain was unable to activate pro-MMP-2 but did degrade fibrin and fibrinogen.[211] The murine MMP-17 catalytic domain was also inhibited by TIMP-1, TIMP-2, or TIMP-3. This later study[211] also showed that MMP-17 has TNF-α convertase activity and could shed pro-TNF-α. MMP-17 also activates ADAMTS-4 (aggrecanase-1).[212]
MMP-18 (collagenase IV)	MMP-18 is a poorly described MMP that degrades collagens I, II, and III.[213] First identified through PCR cloning of human mammary gland DNA, subsequent analysis of mRNA shows wide tissue distribution but absence in brain, skeletal muscle, kidney, liver, and peripheral blood leukocytes.[214] Studies in *Xenopus* suggested a role in amphibian development.[215] mRNA analysis identified the presence of MMP-18 in a variety of cultured human cell lines, including mammary cell lines, prostate cell lines, and human fibroblasts,[216] as well as cartilage.[217] MMP-18 may also be important for macrophage migration through tissue.[218]
MMP-19	MMP-19[219] was identified by PCR cloning from a human liver cDNA library.[220] Northern blot analysis showed higher MMP-19 mRNA expression in placenta, lung, pancreas, ovary, spleen, and intestine, with lower expression in other tissues such as liver and prostate.[220] An identical MMP designated RASI-1 was identified in a cDNA library from inflamed human synovium.[221] MMP-19 is also expressed in normal keratinocytes.[222,223] Recombinant pro-MMP-19 was expressed in *Escherichia coli* and purified from inclusion bodies.[224] The zymogen form of MMP-19 could be activated by trypsin and was inhibited by TIMP-2.[220] MMP-19 also cleaves several FRET[d] peptides,[220] with sequences consistent with an enzyme with a close relationship to the stromelysin group[225–227] of MMPs. Intact MMP-19 has been reported to cleave IGFBP-3,[224] while the recombinant catalytic domain cleaves collagen IV, fibronectin, laminin, and nidogen.[228] The recombinant MMP-19 hemopexin domain binds IGFBP-3.[229] Other studies with the carboxyl-terminal deletion mutant (recombinant catalytic domain), which does not contain the hemopexin domain, demonstrated cleavage of aggrecan at the canonical MMP cleavage site between Asn[341] and Phe[342].[230] Upregulation of MMP-19 is observed in melanoma metastasis.[231]

Matrix Metalloproteinase (MMP)	Characteristics, Specificity, and Function
MMP-20 (enamelysin)	MMP-20[232] was identified by PCR cloning from a porcine enamel organ cDNA library.[233] Human MMP-20 has a domain structure similar to other MMPs, consisting of a pro sequence containing the conserved cysteine residue, a catalytic domain containing a zinc-binding site, and a carboxyl terminal similar to the hemopexin domain observed in other MMPs.[234,235] Porcine MMP-20 showed 49% homology to porcine MMP-1.[234] The recombinant pro-MMP-20 undergoes autocatalytic activation during refolding from inclusion bodies in urea. MMP-20 degrades amelogenin[234,235] and is inhibited by TIMP-2.[234] MMP-20 activates pro-KLK-4.[236,237] Both MMP-20 and KLK-4 are important in the process of enamel development in teeth.[238] MMP-20 also activates KLKs other than KLK-4.[238] While most work has focused on the expression of MMP-20 in developing teeth, expression of MMP-20 in oral tumors has been reported.[239,240] MMP-20 degrades a number of proteins other than amelogenin and pro-KLKs, including fibronectin, collagen IV, laminin 1, laminin 5, and tenascin C.[239]
MMP-21 (*Xenopus* matrix metalloproteinase [XMMP])	MMP-21[241] was described in *Xenopus* embryos.[242] A human homolog/ortholog[243] to XMMP was identified in a cDNA library from human ovary.[244] Subsequent work has shown expression in macrophages and fibroblasts.[245] Recent interest has focused on MMP-21 expression in human tumors.[246]
MMP-22 (chicken matrix metalloproteinase [CMMP])	MMP-22[247] shows limited sequence identity with other MMPs.[248] There is a unique cysteine residue in catalytic domain; a similar cysteine residue has been reported in MMP-21 and MMP-18. A recombinant form missing the N-terminal region was observed to undergo autocatalytic activation and degraded gelatin and casein with a rate similar to that observed with recombinant MMP-1; however, the digestion products suggested a difference in specificity between MMP-1 and MMP-22. A human homolog for MMP-22 has not been reported.
MMP-23 (cysteine array matrix metalloproteinase [CA-MMP])	MMP-23 was identified by PCR cloning of a human ovary cDNA library.[249] Earlier work had identified several isoforms of an MMP that were designated MMP-20/21.[250] A murine homolog, CA-MMP was subsequently identified.[251,252] A rat MMP-23 has also been identified.[253] The recombinant human MMP-23 had low activity in the hydrolysis of one synthetic substrate but lacked activity against two other peptide substrates or gelatin.[249] The murine protein had efficient activity in the hydrolysis of gelatin.[251] It is noted that there are other examples of difference in the activity of orthologs.[254,255]
MMP-24 (MT5-MMP)	MMP-24[256] was identified by PCR cloning of a cDNA library from human brain.[257] MMP-24 can activate pro-MMP-2 (progelatinase A).[258] Murine MMP-24 truncated in transmembrane domain has been expressed in MDCK cells.[259] The purified protein activates pro-MMP-2 in a process requiring TIMP-2; this study[259] also demonstrated that recombinant MMP-24 could degrade gelatin, ECM proteoglycans (chondroitin sulfate proteoglycans, dermatan sulfate proteoglycans), and fibronectin but was not active in the degradation of laminin or collagen I. The recombinant MMP-24 is subject to rapid autolysis under physiological conditions, perhaps representing a control mechanism. The convertase furin can remove MMP-25 from the membrane by cleavage in the stem region, perhaps representing another control mechanism.[260]

(Continued)

Matrix Metalloproteinase (MMP)	Characteristics, Specificity, and Function
MMP-25 (MT6-MMP; leukolysin)	It would seem MMP-25[261] was described as leukolysin in 1970.[262] However, the first unambiguous identification of MMP-25 in leukocytes was obtained by use of an expressed sequence tag (EST) library.[263] A C-terminal truncated form of the enzyme was expressed and shown to have activity in the degradation of gelatin.[263] MMP-25 activates pro-MMP-2 (progelatinase A).[264,265] While the expression of MMP-25 was originally considered to be confined to leukocytes, MMP-26 has been identified in lung, spleen, colon carcinoma, glioblastoma, and astrocytoma.[264,266,267] As with MMP-17, MMP-25 is attached to membrane via a GPI linkage.[267–269] A homodimer form of MMP-25[267,269] has been identified on the surface of colon cancer cells and HL-60 cells. The homodimer is formed by a disulfide bond joining the stem domains of proximate MMP-25 monomers.[269] The dimer form is active and degrades α_1-proteinase inhibitor.[270] Studies with recombinant MMP-25 catalytic domain[271] demonstrated degradation of collagen IV, gelatin, fibronectin, and fibrin, but not laminin. The recombinant MMP-25 domain was unable to activate pro-MMP-2,[271] differing from results obtained with the intact protein.[264,265] It has been suggested that MMP-25 is responsible for the degradation of myelin basic protein in the etiology of multiple sclerosis.[272,273]
MMP-26 (matrilysin 2)	MMP-26[274] is also known as *endometase*, stemming from its discovery in human endometrial tumor.[275] It is similar to matrilysin (MMP-7) in that it is smaller (28 kDa zymogen; 19 kDa active enzyme) than the other MMPs as a result of a lack of a hemopexin domain.[276] MMP-26 degrades α_1-antiprotease inhibitor and certain ECM proteins.[275] Pro-MMP-26, differing from other MMPs, is not activated by organic mercurials.[277,278] Recombinant pro-MMP-26 underwent autocatalytic activation with a single peptide bond cleavage;[278,279] further proteolysis resulted in inactivation of the enzyme.[278] Autodigestion of pro-MMP-26 has been observed during the folding process of the recombinant enzyme from inclusion bodies expressed in *E. coli*.[279] MMP-26 cleaves a variety of proteins, with specificity determined by both P and P' sequences.[280] MMP-26 cleaves fibronectin, vitronectin, fibrinogen, IGFBP, and α_1-antiproteinase inhibitor.[279]
MMP-27	MMP-27 is a poorly described MMP. Studies in the mouse[281] show substantial mRNA expression in liver and spleen, with less expression in other tissues. A later study in the rat[282] found low levels of MMP-27 mRNA expression in bone and kidney. We could not find an original citation for the identification of MMP-27. The earliest paper described the expression of MMP-27 (mRNA) in B lymphocytes.[283] A more recent paper[284] showed that a C-terminal domain in MMP-27 provided for retention in the endoplasmic reticulum and prevented access to the secretion pathway; a mutant missing the C-terminal extension was secreted.
MMP-28 (epilysin)	MMP-28 (epilysin)[285] was identified by PCR cloning of a cDNA library obtained from epithelial cells.[286] There has been particular interest the expression of MMP-28 in keratinocytes and during wound healing.[287–289] MMP-28 is also expressed in macrophages.[290] Other work has suggested that MMP-28 is confined to action within the ECM.[291] MMP-28 is also expressed in tumors.[292,293]

| Matrix Metalloproteinase (MMP) | Characteristics, Specificity, and Function |

Note: Also known as *matrix metallopeptidases,* a group (clan) of proteolytic enzymes that use zinc in the catalytic process. (From Tallant, C., et al., *Biochim. Biophys. Acta* 1803, 20–28, 2010; Fanjul-Fernández, M., et al., *Biochim. Biophys. Acta* 1803, 3–19, 2010.) MMPs are expressed as a precursor of zymogen forms that can be activated by a variety of processes. Activation by nonenzymatic mechanisms with oxidizing agents such as hypochlorite or cysteine modification with mercuric chloride are thought to be based on the disruption of interaction between a cysteine residue in the propeptide and a zinc ion at the active site (from Bläser, J., et al., *Eur. J. Biochem.* 202, 1223–1230, 1991; Shetty, V., et al., *J. Am. Soc. Mass Spectrom.* 18, 1544–1551, 2007), although other mechanisms have been suggested. (From Chen, L.-C., et al., *Biochemistry* 32, 10289–10295, 1993; Rosenblum, G., et al., *J. Am. Chem. Soc.* 129, 13566–13574, 2007.) While hypochlorite can activate MMPs (From Michaelis, J., et al., *Arch. Biochem. Biophys.* 292, 555–562, 1992; Fu, X., et al., *J. Biol. Chem.* 276, 41279–41287, 2001.), hypochlorite can also cause the inactivation of MMP-7 by modification of a tryptophan adjacent to a glycine residue, resulting in a unique condensation product. (From Fu, X., et al., *J. Biol. Chem.* 279, 6209–6212, 2004.) The reader is directed to the review by Sternlicht and Werb (*Annu. Rev. Cell Dev. Biol.* 17, 463–516, 2001).

[a] While the primary function of α_1-antiproteinase inhibitor is the control of proteases in biological fluids, there are several studies that show that the intact and latent serpin has biological activities unrelated to the antiprotease function. Both native and latent α_1-antitrypsin inhibit the inflammatory response (LPS-stimulated synthesis and release of TNF-α). (From Janciauskiene, S., et al., *Biochem. Biophys. Res. Commun.* 321, 592–600, 2004.) Native α_1-antitrypsin inhibited the proliferation of breast tumor cell line (MDA-MB 468), while a C-terminal fragment of α_1-antitrypsin increased the proliferation of the same cell line. (From Zelvyte, I., et al., *Eur. J. Cancer Prev.* 12, 117–124, 2003.)

[b] α_1-Proteinase inhibitor is also degraded by some exogenous proteases of interest regarding its function in the interstitial space: a protease from dust mite (from Kalsheker, N.A., et al., *Biochem. Biophys. Res. Commun.* 221, 59–61, 1996) and German cockroach frass (from Hughes, V.S., et al., *Exp. Lung Res.* 33, 135–150, 2007).

[c] MMP-6 is identical to MMP-3. (From Wilhelm, S.M., et al., *J. Biol. Chem.* 268, 21906–21913, 1993.)

[d] This is an assay used extensively for MMPs. It is based on the presence of a fluorophore on (usually) the N-terminal of a peptide and a quencher at the C-terminus; hydrolysis of an internal peptide bond relieves quenching of the fluorophore with a concomitant increase in fluorescence. (From Matayoshi, E.D., et al., *Science* 247, 954–958, 1990.) This is not a sensitive assay but allows recognition of amino acid residues on both sides of the scissile peptide bond. (From Schechter, I., et al., *Biochem. Biophys. Res. Commun.* 27, 157–162, 1967.)

[e] There is some confusion between macrophage elastase, which is an MMP, and neutrophil elastase (Table 8.1).

[f] The cascade concept is found in a number of biological systems, possibly dating to the use of the term *cascade* to describe the process of blood coagulation. (From MacFarlane, R.G., *Nature* 202, 498–499, 1964.) Implicit in the coagulation hypothesis is the ability to use a cascade to amplify a biological signal. (From Teijaro, J.R, et al., *Proc. Natl. Acad. Sci. USA* 111, 3799–3804, 2014.) It is not clear that amplification of MMP systems occurs with homeostasis, but is amplified with the extravasation of tumors and in inflammation. (From Eberhardt, W., et al., *J. Immunol.* 165, 5788–5797, 2000.)

REFERENCES FOR APPENDIX

1. Houck, J.C., Sharma, V.K., Patel, Y.M., and Gladner, J.A., Induction of collagenolytic and proteolytic activities by anti-inflammatory drugs in the skin and fibroblast, *Biochem. Pharmacol.* 17, 2081–2090, 1968.

2. Bauer, E.A., Eisen, A.Z., and Jeffrey, J.J., Immunologic relationship of a purified human skin collagenase to other human and animal collagenases, *Biochim. Biophys. Acta* 206, 152–160, 1970.

3. Fields, G.B., Van Wart, H.E., and Birkedal-Hansen, H., Sequence specificity of human skin fibroblast collagenase: Evidence for the role of collagen structure in determining the collagenase cleavage site, *J. Biol. Chem.* 262, 6221–6226, 1987.

4. Springman, E.B., Angleton, E.L., Birkedal-Hansen, H., and Van Wart, H.E., Multiple modes of activation of latent human fibroblast collagenase: Evidence for the role of a Cys^{73} active site zinc complex in latency and a "cysteine switch" mechanism for activation, *Proc. Natl. Acad. Sci. USA* 87, 364–368, 1990.

5. Brownell, J., Earley, W., Kunec, E., et al., Comparison of native matrix metalloproteinases and their recombinant catalytic domains using a novel radiometric assay, *Arch. Biochem. Biophys.* 314, 120–125, 1994.

6. Cawston, T.E., Matrix metallopeptidase-1/interstitial collagenase, in *Handbook of Proteolytic Enzymes*, 3rd edn., eds. N.D. Rawlings and G. Salvesen, Chapter 152, pp. 718–725, Elsevier, Amsterdam, the Netherlands, 2013.

7. Stetler-Stevenson, W.G., Talano, J.A., Gallagher, M.E., et al., Inhibition of human type IV collagenase by a highly conserved peptide sequence derived from its prosegment, *Am. J. Med. Sci.* 302, 163–170, 1991.

8. Fowlkes, J.L., Enghild, J.J., Suzuki, K., and Nagase, H., Matrix metalloproteinases degrade insulin-like growth factor-binding protein-3 in dermal fibroblast cultures, *J. Biol. Chem.* 269, 25742–25746, 1994.

9. Birkedal-Hansen, H., Taylor, R.E., Bhown, A.S., et al., Cleavage of bovine skin type III collagen by proteolytic enzymes: Relative resistance of the fibrillar form, *J. Biol. Chem.* 260, 16411–16417, 1985.

10. Welgus, H.G., Jeffrey, J.J., Stricklin, G.P., and Eisen, A.Z., The gelatinolytic activity of human skin fibroblast collagenase, *J. Biol. Chem.* 257, 11534–11539, 1982.

11. Adhikari, A.S., Chai, J., and Dunn, A.R., Mechanical load induces a 100-fold increase in the rate of collagen proteolysis by MMP-1, *J. Am. Chem. Soc.* 133, 1686–1689, 2013.

12. Fasciglione, G.F., Magda, G., Tsukada, H., et al., The collagenolytic action of MMP-1 is regulated by the interaction between the catalytic domain and the hinge region, *J. Biol. Inorg. Chem.* 17, 663–672, 2012.

13. Montfort, I. and Perez-Tamayo, R., Distribution of collagenases in normal rat tissues, *J. Histochem. Cytochem.* 23, 910–920, 1975.

14. Casimiro, S., Mohammed, K.S., Pires, R., et al., RANKL/RANK/MMP-1 molecular triad contributes to the metastatic phenotype of breast and prostate cancer cells *in vitro*, *PLoS One* 8(5), e63153, 2013.

15. Sottrup-Jensen, L. and Birkedal-Hansen, H.Y., Human fibroblast collagenase–α-macroglobulin interactions: Localization of cleavage sites in the bait regions of five mammalian α-macroglobulins, *J. Biol. Chem.* 264, 393–401, 1989.

16. Sudbeck, B.D., Jeffrey, J.J, Welgus, H.G., et al., Purification and characterization of bovine interstitial collagenase and tissue inhibitor of metalloproteinases, *Arch. Biochem. Biophys.* 293, 370–376, 1992.

17. Mast, A.E., Enghild, J.J., Nagase, H., et al., Kinetics and physiologic relevance of the inactivation of α_1-proteinase inhibitor, α_1-antichymotrypsin, and antithrombin III by matrix metalloproteinase-1 (tissue collagenase), -2 (72 kDa gelatinase/Type IV collagenase), and -3 (stromelysin), *J. Biol. Chem.* 266, 15810–15816, 1991.

18. Desrochers, P.E., Jeffrey, J.J., and Weiss, S.J., Interstitial collagenase (matrix metalloproteinase-1) expresses serpinase activity, *J. Clin. Invest.* 87, 2258–2265, 1991.
19. Janciauskiene, S., Zelvyte, I., Jansson, L., and Stevens, T., Divergent effects of α-1-antitrypsin on neutrophil activation *in vitro*, *Biochem. Biophys. Res. Commun.* 315, 288–296, 2004.
20. Moraga, F., Lindgren, S., and Janciauskiene, S., Effects of noninhibitory α-1-antitrypsin on primary human monocyte activation *in vitro*, *Arch. Biochem. Biophys.* 386, 221–226, 2001.
21. Bedair, H., Liu, T.T., Kaar, J.L., et al., Matrix metalloproteinase-1 therapy improves muscle healing, *J. Appl. Physiol.* 102, 2338–2345, 2007.
22. Murphy, G., Matrix metallopeptidase-2 (Gelatinase A), in *Handbook of Proteolytic Enzymes*, 3rd edn., eds. N.D. Rawlings and G. Salvesen, Chapter 156, pp. 747–753, Elsevier, Amsterdam, the Netherlands, 2013.
23. Fujimoto, N., Mouri, N., Iwata, K., et al., A one-step sandwich enzyme immunoassay for human matrix metalloproteinase 2 (72-kDa gelatinase/type IV collagenase) using monoclonal antibodies, *Clin. Chim. Acta* 221, 91–103, 1993.
24. Florentini, C., Bodei, S., Bedussi, F., et al., GPNMB/OA protein increases the invasiveness of human metastatic prostate cancer cell lines DU145 and PC3 through MMP-2 and MMP-9 activity, *Exp. Cell Res.* 323, 100–111, 2014.
25. Liu, W.H., Chen, Y.J., Chien, J.H., and Chang, L.S., Amsacrine suppresses matrix metalloproteinase-2 (MMP-2)/MMP-9 expression in human leukemia cells, *J. Cell. Physiol.* 229, 588–598, 2014.
26. Uwafuji, S., Goi, T., Naruse, T., et al., Protein-bound polysaccharide K reduced the invasive ability of colon cancer cell lines, *Anticancer Res.* 33, 4841–4845, 2013.
27. Lipari, L. and Gerbino, A., Expression of gelatinases (MMP-2, MMP-9) in human articular cartilage, *Int. J. Immunopathol. Pharmacol.* 26, 817–823, 2013.
28. Marbaix, E., Donnez, J., Courtoy, P.J., and Eeckhout, Y., Progesterone regulates the activity of collagenase and related gelatinases A and B in human endometrial explants, *Proc. Natl. Acad. Sci. USA* 89, 11789–11793, 1992.
29. Li, Z., Li, L., Zielke, H.R., et al., Increased expression of 72-kd type IV collagenase (MMP-2) in human aortic atherosclerotic lesions, *Am. J. Pathol.* 148, 121–128, 1996.
30. Nakoman, C., Resmi, H., Ay, O., et al., Effects of basic fibroblast factor (bFGF) on MMP-2, TIMP-2 and type-1 collagen in human lung carcinoma, *Biochimie* 87, 343–351. 2005.
31. Maymon, E., Romero, R., Pacora, P., et al., A role for the 72 kDa gelatinase (MMP-2) and its inhibitor (TIMP-2) in human parturition, premature rupture of membranes and intraamniotic infection, *J. Perinatal Med.* 29, 308–316, 2001.
32. Brinckerhoff, C.E., Rutter, J.L., and Benbow, U., Interstitial collagenases as markers of tumor progression, *Clin. Cancer Res.* 6, 4823–4830, 2000.
33. Xu, J., Rodriguez, D., Petitclerc, E., et al., Proteolytic exposure of a cryptic site within collagen type IV is required for angiogenesis and tumor growth *in vivo*, *J. Cell Biol.* 154, 1069–1079, 2001.
34. Pearce, W.H. and Shively, V.P., Abdominal aortic aneurysm as a complex multifactorial disease: Interactions of polymorphisms of inflammatory genes, features of autoimmunity, and current status of MMPs, *Ann. N.Y. Acad.* 1085, 117–132, 2006.
35. Willenbrock, F., Crabbe, T., Slocombe, P.M., et al., The activity of the tissue inhibitors of metalloproteinases is regulated by C-terminal domain interactions: A kinetic analysis of the inhibition of gelatinase A, *Biochemistry* 32, 4330–4337, 1993.
36. Bernardo, M.M. and Fridman, R., TIMP-2 (tissue inhibitor of metalloproteinase-2) regulates MMP-2 (matrix metalloproteinase-2) activity in the extracellular environment after pro-MMP-2 activation by MT1 (membrane type 1)-MMP, *Biochem. J.* 374, 739–745, 2003.

37. Yu, A.E., Hewitt, R.E., Kleiner, D.E., and Stetler-Stevenson, W.G., Molecular regulation of cellular invasion: Role of gelatinase A and TIMP-2, *Biochem. Cell Biol.* 74, 823–831, 1996.

38. Ali, M.A., Fan, X., and Schulz, R., Cardiac sarcomeric proteins: Novel intracellular targets of matrix metalloproteinase-2 in heart disease, *Trends Cardiovasc. Med.* 21, 112–128, 2011.

39. Jacob-Ferreira, A.L. and Schulz, R., Activation of intracellular matrix metalloproteinase-2 by reactive oxygen–nitrogen species: Consequences and therapeutic strategies in heart, *Arch. Biochem. Biophys.* 540, 82–93, 2013.

40. Steffensen, B., Wallon, U.M., and Overall, C.M., Extracellular matrix binding properties of recombinant fibronectin type II-like modules of 72-KDa gelatinase/type IV collagenase: High affinity binding to matrix type I collagen but not native type IV collagen, *J. Biol. Chem.* 270, 11555–11566, 1995.

41. Hornebeck, W., Bellon, G., and Emonard, H., Fibronectin type II (FnII)-like modules regulate gelatinase A activity, *Pathol. Biol.* 53, 405–410, 2005.

42. Mikhailova, M., Xu, X., Robichaud, T.K., et al., Identification of collagen binding domain residues that govern catalytic activities of matrix metalloproteinase-2 (MMP-2), *Matrix Biol.* 31, 380–388, 2012.

43. Azzam, H.S. and Thompson, E.W., Collagen-induced activation of M_r 72,000 type IV collagenase in normal and malignant human fibroblast cells, *Cancer Res.* 52, 4540–4544, 1992.

44. Sato, H. and Takino, T., Coordinate action of membrane-type matrix metalloproteinase-1 (MT1-MMP) and MMP-2 enhances pericellular proteolysis and invasion, *Cancer Sci.* 101, 843–847, 2010.

45. O'Reilly, M.S., Wiederschain, D., Stetler-Stevenson, W.G., et al., Regulation of angiostatin production by matrix metalloproteinase-2 in a model of concomitant resistance, *J. Biol. Chem.* 274, 29568–29571, 2006.

46. Chung, A.W., Hsiang, Y.N., Matzke, L.A., et al., Reduced expression of vascular endothelial growth factor paralleled with the increased angiostatin expression resulting from the upregulated activities of matrix metalloproteinase-2 and -9 in human type 2 diabetic arterial vasculature, *Circ. Res.* 99, 140–148, 2006.

47. Guo, H., Liu, L., Shi, Y., et al., Chinese yellow wine and red wine inhibit matrix metalloproteinase-2 and improve atherosclerotic plaque in LDL receptor knockout mice, *Cardiovasc. Ther.* 28, 161–168, 2010.

48. Walter, A., Etienne-Selloum, N., Sarz, M., et al., Angiotensin II induces the vascular expression of VEGF and MMP-2 *in vivo*: Preventive effect of red wine polyphenols, *J. Vasc. Res.* 45, 386–394, 2008.

49. Knäuper, V., Will, H., López-Otin, C., et al., Cellular mechanisms for human procollagenase-3 (MMP-13) activation: Evidence that MT1-MMP (MMP-14) and gelatinase a (MMP-2) are able to generate active enzyme, *J. Biol. Chem.* 271, 17124–17131, 1996.

50. Galis, Z.S., Krankhöfer, R., Fenton, J.W., II, and Libby, P., Thrombin promotes activation of matrix metalloproteinase-2 produced by cultured vascular smooth muscle cells, *Arterioscler. Thromb. Vasc. Biol.* 17, 483–489, 1997.

51. Lafleur, M.A., Hollenberg, M.D., Atkinson, S.J., et al., Activation of pro-(matrix metalloproteinase-2) (pro-MMP-2) by thrombin is membrane-type-MMP-dependent in human umbilical vein endothelial cells and generates a distinct 63 kDa active species, *Biochem. J.* 357, 107–115, 2001.

52. Wang, Z., Kong, L., Kang, J., et al., Thrombin stimulates mitogenesis in pig cerebrovascular smooth muscle cells involving activation of pro-matrix metalloproteinase-2, *Neurosci. Let.* 452, 199–203, 2009.

53. Koo, B.H., Han, J.H., Jeom, Y.I., et al., Thrombin-dependent MMP-2 activity is regulated by heparan sulfate, *J. Biol. Chem.* 285, 41270–41279, 2010.

54. Pekovich, S.R., Bock, P.E., and Hoover, R.L., Thrombin–thrombomodulin activation of protein C facilitates the activation of progelatinase A, *FEBS Lett.* 494, 129–132, 2001.
55. Okada, Y., Morodomi, T., Enghild, J.J., et al., Matrix metalloproteinase 2 from human rheumatoid synovial fibroblasts: Purification and activation of the precursor and enzymatic properties, *Eur. J. Biochem.* 194, 721–739, 1990.
56. Guo, X.T., Wang, J.F., Zhang, L.Y., et al., Quantitative assessment of the effects of MMP-2 polymorphisms on lung carcinoma risk, *Asian Pac. J. Cancer Prev.* 13, 2853–2856, 2012.
57. Ortak, H., Demir, S., Ates, Ö., et al., The role of MMP2 (−1306C>T) and TIMP2 (-418 G>C) promoter variants in age-related macular degeneration, *Ophthalmic Genet.* 34, 217–222, 2013.
58. Kaminska, A., Banas-Lezanska, P., Przybylowska, K., et al., The protective role of the -735C/T and the -1306C/T polymorphisms of the MMP-2 gene in the development of primary open-angle glaucoma, *Ophthalmic Genet.* 35, 41–46, 2014.
59. Nie, S.W., Wang, X.F., and Tang, Z.C., Correlations between MMP-2/MMP-9 promoter polymorphisms and ischemic stroke, *Int. J. Clin. Exp. Med.* 7, 400–404, 2014.
60. Nagase, H., Matrix metalloproteinase 3/Stromelysin 1, in *Handbook of Proteolytic Enzymes*, 3rd edn., eds. N.D. Rawlings and G. Salvesen, Chapter 158, pp. 763–774, Elsevier, Amsterdam, the Netherlands, 2013.
61. Sapolsky, A.I., Malemud, C.J., Norby, D.P., et al., Neutral proteinases from articular chondrocytes in culture: 2. Metal-dependent latent neutral proteoglycanase, and inhibitory activity, *Biochim. Biophys. Acta* 658, 138–147, 1981.
62. Galloway, W.A., Murphy, G., Sandy, J.D., et al., Purification and characterization of a rabbit bone metalloproteinase that degrades proteoglycan and other connective-tissue components, *Biochem. J.* 209, 741–752, 1983.
63. Gowen, M., Wood, D.D., Ihrie, E.J., et al., Stimulation by human interleukin 1 of cartilage breakdown and production of collagenase and procollagenase and proteoglycanase by human chondrocytes but not by human osteoblasts *in vitro*, *Biochim. Biophys. Acta* 797, 186–193, 1984.
64. Okada, Y., Harris, E.D., Jr., and Nagase, H., The precursor of a metallopeptidase from human rheumatoid synovial fibroblasts: Purification and mechanisms of activation by endopeptidases and 4-aminophenylmercuric acetate, *Biochem. J.* 254, 731–741, 1988.
65. Machida, C.M., Scott, J.D., and Ciment, G., NGF-induction of the metalloproteinase–transin/stromelysin in PC12 cells: Involvement of multiple protein kinases, *J. Cell Biol.* 114, 1037–1048, 1991.
66. Fang, Q., Liu, X., Al-Mugotir, M., et al., Thrombin and TNF-α/IL-1β synergistically induce fibroblast-mediated collagen gel degradation, *Am. J. Respir. Cell Mol. Biol.* 35, 714–721, 2006.
67. Okada, Y. and Nakanishi, I., Activation of matrix metalloproteinase 3 (stromelysin) and matrix metalloproteinase 2 ("gelatinase") by human neutrophil elastase and cathepsin G, *FEBS Lett.* 249, 353–356, 1989.
68. Beaufort, N., Plaza, K., Utzschneider, D., et al., Interdependence of kallikrein-related peptidases in proteolytic networks, *Biol. Chem.* 391, 581–587, 2010.
69. Geurts, N., Martens, E., Van Aelst, I., et al., β-Hematin interaction with the hemopexin domain of gelatinase B/MMP-9 provokes autocatalytic processing of the propeptide, thereby priming activation by MMP-3, *Biochemistry* 47, 2689–2699, 2008.
70. Johnson, L.L., Pavlovsky, A.G., Johnson, A.R., et al., A rationalization of the acidic pH dependence for stromelysin-1 (matrix metalloproteinase-3) catalysis and inhibition, *J. Biol. Chem.* 275, 11026–11933, 2000.
71. Gunja-Smith, Z., Nagase, H., and Woessner, J.F., Jr., Purification of the neutral proteoglycan-degrading metalloproteinase from human articular cartilage and its identification as stromelysin matrix metalloproteinase-3, *Biochem. J.* 258, 115–119, 1989.

72. Okada, Y., Konomi, H., Yada, T., et al., Degradation of type IX collagen by matrix metalloproteinase-3 (stromelysin) from human rheumatoid synovial cells, *FEBS Lett.* 244, 473–476, 1989.

73. Wu, J.J., Lark, M.W., Chun, L.E., and Eyre, D.R., Sites of stromelysin cleavage in collagen type II, IX, X, and XI of cartilage, *J. Biol. Chem.* 266, 5625–5628, 1991.

74. Wilhelm, S.M., Wunderlich, D., Maniglia, C.A., et al., Primary structure and function of stromelysin/transin in cartilage matrix, *Matrix Suppl.* 1, 37–44, 1992.

75. Coppock, H.S., White, A., Aplin, J.D., and Westwood, M., Matrix metalloprotease-3 and -9 proteolyze insulin-like growth factor-binding protein-1, *Biol. Reprod.* 71, 438–443, 2004.

76. Teahan, J., Harrison, R., Izquierdo, M., and Stein, R.L., Substrate specificity of human fibroblast stromelysin: Hydrolysis of substance P and its analogues, *Biochemistry* 28, 8497–8501, 1989.

77. Schure, R., Costa, K.D., Rezaei, R., et al., Impact of matrix metalloproteinases on inhibition of mineralization by fetuin, *J. Periodont. Res.* 46, 357–366, 2013.

78. Lijnen, H.R., Arza, B., Van Hoef, B., Collen, D., and Declerck, P.J., Inactivation of plasminogen activator inhibitor-1 by specific proteolysis with stromelysin-1 (MMP-3), *J. Biol. Chem.* 275, 37645–37650, 2000.

79. Lijnen, H.R., Ugwu, F., Bini, A., and Collen, D., Generation of an angiostatin-like fragment from plasminogen by stromelysin-1 (MMP-3), *Biochemistry* 37, 4699–4702, 1998.

80. Enghild, J.J., Salvesen, G., Brew, K., and Nagase, H., Interaction of human rheumatoid synovial collagenase (matrix metalloproteinase-1) and stromelysin (matrix metalloproteinase 3) with human α_2-macroglobulin and chicken ovostatin: Binding kinetics and identification of matrix metalloproteinase cleavage sites, *J. Biol. Chem.* 264, 8779–8785, 1989.

81. Willenbrock, F. and Murphy, G., Structure–function relationships in the tissue inhibitors of metalloproteinases, *Am. J. Respir. Crit. Care Med.* 150, S165–S170, 1994.

82. Woessner, J.F., MMPs and TIMPs: An historical perspective, in *Matrix Metalloproteinases Protocols*, Vol. 151, eds. I. Clark, Chapter 1, pp. 1–23, Humana Press, Totowa, NJ, 2001.

83. Matrisian, L.M., Matrix metalloproteinase-7/matrilysin, in *Handbook of Proteolytic Enzymes*, 3rd edn., eds. N.D. Rawlings and G. Salvesen, Chapter 161, pp. 785–795, Elsevier, Amsterdam, the Netherlands, 2013.

84. Woessner, J.F., Jr., Matrilysin, *Methods Enzymol.* 248, 485–495, 1995.

85. Miyazaki, K., Hattori, Y., Umenishi, F., et al., Purification and characterization of extracellular matrix-degrading metalloproteinase, matrin (Pump-1), secreted from human rectal carcinoma cell line, *Cancer Res.* 50, 7758–7764, 1990.

86. Remacle, A.G., Golubkov, V.S., Shiryaev, S.A., et al., Novel MT1-MMP small-molecule inhibitors based on insights into hemopexin domain function in tumor growth, *Cancer Res.* 72, 2339–2349, 2012.

87. Correia, A.L., Mori, H., Chen, E.I., et al., The hemopexin domain of MMP-3 is responsible for mammary epithelial invasion and morphogenesis through extracellular interaction with HSP90β, *Genes Dev.* 27, 805–817, 2013.

88. Crabbe, T., Willenbrock, F., Eaton, D., et al., Biochemical characterization of matrilysin: Activation conforms to the stepwise mechanisms proposed for other matrix metalloproteinases, *Biochemistry* 31, 8500–8507, 1992.

89. Rims, C.R. and McGuire, J.K., Matrilysin (MMP-7) catalytic activity regulates β-catenin localization and signaling activation in lung epithelial cells, *Exp. Lung Res.* 40, 126–136, 2014.

90. Fu, X., Kassim, S.Y., Parks, W.C., and Heinecke, J.W., Hypochlorous acid oxygenates the cysteine switch domain of pro-matrilysin (MMP-7): A mechanism for matrix metalloproteinase activation and atherosclerotic plaque rupture by myeloperoxidase, *J. Biol. Chem.*276, 41279–41287, 2001.

91. Fu, X., Kao, J.L., Bergt, C., et al., Oxidative cross-linking of tryptophan to glycine restrains matrix metalloproteinase activity: Specific structural motifs control protein oxidation, *J. Biol. Chem.* 279, 6209–6212, 2004.

92. Bonacci, G., Schopfer, F.J., Batthyany, C.I., et al., Electrophilic fatty acids regulate matrix metalloproteinase activity and expression, *J. Biol. Chem.* 286, 16074–16081, 2011.

93. Wilson, C.L. and Matrisian, L.M., Matrilysin: An epithelial matrix metalloproteinase with potentially novel functions, *Int. J. Biochem. Cell Biol.* 28, 123–136, 1996.

94. Baker, A.H., Edwards, D.R., and Murphy, G., Metalloprotease inhibitors: Biological actions and therapeutic opportunities, *J. Cell Sci.* 115, 3719–3727, 2002.

95. Tscheche, H. and Wenzel, H., Neutrophil collagenase, in *Handbook of Proteolytic Enzymes*, 3rd edn., eds. N.D. Rawlings and G. Salvesen, Chapter 153, pp. 725–738, Elsevier, Amsterdam, the Netherlands, 2013.

96. Capodici, C., Muthukumaran, G., Amoruso, M.A., and Berg, R.A., Activation of neutrophil collagenase by cathepsin G, *Inflammation* 13, 245–258, 1989.

97. Knäuper, V., Wilhelm, S.M., Seperack, P.K., et al., Direct activation of human neutrophil procollagenase by recombinant stromelysin, *Biochem. J.* 295, 581–586, 1993.

98. Okamoto, T., Akaike, T., Nagano, T., et al., Activation of human neutrophil procollagenase by nitrogen dioxide and peroxynitrite: A novel mechanism for procollagenase activation involving nitric oxide, *Arch. Biochem. Biophys.* 342, 262–274, 1997.

99. Saari, H., Suomalainen, K., Lindy, O., et al., Activation of latent human neutrophil collagenase by reactive oxygen species and serine proteases, *Biochem. Biophys. Res. Commun.* 171, 979–987, 1990.

100. Chatham, W.W., Blackburn, W.D., Jr., and Heck, L.W., Additive enhancement of neutrophil collagenase activity by HOCl and cathepsin G, *Biochem. Biophys. Res. Commun.* 184, 560–567, 1992.

101. Michaelis, J., Vissers, M.C., and Winterbourn, C.C., Human neutrophil collagenase cleaves α_1-antitrypsin, *Biochem. J.* 270, 809–814, 1990.

102. Gioia, M., Fasciglione, G.F., Marini, S., et al., Modulation of the catalytic activity of neutrophil collagenase MMP-8 on bovine collagen I: Role of the activation cleavage and of the hemopexin-like domain, *J. Biol. Chem.* 277, 23123–23130, 2002.

103. Brandstetter, H., Grams, F., Glitz, D., et al., The 1.8-A crystal structure of a matrix metalloproteinase 8-barbiturate inhibitor complex reveals a previously unobserved mechanism for collagenase substrate recognition, *J. Biol. Chem.* 276, 17405–17412, 2001.

104. Desrochers, P.E., Mookhtiar, K., Van Wart, H.E., et al., Proteolytic inactivation of α_1-proteinase inhibitor and α_1-antichymotrypsin by oxidatively activated human neutrophil metalloproteinases, *J. Biol. Chem.* 267, 5005–5012, 1992.

105. Sorsa, T., Lindy, O., Konttinen, Y.T., et al., Doxycycline in the protection of serum α_1-antitrypsin from human neutrophil collagenase and gelatinase, *Antimicrob. Agents Chemother.* 37, 592–594, 1993.

106. Lee, H.M., Ciancio, S.G., Tüter, G., et al., Subantimicrobial dose doxycycline efficacy as a matrix metalloproteinase inhibitor in chronic periodontitis patients is enhanced when combined with a non-steroidal anti-inflammatory drug, *J. Periodontol.* 75, 453–463, 2004.

107. Mäkitalo, L., Rintamäki, H., Tervahartinala, T., et al., Serum MMPs 7–9 and their inhibitors during glucocorticoid and anti-TNF-α therapy in pediatric inflammatory bowel disease, *Scand. J. Gastroenterol.* 47, 785–794, 2012.

108. Farr, M., Pieper, M., Calvete, J., and Tschesche, H., The N-terminus of collagenase MMP-8 determines superactivity and inhibition: A relation of structure and function analyzed by biomolecular interaction analysis, *Biochemistry* 38, 7332–7338, 1999.

109. Owen, C.A., Hu, Z., Lopez-Otin, C., and Shapiro, S.D., Membrane-bound matrix metalloproteinase-8 on activated polymorphonuclear cells is a potent tissue inhibitor of metalloproteinase-resistant collagenase and serpinase, *J. Immunol.* 172, 7791–7803, 2004.

110. Sopata, I. and Dancewicz, A.M., Presence of a gelatin-specific proteinase and its latent form in human leucocytes, *Biochim. Biophys. Acta* 370, 510–523, 1974.

111. Triebel, S., Bläser, J., Reinke, H., and Tschesche, H., A 25 kDa α-2-microglobulin-related protein is a component of the 125 kDa form of human gelatinase, *FEBS Lett.* 314, 386–388, 1992.

112. Eisen, A.Z., Sarker, S.K., Newman, K.C., and Goldberg, G.I., Matrix metalloproteinase 9/gelatinase B, in *The Handbook of Proteolytic Enzymes*, 3rd edn., eds. N.D. Rawlings and G. Salvesen, Chapter 157, pp. 754–763, Elsevier, Amsterdam, the Netherlands, 2013.

113. Okada, Y., Gonoji, Y., Naka, K., et al., Matrix metalloproteinase 9 (93-kDa gelatinase/type IV collagenase) from HT 1080 human fibrosarcoma cells, *J. Biol. Chem.* 267, 21712–21719, 1992.

114. Meli, D.N., Christen, S., and Lieb, S.L., Matrix metalloproteinase-9 in pneumococcal meningitis activation via an oxidative pathway, *J. Infect. Dis.* 187, 1411–1415, 2003.

115. Hughes, V.S. and Page, K., German cockroach frass proteases cleave pro-matrix metalloproteinase-9, *Exp. Lung Res.* 33, 135–150, 2007.

116. Kjeldsen, L., Johnson, A.H., Sengeløv, H., and Borregaard, N., Isolation and primary structure of NGAL, a novel protein associated with human neutrophil gelatinase, *J. Biol. Chem.* 268, 10425–10432, 1993.

117. Winberg, J.-O., Kolset, S.O., Berg, E., and Uhlin-Hansen, L., Macrophage secrete matrix metalloproteinase 9 covalently linked to the core protein of chondroitin sulphate proteoglycans, *J. Mol. Biol.* 304, 669–680, 2000.

118. Vandooren, J., Van den Steem, P.E., and Opdenakker, G., Biochemistry and molecular biology of gelatinase B or matrix metalloproteinase-9 (MMP-9): The next decade, *Crit. Rev. Biochem. Mol. Biol.* 48, 222–272, 2013.

119. Yu, Q. and Stamenkovic, I., Cell surface–localized matrix metalloproteinase-9 proteolytically activated TGF-β and promotes tumor invasion and angiogenesis, *Genes Dev.* 14, 163–176, 2000.

120. Chetty, C., Vanamala, S.K., Gondi, C.S., et al., MMP-9 induces CD44 cleavage and CD44 mediated cell migration in glioblastoma xenograft cells, *Cell Signal.* 24, 549–559, 2012.

121. Naor, D., CD44, in *Encyclopedia of Immunology*, Vol. 1, 2nd edn., eds. P.J. Delves and I.M. Raitt, pp. 488–491, Academic Press, San Diego, CA, 1998.

122. Schmidt, S. and Friedl, P., Interstitial cell migration: Integrin-dependent and alternative adhesion mechanisms, *Cell Tissue Res.* 339, 92, 2010.

123. Niyibizi, C., Chan, R., Vu, J.-J., and Eyre, D., A 93 kDa gelatinase (MMP-9) cleavage site in native type V collagen, *Biochem. Biophys. Res. Commun.* 202, 328–333, 1994.

124. Bigg, H.F., Rowan, A.D., Barker, M.D., and Cawston, T.E., Activity of matrix metalloproteinase 9 against native collagenase types I and III, *FEBS J.* 274, 1246–1255, 2007.

125. Christiansen, V.J., Jackson, K.W., Lee, K.N., and McKee, P.A., Effect of fibroblast activation protein and α_2-antiplasmin cleaving enzyme on collagen types I, III, and IV, *Arch. Biochem. Biophys.* 457, 177–186, 2007.
126. Minond, D., Lauer-Fields, J.L., Cudic, M., et al., The roles of substrate thermal stability and P_2 and $P_{1'}$ subsite identity on matrix metalloproteinase triple-helical peptidase activity and collagen specificity, *J. Biol. Chem.* 281, 38302–38313, 2006.
127. Schönbeck, U., Mach, F., and Libby, P., Generation of biologically active IL-1β by matrix metalloproteinases: A novel caspace-1-independent pathway of IL-1β processing, *J. Immunol.* 161, 3340–3346, 1998.
128. Yin, K.J., Cirrito, J.R., Yan, P., et al., Matrix metalloproteinases expressed by astrocytes mediate extracellular amyloid-β peptide catabolism, *J. Neurosci.* 26, 10939–10948, 2006.
129. Senior, R.M., Griffin, G.L., Fliszar, C.J., et al., Human 92- and 72-kilodalton type IV collagenases are elastases, *J. Biol. Chem.* 266, 7870–7875, 1991.
130. Opdenakker, G., Van den Steen, P.E., Dubois, B., et al., Gelatinase B functions as regulator and effector in leukocyte biology, *J. Leukocyte Biol.* 69, 851–859, 2001.
131. Patterson, B.C. and Sang, Q.A., Angiostatin-converting enzyme activities of human matrilysin (MMP-7) and gelatinase B/type IV collagenase (MMP-9), *J. Biol. Chem.* 272, 28823–28825, 1997.
132. Pozzi, A., LeVine, W.F., and Gardner, H.A., Low plasma levels of matrix metalloproteinase 9 permit increased tumor angiogenesis, *Oncogene* 21, 272–281, 2002.
133. Lium Z., Zhou, K, Shapiro, S.D., et al., The serpin α_1-proteinase inhibitor is a critical substrate for gelatinase B/MMP-9 *in vivo*, *Cell* 102, 647–655, 2000.
134. Muroski, M.E., Roycik, M.D., Newcomer, R.G., et al., Matrix metalloproteinase-9/gelatinase B is a putative therapeutic target of chronic obstructive pulmonary disease and multiple sclerosis, *Curr. Pharmaceut. Biotechnol.* 9, 34–46, 2008.
135. Janciauskiene, S., Zelvyte, I., Jansson, L., et al., Divergent effects of α_1-antitrypsin on neutrophil activation, *in vitro*, *Biochem. Biophys. Res. Commun.* 315, 288–296, 2004.
136. Han, Y.-P., Yan, C., and Garner, W.L., Proteolytic activation of matrix metalloproteinase-9 in skin wound healing is inhibited by α-1-antichymotrypsin, *J. Invest. Derm.* 128, 2334–2342, 2008.
137. Reiss, M.J., Han, Y.-P., and Garner, W.L., α1-Antichymotrypsin activity correlates with and may modulate matrix metalloproteinase-9 in human acute wounds, *Wound Rep. Reg.* 17, 418–426, 2009.
138. Zilm, P.S. and Bartold, P.M., Proteomic identification of proteinase inhibitors in the porcine enamel matrix derivative, EMD®, *J. Periodontol. Res.* 46, 111–117, 2011.
139. Fingleton, B., Matrix metallopeptidase-10/stromelysin 2, in *Handbook of Proteolytic Enzymes*, 3rd edn., eds. N.D. Rawlings and G. Salvesen, Chapter 159, pp. 774–778, Elsevier, Amsterdam, the Netherlands, 2013.
140. Sirum, K.L. and Brinckerhoff, C.E., Cloning of the gene for human stromelysin and stromelysin-2: Differential expression in rheumatoid synovial fibroblasts, *Biochemistry* 28, 8691–8698, 1989.
141. Bord, S., Horner, A., Hembry, R.M., and Compton, J.E., Stromelysin-1 (MMP-3) and stromelysin-2 (MMP-10) expression in developing human bone: Potential roles in skeletal development, *Bone* 23, 7–12, 1998.
142. Bodey, B., Bodey, B., Jr., Siegel, S.E., and Kaiser, H.E., Matrix metalloproteinases in neoplasm-induced extracellular matrix remodeling in breast carcinoma, *Anticancer Res.* 21, 2021–2028, 2001.
143. Burbridge, M.F., Cogé, F., Galizzi, J.P., et al., The role of the matrix metalloproteinases during *in vitro* vessel formation, *Angiogenesis* 5, 215–226, 2002.

144. Batra, J., Robinson, J., Soares, A.S., et al., Matrix metalloproteinase-10 (MMP-10) interaction with tissue inhibitors of metalloproteinases TIMP-1 and TIMP-2: Binding studies and crystal structure, *J. Biol. Chem.* 287, 15935–15946, 2012.
145. Batra, J., Soares, A.S., Mehner, C., and Radisky, E.S., Matrix metalloproteinase-10/TIMP-2 structure and analyses define conserved core interactions and diverse exosite interactions in MMP/TIMP complexes, *PLoS One* 8(9), e75836, 2013.
146. Rio, M.-C., Matrix metalloproteinase-11/stromelysin 3, in *Handbook of Proteolytic Enzymes*, 3rd edn., eds. N.D. Rawlings and G. Salvesen, Chapter 160, pp. 779–786, Elsevier, Amsterdam, the Netherlands, 2013.
147. Pei, D., Majmudar, G., and Weiss, S.J., Hydrolytic inactivation of a breast carcinoma cell-derived serpin by serpin stromelysin-3, *J. Biol. Chem.* 269, 25849–25855, 1994.
148. Noël, A., Santavicca, M., Stoll, I., et al., Identification of structural determinants controlling human and mouse stromelysin-3 proteolytic activities, *J. Biol. Chem.* 270, 22866–22872, 1995.
149. Pan, W., Arnone, M., Kendall, M., et al., Identification of peptide substrates for human MMP-11 (stromelysin-3) using phage display, *J. Biol. Chem.* 278, 27820–27827, 2003.
150. Mañes, S., Mira, E., del Mar Barbarcid, M., et al., Identification of insulin-like growth factor-binding protein-1 as a potential physiological substrate for human stromelysin-3, *J. Biol. Chem.* 272, 27506–25712, 1997.
151. Meyer, B.S. and Rademann, J., Extra- and intracellular imaging of human matrix metalloprotease 11 (*h*MMP-11) with a cell-penetrating FRET substrate, *J. Biol. Chem.* 287, 37857–37867, 2012.
152. Tan, J., Buache, E., Alpy, F., et al., Stromal matrix metalloproteinase-11 is involved in the mammary gland postnatal development, *Oncogene*, 33, 4050–4059, 2014.
153. Okada, A., Saez, S., Misumi, Y., et al., Rat stromelysin 3: cDNA cloning from healing skin wound, activation by furin and expression in rat tissues, *Gene* 185, 187–193, 1997.
154. Asch, P.H., Basset, P., Roos, M., et al., Expression of stromelysin 3 in keratoacanthoma and squamous cell carcinoma, *Am. J. Dermatopathol.* 21, 146–150, 1999.
155. Pei, D. and Weiss, S.J., Furin-dependent intracellular activation of the human stromelysin-3 zymogen, *Nature* 375, 244–247, 1995.
156. Kaynar, M. and Shapiro, S.D., Matrix metallopeptidase-12/macrophage elastase, in *Handbook of Proteolytic Enzymes*, 3rd edn., eds. N.D. Rawlings and G. Salvesen, Chapter 163, pp. 800–864, Elsevier, Amsterdam, the Netherlands, 2013.
157. Banda, M.J. and Werb, Z., Mouse macrophage elastase. Purification and characterization as a metalloproteinase, *Biochem. J.* 193, 589–605, 1981.
158. Shapiro, S.D., Kobayashi, D.K., and Ley, T.J., Cloning and characterization of a unique elastolytic metalloproteinase produced by human alveolar macrophages, *J. Biol. Chem.* 268, 23824–23829, 1993.
159. Bhaskaran, R., Palmier, M.O., Lauer-Fields, J.L., et al., MMP-12 catalytic domain recognizes triple helical peptide models of collagen V with exosites and high activity, *J. Biol. Chem.* 283, 21779–21783, 2008.
160. Banda, M.J., Rice, A.G., Griffin, G.L., and Senior, R.M., α_1-Proteinase inhibitor is a neutrophil chemoattractant after proteolytic inactivation by macrophage elastase, *J. Biol. Chem.* 263, 4481–4484, 1988.
161. Cornelius, L.A., Nehring, L.C., Harding, E., et al., Matrix metalloproteinases generate angiostatin: Effects on neovascularization, *J. Immunol.* 161, 6845–6852, 1998.
162. Gronski, T.J., Jr., Martin, R.L., Kobayashi, D.K., et al., Hydrolysis of a broad spectrum of extracellular matrix proteins by human macrophage elastase, *J. Biol. Chem.* 272, 12189–12194, 1997.
163. Banda, M.J., Clark, E.J., Sinha, S., and Travis, J., Interaction of mouse macrophage elastase with native and oxidized human α_1-proteinase inhibitor, *J. Clin. Invest.* 79, 1314–1317, 1987.

164. Le Quément, C., Guénon, I., Gillon, J.Y., et al., MMP-12 induces IL-8/CSCL8 secretion through EGFR and ERK1/2 activation in epithelial cells, *Am. J. Physiol. Lung Cell Mol. Physiol.* 294, L1076–L1084, 2008.

165. Henriet, P. and Eeckhout, Y., Matrix metallopeptidase-13 (collagenase 3), in *Handbook of Proteolytic Enzymes*, 3rd edn., eds. N.D. Rawlings and G. Salvesen, Chapter 154, pp. 734–744, Academic Press/Elsevier, Amsterdam, the Netherlands, 2013.

166. Borden, P., Solymar, D., Sucharczuk, A., et al., Cytokine control of interstitial collagenase and collagenase-3 gene expression in human chondrocytes, *J. Biol. Chem.* 271, 23577–23581, 1996.

167. Haston, J.L., FitzGerald, O., Kane, D., and Smith, K.D., The influence of α_1-acid glycoprotein on collagenase-3 activity in early rheumatoid arthritis, *Biomed. Chromatog.* 17, 361–364, 2003.

168. Barksby, H.E., Milner, J.M., Patterson, A.M., et al., Matrix metalloproteinase 10 promotion of collagenolysis via procollagenase activation: Implications for cartilage degradation in arthritis, *Arthritis Rheum.* 54, 3244–3253, 2006.

169. Austin, K.M., Covic, L., and Kuliopulos, A., Matrix metalloproteases and PAR1 activation, *Blood* 121, 431–439, 2013.

170. Huang, C.-Y., Lin, H.-J., Chen, H.-S., et al., Thrombin promotes matrix metalloproteinase-13 expression through the PKCδ/c-Src/EGFR/P13K/Akt/AP-1 signaling pathway in human chondrocytes, *Mediators Inflamm.* 2013, 326041, 2013.

171. Beekman, B., Drijfhout, J.W., Ronday, H.K., and TeKoppele, J.M., Fluorogenic MMP activity assay for plasma including MMPs complexed to α_2-macroglobulin, *Ann. N.Y. Acad. Sci.* 878, 150–158, 1999.

172. Itoh, Y. and Selki, M., Membrane-type matrix metalloproteinase 1, in *Handbook of Proteolytic Enzymes*, 3rd edn., eds. N.D. Rawlings and G. Salvesen, Chapter 164, pp. 804–814, Elsevier, Amsterdam, the Netherlands, 2013.

173. Sato, H., Takino, T., Okada, Y., et al., A matrix metalloproteinase expressed on the surface of invasive tumor cells, *Nature* 370, 61–65, 1994.

174. Golubkov, V.S., Chekanov, A.V., Shiryaev, S.A., et al., Proteolysis of the membrane type-1 matrix metalloproteinase prodomain: Implications for a two-step proteolytic processing and activation, *J. Biol. Chem.* 282, 36283–36291, 2007.

175. Roghi, C., Jones, L., Gratian, M., et al., Golgi reassembly stacking protein 55 interacts with membrane-type (MT) 1-matrix metalloproteinase (MMP) and furin and plays a role in the activation of the MT1-MMP zymogen, *FEBS J.* 277, 3158–3175, 2010.

176. Holmbeck, K., Bianco, P., Yamada, S., and Birkedal-Hanson, H., MT1-MMP, a tethered collagenase, *J. Cell Physiol.* 200, 11–19, 2004.

177. Sato, H. and Takino, T., Coordinate action of membrane-type matrix metalloproteinase-1 (MT1-MMP) and MMP-2 enhances pericellular proteolysis and invasion, *Cancer Sci.* 101, 843–847, 2010.

178. Ries, C., Egea, V., Karow, M., et al., MMP-2, MT1-MMP, and TIMP-2 are essential for the invasive capacity of human mesenchymal cells: Differential regulation by inflammatory cytokines, *Blood* 109, 4055–4063, 2007.

179. Lafleur, M.A., Tester, A.M., and Thompson, E.W., Selective involvement of TIMP-2 in the second activational cleavage of pro-MMP-2: Refinement of the pro-MMP-2 activation mechanism, *FEBS Lett.* 553, 457–463. 2003.

180. Hernandez-Barrantas, S., Toght, M., Bernardo, M.M., et al., Binding of active (57 kDa) membrane type 1-matrix metalloproteinase (MT1-MMP) to tissue inhibitor of metalloproteinase (TIMP)-2 regulates MT1-MPP processing and pro-MMP-2 activation, *J. Biol. Chem.* 275, 12080–12089, 2008.

181. Strongin, A.Y., Collier, I., Bannikov, G., et al., Mechanism of cell surface activation of 72-kDa type IV collagenase: Isolation of the activated form of the membrane metalloprotease, *J. Biol. Chem.* 270, 5331–5338, 1995.

182. Lambert, E., Dassé, E., Haye, B., and Petitfrère, E., TIMPs as multifacial proteins, *Crit. Rev. Oncology Hematol.* 49, 287–198, 2004.
183. Toole, B.P., Emmprin (CD147), a cell surface regulator of matrix metalloproteinase production and function, *Curr. Top. Dev. Biol.* 54, 371–389, 2003.
184. Schmidt, R., Redecke, V., Breitfeld, Y., et al., EMMPRIN (CD 147) is a central activator of extracellular matrix degradation by *Chlamydia pneumoniae*–infected monocytes: Implications for plaque rupture, *Thromb. Haemost.* 95, 151–158, 2006.
185. Huet, E., Gabison, E.E., Mourah, S., and Menashi, S., Role of emmprin/CD147 in tissue remodeling, *Connect. Tissue Res.* 49, 175–179, 2008.
186. Egawa, N., Koshikawa, N., Tomari, T., et al., Membrane type 1 matrix metalloproteinase (MT1-MMP) cleaves and releases a 22-kDa extracellular matrix metalloproteinase inducer (EMMPRIN) from tumor cells, *J. Biol. Chem.* 281, 37576–37586, 2006.
187. Polette, M., Nawrocki-Raby, B., Gilles, C., et al., Tumour invasion and matrix metalloproteinases, *Crit. Rev. Oncol. Hematol.* 49, 179–186, 2004.
188. Remacle, A.G., Shiryaev, S.A., Golubkov, V.S., et al., Non-destructive and selective imaging of the functionally active, pro-invasive membrane type-1 matrix metalloproteinase (MT1-MMP) enzyme in cancer cells, *J. Biol. Chem.* 288, 20568–20580, 2013.
189. Miller, M.C., Manning, H.B., Jain, A., et al., Membrane type 1 matrix metalloproteinase is a crucial promoter of synovial invasion in human rheumatoid arthritis, *Arthritis Rheum.* 60, 686–697, 2009.
190. Cork, S.M., Kaur, B., Devi, N.S., et al., A proprotein convertase (MMP-14) proteolytic cascade releases a novel 40 kDa vasculostatin from tumor suppressor BAI1, *Oncogene* 31, 5144–5152, 2012.
191. Yama, I. and Seikli, M., Membrane-type-2 metalloproteinase, in *Handbook of Proteolytic Enzymes*, 3rd edn., eds. N.D., Rawlings and G. Salvesen, Chapter 165, pp. 815–817, Elsevier, Amsterdam, the Netherlands, 2013.
192. Will, H. and Hinzmann, B., cDNA sequence and mRNA tissue distribution of a novel human matrix metalloproteinase with a potential transmembrane segment, *Eur. J. Biochem.* 231, 602–608, 1995.
193. Morrison, C.J., Butler, G.S., Biggs, H.F., et al., Cellular activation of MMP-2 (gelatinase A) by MT2-MMP occurs via a TIMP-2 independent pathway, *J. Biol. Chem.* 276, 47402–47410, 2001.
194. Morrison, C.J. and Overall, C.M., TIMP independence of matrix metalloproteinase (MMP)-2 activation by membrane type 2 (MT2)-MMP is determined by contributions of both the MT2-MMP catalytic and hemopexin C domains, *J. Biol. Chem.* 281, 26528–26539, 2006.
195. Kontinnen, Y.T., Ainola, M., Valleala, H., et al., Analysis of 16 different matrix metalloproteinases (MMP-1 to MMP-20) in the synovial membrane: Different profiles in trauma and rheumatoid arthritis, *Ann. Rheum. Dis.* 58, 691–697, 1999.
196. Mohammaed, F.F., Pennington, C.J., Kassiri, Z., et al., Metalloproteinase inhibitor TIMP-1 affects hepatocyte cell cycle via HGF activation in murine liver regeneration, *Hepatology* 41, 857–867, 2005.
197. Bodnar, M., Szylberg, L., Kazmierczak, W., and Marszalek, A., Differentiated expression of membrane type metalloproteinases (MMP-14, MMP-15) and pro-MMP2 in laryngeal squamous cell carcinoma: A novel mechanism, *J. Oral Pathol. Med.* 42, 267–274, 2013.
198. Fu, H.-L. and Friedman, R., Membrane-type 3-matrix metalloproteinase (MMP-16), in *Handbook of Proteolytic Enzymes*, 3rd edn., eds. N.D. Rawlings and G. Salvesen, Chapter 166, pp. 817–822, Elsevier, Amsterdam, the Netherlands, 2013.
199. Shofuda, K.-i., Yasumistui, H., Nishihashi, A., et al., Expression of three membrane-type matrix metalloproteinases (MT-MMPs) in rat vascular smooth muscle cells and characterization of MT3-MMPs with and without transmembrane domain, *J. Biol. Chem.* 272, 9749–9754, 1997.

200. Zucker, S., Pei, D., Cao, J., and Lopez-Otin, C, Membrane type-matrix metalloproteinase, *Curr. Top. Dev. Biol.* 54, 1–74, 2003.
201. Zhao, H., Bernardo, M.M., Osenkowski, P., et al., Differential inhibition of membrane type 3 (MT3)-matrix metalloproteinase (MMP) and MT1-MMP by tissue inhibitor of metalloproteinase (TIMP)-2 and TIMP-3 regulates pro-MMP-2 activation, *J. Biol. Chem.* 279, 8592–8601, 2004.
202. Matsumoto, S., Katoh, M., Saito, S., et al., Identification of soluble type of membrane-type matrix metalloproteinase-3 formed by alternative spliced mRNA, *Biochim. Biophys. Acta* 1354, 159–170, 1997.
203. Shimada, T., Nakamura, H., Ohuchi, E., et al., Characterization of a truncated recombinant form of human membrane type 3 matrix metalloproteinase, *Eur. J. Biochem.* 262, 907–914, 1999.
204. Itoh, Y. and Seikli, M., Membrane-type matrix metalloproteinase 4, in *Handbook of Proteolytic Enzymes*, 3rd edn., eds. N.D. Rawlings and G. Salvesen, Chapter 167, pp. 823–826, Elsevier, Amsterdam, the Netherlands, 2013.
205. Puente, X.S., Pendás, A.M., Llano, E., et al., Molecular cloning of a novel membrane-type matrix metalloproteinase from a human breast carcinoma, *Cancer Res.* 56, 944–949, 1996.
206. Kajita, M., Kinoh, H., Ito, N., et al., Human membrane type-4 matrix metalloproteinase (MT4-MMP) is encoded by a novel major transcript: Isolation of complementary DNA clones for human and mouse *mt4-mmp* transcripts, *FEBS J.* 457, 353–356, 1999.
207. Itoh, Y., Kajita, M., Kinoh, H., et al., Membrane type 4 matrix metalloproteinase (MT4-MMP, MMP-17) is a glycosylphosphatidylinositol-anchored proteinase, *J. Biol. Chem.* 274, 34260–34266, 1999.
208. Paulick, M.G., Forstner, M.B., Groves, J.T., and Bertozzi, C.R., A chemical approach to unraveling the biological function of the glycosylphosphatidylinositol anchor, *Proc. Natl. Acad. Sci. USA* 104, 20332–20337, 2007.
209. Wang, Y., Johnson, A.R., Ye, Q.-Z., et al., Catalytic activities and substrate specificity of the human membrane type 4 matrix metalloproteinase catalytic domain, *J. Biol. Chem.* 274, 33043–33049, 1999.
210. Kolkenbrock, H., Essers, L., Ulrich, N., and Will, H., Biochemical characterization of the catalytic domain of membrane-type 4 matrix metalloproteinase, *Biol. Chem.* 380, 1103–1108, 1999.
211. English, W.R., Puente, X.S., Freije, J.M.P., et al., Membrane type 4 matrix metalloproteinase (MMP17) has tumor necrosis factor-α convertase activity but does not activate pro-MMP2, *J. Biol. Chem.* 275, 14046–14055, 2000.
212. Gao, G., Plaas, A., Thompson, V.P., et al., ADAMTS4 (aggrecanase-I) activation on the cell surface involves C-terminal cleavage by glycosylphosphatidylinositol-anchored membrane type-4 matrix metalloproteinase and binding of the activated proteinase to chondroitin sulfate and heparan sulfate on syndecan-1, *J. Biol. Chem.* 279, 10042–10051, 2004.
213. Sang, Q.A. and Shi, Y.-B., Matrix metallopeptidase-18 (collagenase 4), in *Handbook of Proteolytic Enzymes*, 3rd edn., eds. N.D. Rawlings and G. Salvesen, Chapter 155, pp. 744–747, Elsevier, Amsterdam, the Netherlands, 2013.
214. Cossins, J., Dudgeon, T.J., Catlin, G., et al., Identification of MMP-18, a putative novel human matrix metalloproteinase, *Biochem. Biophys. Res. Commun.* 228, 494–498, 1996.
215. Stolow, M.A., Bauzon, D.D., Li, J., et al., Identification and characterization of a novel collagenase in *Xenopus laevis*: Possible roles during frog development, *Molec. Biol. Cell* 7, 1471–1483, 1996.
216. Grant, G.M., Giambernardi, T.A., Grant, A.M., and Klebe, R.J., Overview of expression of matrix metalloproteinases (MMP-17, MMP-18, and MMP-20) in cultured human cells, *Matrix Biol.* 18, 145–148, 1999.

217. Foos, M.J., Hickox, J.R., Mansour, P.G., et al., Expression of matrix metalloproteases and tissue inhibitor of metalloprotease genes in human anterior cruciate ligament, *J. Orthopaedic Res.* 19, 642–649, 2001.

218. Tomlinson, M.L., Garcia-Morales, C., Abu-Elmagd, M., and Wheeler, G.N., Three main metalloproteinases are required *in vivo* for macrophage migration during embryonic development, *Mech. Dev.* 125, 1059–1070, 2008.

219. Fanjul-Fernández, M. and López-Otín, C., Matrix metalloproteinase 19, in *Handbook of Proteolytic Enzymes*, 3rd edn., eds. N.D. Rawlings and G. Salvesen, Chapter 170, pp. 830–835, Elsevier, Amsterdam, the Netherlands, 2013.

220. Pendás, A.M., Knäuper, V., Puente, X.S., et al., Identification and characterization of a novel human matrix metalloproteinase with unique structural characteristics, chromosomal location, and tissue distribution, *J. Biol. Chem.* 272, 4281–4286, 1997.

221. Kolb, C., Mauch, S., Peter, H.-H., et al., The matrix metalloproteinase RASI-1 is expressed in synovial blood vessels of a rheumatoid arthritis patient, *Immunol. Lett.* 57, 83–88, 1997.

222. Impola, U., Toriseva, M., Suomela, S., et al., Matrix metalloproteinase-19 is expressed by proliferating epithelium but disappears with neoplastic dedifferentiation, *Int. J. Cancer* 103, 709–716, 2003.

223. Sadowski, T., Dietrich, S., Müller, M., et al., Matrix metalloproteinase-19 expression normal and diseased skin: Dysregulation by epidermal proliferation, *J. Invest. Derm.* 121, 989–996, 2003.

224. Sadowski, T., Dietrich, S., Koschinsky, F., and Sedlacek, R., Matrix metalloproteinase 19 regulates insulin-like growth factor-mediated proliferation, migration, and adhesion in human keratinocytes through proteolysis of insulin-like growth factor binding protein-3, *Mol. Biol. Cell.* 14, 4569–4580, 2003.

225. Evans, C.H., The role of proteases in cartilage destruction, *Agents Actions Suppl.* 32, 137–152, 1991.

226. Stockman, B.J., Waldon, D.J., Gates, J.A., et al., Solution structures of stromelysin complexed to thiadiazole inhibitors, *Protein Sci.* 7, 2291–2286, 1998.

227. Schache, M. and Baird, P.N., Assessment of the association of matrix metalloproteinases with myopia, refractive error and ocular biometric measures in an Australian cohort, *PLoS One* 7(10), e47181, 2012.

228. Stracker, J.O., Hutton, M., Stewart, M., et al., Biochemical characterization of the catalytic domain of human matrix metalloproteinase 19, *J. Biol. Chem.* 275, 14809–14816, 2000.

229. Mysliwy, J., Dingley, A.J., Sedlacek, R., and Grötzinger, J., Structural characterization and binding properties of the hemopexin-like domain of matrix metalloproteinase-19, *Protein Expr. Purif.* 46, 406–413, 2006.

230. Stracke, J.O., Fosang, A.J., Last, K., et al., Matrix metalloproteinases 19 and 20 cleave aggrecan and cartilage oligomeric matrix protein (COMP), *FEBS Lett.* 478, 53–56, 2000.

231. Müller, M., Beck, I.M., Gadesmann, J., et al., MMP19 is upregulated during melanoma progression and increases invasion of melanoma cells, *Mod. Pathol.* 23, 511–521, 2010.

232. Bartlett, J.D., Matrix metalloproteinase-20/enamelysin, in *Handbook of Proteolytic Enzymes*, 3rd edn., eds. N.D. Rawlings and G. Salvesen, Chapter 171, pp. 835–840, Elsevier, Amsterdam, the Netherlands, 2013.

233. Yang, M., Murray, M.T., and Kurkinen, M., A novel matrix metalloproteinase gene (XMMP) encoding vitronectin-like motifs is transiently expressed in *Xenopus laevis* embryo development, *J. Biol. Chem.* 272, 13527–13533, 1997.

234. Llano, E., Pendás, A.M., Knäuper, V., et al., identification and structural and functional characterization of human enamelysin (MMP-20), *Biochemistry* 36, 15101–15108, 1997.

235. Ryu, O.H., Fincham, A.G., Hu, C.-C., et al., Characterization of recombinant pig enamelysin activity and cleavage of recombinant pig and mouse amelogenins, *J. Dent. Res.* 78, 743–750, 1999.
236. Ryu, O.H., Hu, J.C.C., Yamakoshi, Y., et al., Porcine kallikrein-4 activation, glycosylation, activity and expression in prokaryotic and eukaryotic hosts, *Eur. J. Oral Sci.* 110, 358–365, 2002.
237. Yamakoshi, Y., Simmer, J.P., Bartlett, J.D., et al., MMP20 and KLK4 activation and inactivation *in vitro, Arch. Oral. Biol.* 58, 1569–1577, 2013.
238. Lu, Y., Papagerakis, P., Yamakoshi, Y., et al., Functions of KLK4 and MMP-20 in dental enamel formation, *Biol. Chem.* 389, 695–700, 2008.
239. Väänänen, A., Srinivas, R., Parikka, M., et al., Expression and regulation of MMP-20 in human tongue carcinoma cells, *J. Dent. Res.* 80, 1884–1889, 2001.
240. Liu, Y., Li, Y., Liu, Z., et al., Prognostic significance of matrix metalloproteinase-20 overexpression in laryngeal squamous cell carcinoma, *Acta Otolaryngol.* 131, 769–773, 2011.
241. Yang, M. and Kurkinen, M., Matrix metalloproteinase 21, in *Handbook of Proteolytic Enzymes*, 3rd edn., eds. N.D. Rawlings and G. Salvesen, Chapter 172, pp. 840–841, Elsevier, Amsterdam, the Netherlands, 2013.
242. Yang, M., Murray, M.T., and Kurkinen, M., A novel matrix metalloproteinase gene (XMMP) encoding vitronectin-like motifs is transiently expressed in *Xenopus laevis* early embryo development, *J. Biol. Chem.* 272, 13527–13533, 1997.
243. Dixon, K.H., Cowell, I.G., Xia, C.L., et al., Control of expression of the human glutathione S-transferase pi gene differs from its rat orthologue, *Biochem. Biophys. Res. Commun.* 163, 815–822, 1989.
244. Ahokas, K., Lohi, J., Lohi, H., et al., Matrix metalloproteinase-21, the human orthologue for XMMP, is expressed during fetal development and in cancer, *Gene* 301, 31–41, 2002.
245. Skoog, T., Ahokas, K., Oramark, C., et al., MMP-21 is expressed by macrophages and fibroblasts *in vivo* and in culture, *Exp. Dermatol.* 15, 775–783, 2006.
246. Pu, Y., Wang, L., Wu, H., et al., High MMP-21 expression in metastatic lymph nodes predicts unfavorable overall survival for oral squamous cell carcinoma patients with lymphatic metastasis, *Oncol. Rep.* 31, 2644–2650, 2014.
247. Yang, M. and Kurkinen, M., Chicken matrix metalloproteinase 22, in *Handbook of Proteolytic Enzymes*, 3rd edn., eds. N.D. Rawlings and G. Salvesen, Chapter 173, pp. 842–843, Elsevier, Amsterdam, the Netherlands, 2013.
248. Yang, M. and Kurkinen, M., Cloning and characterization of a novel matrix metalloproteinase (MMP), CMMP from chicken embryo fibroblasts, *J. Biol. Chem.* 273, 17893–17900, 1998.
249. Velasco, G., Pendás, A.M., Fueyo, A., et al., Cloning and characterization of human MMP-23, a new matrix metalloproteinase predominantly expressed in reproductive tissues and lacking conserved domains in other family members, *J. Biol. Chem.* 274, 4570–4576, 1999.
250. Guruajen, R., Grenet, J., Lahti, J.M., and Kidd, V.J., Isolation and characterization of two novel metalloproteinase genes linked to the *Cdc2L* locus on human chromosome 1p36.3, *Genomics* 52, 101–106, 1998.
251. Pei, D., CA-MMP: A matrix metalloproteinase with a novel cysteine array, but without the classic cysteine switch, *FEBS Lett.* 457, 262–270, 1999.
252. Pei, D., Kang, T., and Qi, H., Cysteine array matrix metalloproteinase (CA-MMP)/MMP-23 is a type II transmembrane matrix metalloproteinase regulated by a single cleavage for both secretion and activation, *J. Biol. Chem.* 275, 33988–33997, 2000.
253. Ohnishi, J., Ohnishi, E., Jin, M., et al., Cloning and characterization of a rat ortholog of MMP-23 (matrix metalloproteinase-23), a unique type of membrane-anchored matrix metalloproteinase and conditioned switching of its expression during the ovarian follicular development, *Mol. Endocrinol.* 15, 747–764, 2001.

254. Dixon, K.H., Cowell, I.G., Xia, C.L., et al., Control of expression of the human glutathione S-transferase pi gene differs from its rat orthologue, *Biochem. Biophys. Res. Commun.* 163, 815–822, 1989.
255. Sesardic, D., Boobis, A.R., Murrya, B.P., et al., Furafylline is a potent and selective inhibitor of cytochrome P450IA2 in man, *Br. J. Clin. Pharmacol.* 29, 651–663, 1990.
256. Pei, D., Membrane-type matrix metalloproteinase-5, in *Handbook of Proteolytic Enzymes*, 3rd edn., eds. N.D. Rawlings and G. Salvesen, Chapter 169, pp. 826–828, Elsevier, Amsterdam, the Netherlands, 2013.
257. Liano, E., Pendás, A.M., Freije, J.P., et al., Identification and characterization of human MT5-MMP, a new membrane-bound activator of progelatinase A overexpressed in brain tumors, *Cancer Res.* 59, 2570–2576, 1999.
258. Pei, D., Identification and characterization of the fifth membrane-type matrix metalloproteinase MT5-MMP, *J. Biol. Chem.* 274, 8925–8932, 1999.
259. Wang, X., Yi, J., Lei, J., and Pei, D., Expression, purification and characterization of recombinant mouse MT5-MMP protein products, *FEBS Lett.* 462, 261–266, 1999.
260. Wang, X. and Pei, D., Shedding of membrane type matrix metalloproteinase 5 by a furin-type convertase, *J. Biol. Chem.* 276, 35953–35960, 2001.
261. Pei, D., Membrane-type matrix metalloproteinase-6, in *Handbook of Proteolytic Enzymes*, 3rd edn., eds. N.D. Rawlings and G. Salvesen, Chapter 170, pp. 828–830, Elsevier, Amsterdam, the Netherlands, 2013.
262. Wenk, K. and Blobel, H., Investigations on staphylococcal "leucocidins" of varying origins, *Zentralbl. Bakteriol. Orig.* 213, 479–487, 1972.
263. Pei, D., Leukolysin/MMP-25/MT6-MMP: A novel matrix metalloproteinase specifically expressed in the leukocyte linage, *Cell Res. Cell Res.* 9, 291–303, 1999.
264. Velasco, G., Cal, S., Merios-Suarez, A., et al., Human MT6-matrix metalloproteinase: Identification, progelatinase A activation, and expression in brain tumors, *Cancer Res.* 60, 877–882, 2000.
265. Nie, J. and Pei, D., Direct activation of pro-matrix metalloproteinase-2 by leukolysin/membrane-type 6 matrix metalloproteinase/matrix metalloproteinase 25 at the Asn[109]–Tyr bond, *Cancer Res.* 63, 6758–6762, 2003.
266. Nuti, E., Casalini, F., Santamaria, S., et al., Synthesis and biological evaluation in U87MG glioma cells of (ethynylthiophene)sulfonamido-based hydroxamates as matrix metalloproteinase inhibitors, *Eur. J. Med. Chem.* 46, 2617–2629, 2011.
267. Sun, Q., Weber, C.R., Sohail, A., et al., MMP25 (MT6-MMP) is highly expressed in human colon cancer, promotes tumor growth, and exhibits unique biochemical properties, *J. Biol. Chem.* 282, 21998–22010, 2007.
268. Kojima, S.-I., Itoh, Y., Matsumoto, S.-I., et al., Membrane-type 6 matrix metalloproteinase (MT6-MMP, MMP-25) is the second glycosyl-phosphatidyl-inositol (GPI) anchored MMP, *FEBS Lett.* 480, 142–146, 2000.
269. Zhao, H., Sohail, A., Sun, Q., et al., Identification and role of the homodimerization interface of the glycosylphosphatidylinositol-anchored membrane type 6 matrix metalloproteinase (MMP 25), *J. Biol. Chem.* 283, 35023–35032, 2008.
270. Nie, J. and Pei, D., Rapid inactivation of α_1-proteinase inhibitor by neutrophil specific leukolysin/membrane-type matrix, *Exp. Cell Res.* 296, 145–150, 2004.
271. English, W.R., Velasco, G., Stracke, J.O., et al., Catalytic activities of membrane-type 6 matrix metalloproteinase (MMP25), *FEBS Lett.* 491, 137–142, 2001.
272. Shiryaev, S.A., Savinov, S.Y., Cieplak, P., et al., Major metalloproteinase proteolysis of the myelin basic protein isoforms is a source of immunogenic peptides in autoimmune multiple sclerosis, *PLoS One* 4(3), e4952, 2009.
273. Shiryaev, S.A., Remacle, A.C., Savinov, A.Y., et al., Inflammatory proprotein convertase-matrix metalloproteinase proteolytic pathway in antigen-presenting cells as a step to autoimmune multiple sclerosis, *J. Biol. Chem.* 284, 30615–30626, 2009.

274. Sang, Q.Y.A., Matrix metalloproteinase-26/matrilysin 2 (*Homo sapiens*), in *Handbook of Proteolytic Enzymes*, 3rd edn., eds. N.D. Rawlings and G. Salvesen, Chapter 162, pp. 795–800, Elsevier, Amsterdam, the Netherlands, 2013.

275. Park, H.I., Ni, J., Gerkema, F.E., et al., Identification and characterization of human endometase (matrix metalloproetinase-26) from endometrial tumor, *J. Biol. Chem.* 275, 20540–20544, 2000.

276. Benoit de Coignac, A., Elson, G., Delneste, Y., et al., Cloning of MMP-26: A novel matrilysin-like proteinase, *Eur. J. Biochem.* 267, 3323–3329, 2000.

277. Marcenko, G.H., Ratnikov, B.I., Rozanov, D.V., et al., Characterization of matrix metalloproteinase-26, a novel metalloproteinase widely expressed in cancer cells of epithelial origin, *Biochem. J.* 356, 705–718, 2001.

278. Marchenko, N.D., Marchenko, G.N., and Strongin, A.Y., Unconventional activation mechanisms of MMP-26, a human matrix metalloproteinase with a unique PHCGXXD cysteine switch motif, *J. Biol. Chem.* 277, 18967–18972, 2002.

279. Park, H.L., Turk, B.E., Gerkema, F.E., et al., Peptide substrate specificities and protein cleavage sites of human endometase/matrilysin-2/matrix metalloproteinase-26, *J. Biol. Chem.* 277, 35168–35175, 2002.

280. Schechter, I. and Berger, A., On the size of the active site in proteases: I. Papain, *Biochem. Biophys. Res. Commun.* 27, 157–162, 1967.

281. Nuttad, R.K., Sampieri, C.L., Pennington, C.J., et al., Expression analysis of the entire MMP and TIMP gene families during mouse tissue development, *FEBS Lett.* 563, 129–134, 2004.

282. Bernal, F., Hartung, H.-P., and Kieseier, B.C., Tissue mRNA expression in rat of newly described matrix metalloproteinases, *Biol. Res.* 38, 267–271, 2005.

283. Bar-Or, A., Nuttall, R.K., Duddy, M., et al., Analyses of all matrix metalloproteinase members in leukocytes emphasize monocytes as major inflammatory mediators in multiple sclerosis, *Brain* 126, 2738–2749, 2003.

284. Cominelli, A., Halbout, M., N'Kuli, F., et al., A unique C-terminal domain allows retention of matrix metalloproteinase-27 in the endoplasmic reticulum, *Traffic* 15, 401–417, 2014.

285. Lohi, J., Parks, W.C., and Manicone, M., Matrix metalloproteinase-28/epilysin, in *Handbook of Proteolytic Enzymes*, 3rd edn., eds. N.D. Rawlings and G. Salvesen, Chapter 175, pp. 845–850, Elsevier, Amsterdam, the Netherlands, 2013.

286. Lohi, J., C.L., Wilson, J.D., and Parks, W.C., Epilysin, a novel human matrix metalloproteinase (MMP-28) expressed in testes and keratinocytes and in response to injury, *J. Biol. Chem.* 276, 10134–10144, 2001.

287. Saarialho, U., Kekelä., E., Jahkola, T., et al., Epilysin (MMP-28) expression is associated with cell proliferation during epithelial repair, *J. Invest. Dermatol.* 139, 14–21, 2002.

288. Reno, F., Sabbatini, M., Stella, M.D., et al., Effect of *in vitro* mechanical compression on epilysin (matrix metalloproteinase-28) expression in hypertrophic scars, *Wound Rep. Reg.* 13, 255–261, 2005.

289. Illman, S.A., Lohi, J., and Keski-Oja, J., Epilysin (MMP-28): Structure, expression and potential functions, *Exp. Dermatol.* 17, 897–907, 2008.

290. Manicone, A.M., Birkland, T.P., Lin, M., et al., Epilysin (MMP-28) restrains early macrophage recruitment in *Pseudomonas aeruginosa* pneumonia, *J. Immunol.* 182, 3866–3876, 2009.

291. Rodgers, U.R., Kevorkian, L., Surridge, A.K., et al., Expression and function of matrix metalloproteinase (MMP)-28, *Matrix Biol.* 28, 263–272, 2009.

292. Marchenko, G.N. and Strongin, A.Y., MMP-28, a new human matrix metalloproteinase with an unusual cysteine-switch sequence is widely expressed in tumors, *Gene* 265, 87–93, 2001.

293. Lin, M.H., Liu, S.Y., Su, H.J., and Liu, Y.C., Functional role of matrix metalloproteinase-28 in the oral squamous cell carcinoma, *Oral Oncol.* 42, 907–913, 2006.

8 Coagulation Factors in the Interstitial Space

8.1 COAGULATION FACTORS AND THEIR REGULATION IN INTERSTITIAL SPACE

The great majority of research on blood coagulation is focused on events occurring within the vascular space involved in thrombosis and hemostasis. Comparatively little work is directed toward the interaction of the various components of coagulation present in the interstitial space. It is acknowledged that perivascular components, such as tissue factor, fall into a gray area in having a role in vascular hemostasis and in the interstitial space. In the past two decades, there has been an increased interest in the possible role of coagulation proteins in interstitial fibrosis and in the role of thrombin in the brain and other organs mediated through action on protease-activated receptors.[1] The following discussion will show that, with the exception of blood platelets, the various components of coagulation are present in the interstitial space.

Conventional wisdom would suggest that the coagulation factors present in the interstitium are mostly derived from extravasation from the intravascular space and return to the vascular space via the lymphatic system. However, a closer examination of the literature shows that there is substantial local synthesis of coagulation factors contributing to protein content in the interstitial space. As discussed in Chapter 1 (Section 1.3), endothelial cells and epithelial cells exhibit polarity in secretion. Endothelial cells can secrete proteins from the apical or luminal surface into the circulation and from the basolateral or abluminal surface into the extracellular matrix (ECM)/interstitial space. Pillai and coworkers[2] studied *directional secretomes* in differentiated human bronchial epithelial cells in culture. They reported 69 proteins in apical secretion, 13 in basolateral secretion, and 25 showing both apical and basolateral secretion.

There are a few examples of the local tissue synthesis of blood coagulation factors and secretion into the interstitial space; the examples selected are large proteins that are thought to pass from the vascular space to the interstitium with difficulty.[3] In general, there is a relationship between protein size and rate of extravasation. However, that is based on a globular shape; asymmetric proteins such as fibrinogen, which has a relatively large diffusion coefficient and large axial ratio, behave as much larger proteins and therefore show a lower concentration than would be expected only from consideration of the molecular weight. Similar asymmetry is likely for von Willebrand factor (vWF), factor VIII, and factor V. Basolateral secretion of fibrinogen has been demonstrated in pulmonary epithelium.[4] The possibility of basolateral secretion of factor VIII has not been demonstrated in native endothelial cells but is suggested from the secretion of factor VIII in retroviral transduced gut epithelial cells,[5] as well as from the studies of Shovlin and coworkers on factor VIII expression in the pulmonary endothelium.[6] Factor V expression has been reported in mesangial cells within the glomerulus,[7] in association with fibrin deposition and increased ECM formation.[8] It is important to recognize that the polarity of secretion in endothelial cells is influenced by external stimuli.[9,10]

There is a cellular phase of blood coagulation in addition to the humoral phase. Platelets are critical for normal blood coagulation in the vascular space and are either absent or present at low concentration[11–13] in the interstitium. However, the requirement for blood platelets is not absolute and it has been observed that lymph clots without the addition of plalelets[12,13] but does not undergo clot retraction.[12] Other cellular elements that have been demonstrated to participate in coagulation, such as leukocytes and macrophages, have been shown to migrate into the interstitial space.[14,15] Platelets have also been shown to enter the interstitial space by diapedesis, but there is a change in morphology and perhaps function.[16]

8.2 COAGULATION FACTORS IN LYMPH AND INTERSTITIAL FLUID

Over the past 70 years, there have been several reports on the concentration of coagulation factors in lymph, synovial fluid, and interstitial fluid. Table 8.1 contains information on the concentration of the various coagulation factors in several extravascular fluids. It is acknowledged that the data presented were obtained by a number of laboratories over a relatively long time period using various assay systems. One of the authors (RLL) is of sufficient age to be familiar with (1) the several laboratories that reported these results and (2) the various assay systems and their relationship to current technology. As such, he is comfortable with the quality of the data.

Early work by Brinkhous and Walker[17] showed that the concentration of prothrombin in lymph depends on the specific lymph channel; the prothrombin concentration was 93% of normal plasma in the portal lymphatic, 47% in the thoracic lymphatic, and 8% in the femoral (peripheral) channel. As can be seen in Table 8.1, the lowest value (8% of normal clottable fibrinogen) for fibrinogen was obtained by Miller and coworkers[18] from peripheral afferent lymph. This value is consistent with the concentration of fibrinogen (5%) obtained for dog hind paw lymph.[19] Bell and coworkers[19,20] discuss the potential heterogeneity of lymph dependent on tissue source. However, they suggest that the dog hind paw would be similar to muscle or tendon. These investigators also note[19,20] that the interstitial space available for fibrinogen is less than that for albumin, reflecting the gel properties of hyaluronan and ECM components such as collagen.[20] The age of the subject also influences the distribution of plasma proteins.[21] An additional factor is the degradation of some proteins during extravasation, interstitial transport, and passage through the lymphatic system. Consider the results of Brinkhous and Walker,[17] where the concentration of prothrombin was 93% in the portal lymphatic and 7% in the femoral. The portal lymphatic is one of three hepatic lymphatics; 80% of hepatic lymph flow is through the portal lymphatic[22] and the liver is the primary site of prothrombin synthesis. Prothrombin is somewhat more sensitive to inactivation by proteolysis than other

TABLE 8.1

Coagulation Factors in the Interstitial Space, Lymph, and Synovial Fluid

Coagulation Factor	Lymph	Interstitial Fluid	Synovial Fluid
Fibrinogen	28%[a,1]		ND[c,e,l,2]
	5%[b,c,3]		
	25%[b,d,3]		
	22%[f,g,4]		
	51%[c,f,5]		
	38%[c,f,6]		
	42%[c,f,7]		
Prothrombin	26%[a,1]	35%[c,8]	21%[c,k,9]
	47%[b,c,3]		24%[c,l,2]
	50%[b,d,3]		22%[c,k,10]
	50%[f,g,4]		29%[c,l,10]
	48%[c,f,5]		7%[c,n,10]
	93%[c,i,5]		
	8%[c,j,5]		
	57%[c,f,7]		
Factor V	8%[a,1]	15%[c,8]	<1%[c,k,9]
	ND[b,c,e,3]		5%[c,k,2]
	22%[b,d,3]		
	18%[f,g,4]		
	27%[c,f,6]		
Factor VII	17%[a,1]	27%[c,8]	34%[c,l,2]
	29%[b,c,3]		
	5%[b,d,3]		
	43%[f,g,4]		
Factor VIII	8%[a,1]		<1%[c,k,9]
	4%[b,c,3]		56%[c,l,2]
	28%[f,g,4]		
	24.7%[c,f,6]		
Factor IX	13%[b,c,3]		10%[c,k,9]
	9%[b,d,3]		19%[c,k,10]
	23%[f,g,4]		44%[c,l,10]
	60%[c,f,6]		21%[c,n,10]
Factor X	24%[a,1]		49%[c,l,2]
	25%[b,c,3]		26%[c,k,10]
	28%[b,d,3]		28%[c,l,10]
	75%[f,g,4]		8%[c,n,10]
	8%[h,c,11]		
Factor XI	23%[a,1]		32%[c,k,9]
Factor XII	27%[b,c,3]		46%[c,l,2]
Factor XIII	33%[f,g,4]		26%[c,l,2]
Protein C	24%[b,d,3]		16%[c,l,2]

(Continued)

TABLE 8.1 (CONTINUED)
Coagulation Factors in the Interstitial Space, Lymph, and Synovial Fluid

Coagulation Factor	Lymph	Interstitial Fluid	Synovial Fluid
Protein S	11%[b,d,3]		
Protein Z			
Platelets			
Antithrombin	38%[a,1]		74%[d,k,9]
	66%[b,d,3]		51%[c,l,2]
	78%[f,c,4]		46%[c,k,10]
			45%[c,l,10]
			12%[c,m,10]
TFPI	40%[a,1]		
α_2-Macroglobulin			13%[d,k,9]
von Willebrand factor			<1%[d,k,9]

Note: Results are expressed as a percentage of plasma values. It is acknowledged that different assay systems are used, but this does not affect the quality of the data.

[a] Rabbit limb lymph.
[b] Human femoral lymph.
[c] Activity.
[d] Antigen.
[e] ND, not detected.
[f] Canine thoracic lymph.
[g] Activity samples were taken over a 24-hour period after cannulation of the thoracic duct. The results are expressed graphically. The information shown in Table 8.1 is an average of the several data points obtained during the 24-hour period.
[h] Human peripheral lymph (subcutaneous lymph channel in dorsum of the foot).
[i] Canine portal lymph.
[j] Canine femoral lymph.
[k] Human synovial fluid (chronic osteoarthritis).
[l] Human synovial fluid (rheumatoid arthritis).
[m] Normal (cadaver) synovial fluid.

REFERENCES FOR TABLE 8.1

1. Le, D.T., Borgs, P., Toneff, T.W., et al., Hemostatic factors in rabbit limb lymph: Relationship to mechanisms regulating extravascular coagulation, *Am. J. Physiol.* 274, H769–H776, 1998.
2. Carmassi, F., de Negri, F., Morale, M., et al., Fibrin degradation in the synovial fluid of rheumatoid arthritis patients: A model for extravascular fibrinolysis, *Sem. Thromb. Hemost.* 22, 489–496, 1996.

3. Miller, G.J., Howarth, D.J., Attfield, J.C., et al., Haemostatic factors in human peripheral afferent lymph, *Thromb. Haemost.* 83, 427–432, 2000.
4. Müller, N. and Danckworth, H.-P., Gerrinungs physiologische Befunde der Gewebsflüssigkeit: I. Mitteilung: Die Faktoren des Gerinnugs-Systems in der Ductus-throacicus-Lymphe, *Zeitschrift Lymphol.* 4, 11–17, 1980.
5. Brinkhous, K.M. and Walker, S.A., Prothrombin and fibrinogen in lymph, *Am. J. Physiol.* 132, 666–669, 1941.
6. Leandoer, L., Bergentz, S.E., and Nilsson, I.M., Coagulation factors and components of the fibrinolytic system in lymph and blood in dogs, *Thromb. Diath. Haemorrh.* 19, 129–135, 1968.
7. Fantl, P. and Nelson, J.E., Coagulation in lymph, *J. Physiol.* 122, 33–37, 1953.
8. Witte, S., Intra- und extravasle Verteilung von Gerinnungsproteinen Wechselwirkung mit Gefäszwand, *Behring Inst. Mitt.* 73, 13–28, 1983.
9. Chang, P., Aronson, D.L., Borenstein, D.G., and Kessler, C.M., Coagulant proteins and thrombin generation in synovial fluid: A model for extravascular coagulation, *Am. J. Hematol.* 50, 79–83, 1995.
10. Furmaniak-Kazmierczak, E., Cooke, T.D.V., Manuel, R., et al., Studies of thrombin-induced proteoglycan release in the degradation of human and bovine cartilage, *J. Clin. Invest.* 94, 472–480, 1994.
11. Roberts, H.R., Lechler, E., Webster, W.P., and Penick, G.D., Survival of transfused factor X in patients with Stuart disease, *Thromb. Diath. Haemorrh* 13, 305–313, 1965.

vitamin K–dependent clotting factors. The other coagulation factors with low concentrations in peripheral lymphatics are factor V and factor VIII, both of which are sensitive to inactivation by proteolysis. Witte[23] described the consumption of coagulation factors in the interstitial space. Miller and coworkers[18] reported a much higher value (26%) for fibrinogen antigen, which would be consistent with the proteolytic degradation of fibrinogen.[24] Furthermore, Bell and coworkers[19] observed that while the amount of fibrinogen in peripheral lymph was relatively low (5%), there were substantial amounts of albumin (23%) and immunoglobulin (17%), which are more resistant to proteolysis.

Witte[23] reported that coagulation factors were distributed into the interstitial space on the basis of molecular weight. Witte[23] used proteins labeled with fluorescein to study the physical process of extravasation, and evidence was obtained to show that fibrinogen, fibronectin, and peptides derived from a factor VIII digest had an affinity for the vascular wall. Witte[23] also measured coagulation factor activity in plasma and in skin blister fluid. Measurement of proteins in skin blisters is considered to be reliable assay for interstitial fluid.[25-27]

8.3 PROTHROMBIN

Prothrombin is present in lymph at concentrations adequate to support thrombin generation (Table 8.1) and the majority is likely derived from extravasation. Liver is the primary site of prothrombin biosynthesis, but there is considerable evidence to support the biosynthesis of prothrombin in at least one other tissue. Prothrombin synthesis has been reported in brain,[28,29] but it is thought that prothrombin in cerebrospinal fluid is derived from a vascular source.[5] Dihanich and coworkers[28] suggested that the expression of prothrombin mRNA in brain tissue supports a role for prothrombin (thrombin) in regulatory processes in the brain. Arai and coworkers[29] demonstrated the expression of prothrombin mRNA in brain cells, neuroblastoma cells, cultured human astrocytes, oligodendrocytes, and microglial cells. These investigators also showed that prothrombin and thrombin were present in neurofibrillary tangles and suggested that thrombin was involved in tau proteolysis. Weinstein and coworkers[30] observed a colocalization of prothrombin mRNA and PAR-1 mRNA in mesencephalic dopaminergic neurons. An increase in prothrombin mRNA after cerebral ischemia with constant expression of protease nexin-1 and PAR receptors has been reported.[31] It has been noted that high concentrations of thrombin increase neural damage, while low concentrations of thrombin prevent cell necrosis.[32] Other investigators have suggested that prothrombin[33] and thrombin[34] in the central nervous system can be derived from the circulation.

8.4 FIBRINOGEN

While there are substantial amounts of fibrinogen in the interstitial fluid and the lymph, there is little evidence of fibrin formation in the interstitium. Fibrin is deposited in the dermal interstitium in delayed-type hypersensitivity.[35] Fibrin formation, measured by the release of fibrinopeptide A, occurs in cutaneous allergic reactions, as studied with a skin chamber model.[36] While the skin chamber model appears to be used mostly for the study of neutrophil migration,[37] it has been used to obtain wound fluid for the study of matrix metalloproteinase (MMP) expression.[38] Wound fluid is derived from interstitial fluid,[39] and while components such as vasoactive peptides, which result in greater vascular permeability, may enhance extravasation, it may be a good model for studying interstitial fluid. There is also considerable evidence to support a role for fibrinogen in the ECM.[40] Simpson-Hadaris and Rybarczyk[40] suggested that a conformationally altered fibrinogen, not fibrin, was incorporated into the ECM of a developing tumor. Zammaron and coworkers[41] reported that the binding of fibrinogen to a surface exposes fibrin epitopes. This suggests that the incorporation of fibrinogen into the ECM is similar to the process of forming a fibrin clot. There is also evidence to support the local synthesis of fibrinogen by tumor cells.[40,42] Rybarczyk and coworkers[43] presented evidence for the presence of fibrinogen in the ECM secreted by fibroblasts and epithelial cells.

8.4.1 FIBRINOGEN AND HYALURONAN

Early work reported that acacia[44] or poly(ethylene) glycol[45] enhanced fibrin polymerization. Both were used to enhance the visual end point in the determination of thrombin concentration by a manual fibrinogen clotting assay. There is no evidence that there is specific binding of acacia, a complex polysaccharide, or poly(ethylene) glycol to fibrinogen. As with acacia, hyaluronan is a complex polysaccharide, while poly(ethylene) glycol is similar to polysaccharides in solution characteristics. While some early work suggested an interaction of hyaluronan and fibrin,[46,47] it was not until the work of Leboeuf and coworkers[48] that it became apparent that there is a relatively specific interaction between hyaluronan and fibrinogen. Leboeuf and coworkers[48] studied the binding to fibrinogen of hyaluronan in solution and in solid-phase binding. The binding is of relatively high affinity ($K_d \approx 4.5 \times 10^8$). However, these data were obtained from solid-phase binding studies using fibrinogen bound to a glass fiber filter. Binding studies using hyaluronan bound to Sepharose® suggest that the interaction is sensitive to ionic strength, with approximately 30% of radiolabeled fibrinogen released at 0.15 M NaCl and an additional 20% released at 0.3 M NaCl. Lysozyme, a basic protein, was bound less tightly than fibrinogen. Studies from another laboratory demonstrated that hyaluronan binding to lysozyme is highly sensitive to ionic strength.[49] Smaller hyaluronan fragments (MW ~ 3000) were less effective than larger polymers (80 kDa). Subsequent work[50] demonstrated that hyaluronan, as observed with acacia and poly(ethylene) glycol, enhanced fibrin polymerization and the quality of the final fibrin product. In more recent work, Rinaudo[51] showed that the addition of fibrinogen to hyaluronan promotes non-Newtonian behavior when hyaluronan exceeds the critical overlap concentration. It would seem that interaction of hyaluronan and fibrinogen may have a role in the development of fibrosis[52] and that the interaction of fibrinogen and hyaluronan with CD44 receptors may be important in this process.[53,54] Raman and coworkers[54] studied the interaction of CD44s (the standard CD44 isoform and a variant, CD44v) with hyaluronan and fibrin using atomic force microscopy. Fibrinogen was coupled to the cantilever[55] by chemical cross-linking and the force of interaction was measured with a CD44 receptor embedded in phospholipid bilayer. Raman and coworkers[54] observed that the binding of fibrin with the CD44 receptor was tighter than fibrinogen, but the binding of hyaluronan with CD44 was at least two orders of magnitude tighter than either fibrin or fibrinogen. It can be concluded that there is a specific interaction of fibrinogen with hyaluronan in the interstitial space that may influence fibrinogen function, but further studies are necessary to determine the significance of this interaction in the interstitial space.

8.5 FACTOR VII, FACTOR VIIA, AND TISSUE FACTOR

Some time ago, fibrin formation in plasma was thought to result from two cascade pathways, the *extrinsic system* and the *intrinsic system* (Figure 8.1). The extrinsic system required the participation of tissue factor, a material considered outside or *extrinsic* to blood, while the intrinsic system only required substances present in blood. The two systems converged at the formation of factor Xa and the subsequent formation of prothrombinase. Current work would suggest that the two systems are connected and cannot be considered in isolation, and may be considered the tissue factor and contact activation pathways. However, it seems reasonable to suggest that the tissue factor pathway is involved, together with blood platelets, in the initial hemostatic response, while the contact activation pathway is involved in the amplification phase of thrombin formation.[56]

Tissue factor is a cofactor for factor VIIa in the activation of factor X in the initiation of the extrinsic coagulation pathway.[57] Factor VII is bound to tissue factor, has a low level of activity, and is converted to factor VIIa, perhaps by factor Xa.[58] Factor VIIa passes from the vascular system to the interstitial space,[59] but it is not clear that this has any relevance to the function of the extrinsic coagulation pathway

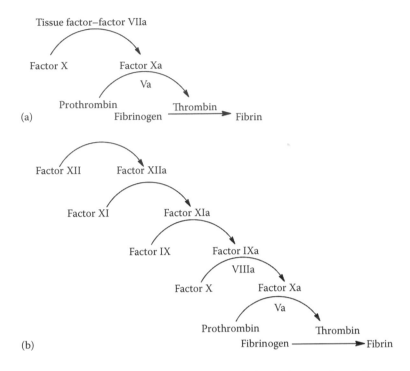

FIGURE 8.1 Classical mechanism for blood coagulation in human plasma. These are the mechanisms proposed in 1964 for the process of blood coagulation. (From Davie, E.W. and Ratnoff, O.D., *Science* 145, 1310–1312, 1964; MacFarlane, R.G., *Nature* 202, 498–499, 1964.) It is recognized that there is interaction between the extrinsic (A) and intrinsic (B) pathways as well as positive and negative feedback.

in the interstitial space. Table 8.1 shows that prothrombin and factor X are present in lymph. McBane and coworkers[60] reported the presence of prothrombin in smooth muscle, and Gentry and coworkers[61] demonstrated the presence of extrinsic system components in human ovarian follicular fluid.

The function of active tissue factor in the interstitium is not clear. The perivascular location of tissue factor does suggest a role in the hemostatic response. Jacob and coworkers[62] studied the distribution of several coagulation factors in the human myocardium using immunohistochemical techniques. In their studies on the human myocardium, Jacob and coworkers[62] found that albumin was distributed throughout the interstitial space, while tissue factor was found around arterioles and capillaries but was absent from the venules and small veins. Hoffman and coworkers[63] reported that factor VII is bound to tissue factor in the dermal interstitium. This observation, together with later work by Gopalakrishnan and coworkers,[59] would suggest that a hemostatic mechanism is "primed" in the interstitial space. Hoffman and coworkers[63] used immunohistochemistry to demonstrate the presence of tissue factor around dermal blood vessels and in the squamous epithelium; the combined use of a monospecific antibody and a modified factor VIIa suggested that factor VII/VIIa was bound to the perivascular tissue factor. It is possible, however, that this is *cryptic* tissue factor. In addition to expression on endothelial cells and epithelial cells, tissue factor is expressed on neutrophils[64] and monocyte/macrophages[65] that can be found in the interstitial space.

8.5.1 Regulation of Tissue Factor in Interstitial Space and Cryptic Tissue Factor

GRP78 (78 kDa glucose-regulated protein) is a molecular chaperone involved in the processing of glycoproteins found on the surface of endothelial cells and monocyte/macrophages[66] that binds tissue factor and decreases cell surface tissue factor activity.[67] It is not unreasonable to suggest that the binding of tissue factor to GRP78 is responsible for cryptic tissue factor.[68,69]

Tissue factor can be present in a cryptic or inactive form or an active form.[70–72] The presence of cryptic tissue factor is not limited to a cell type.[73] The *in vitro* activation of cryptic tissue factor can be achieved by treatment with detergent, which is suggested to influence phospholipid distribution or asymmetry in the membrane.[72] Other investigators have suggested a role for disulfide formation exchange.[74] More recent work[75] has suggested a synergy between phosphatidylserine exposure and disulfide exchange catalyzed by protein disulfide isomerase in the activation of cryptic tissue factor. The binding of tissue factor to GRP78[66–69] as described is another explanation for the presence of cryptic tissue factor.

In vivo activation of cryptic tissue factor can occur by cell activation[73,74–78] and likely takes place during inflammation. Tissue factor activity increases during inflammation[76] and it is suggested that the activation (decryption) of cryptic tissue factor is due to this increased activity.[73] Kothari and coworkers[73] showed that monoclonal antibodies did not distinguish between cryptic and active tissue factor. Therefore, immunoreactivity does not distinguish between cryptic and active tissue factor. Factor VIIa will bind to both procoagulant active tissue factor and cryptic tissue factor.[75] The binding of factor VIIa is of higher affinity to active tissue factor than to cryptic tissue factor[75] and is more rapid.[73] The binding of factor VIIa to cryptic tissue factor results in cell signaling via PAR-2 activation.[77] Camerer and Trejo[78] suggested that the action of cryptic tissue factor may be directed toward cell signaling rather than coagulation, which may be of great importance in the interstitial space.

8.5.2 Activity of Tissue Factor, Factor VII/VIIa, and Tissue Factor–Factor VIIa Not Related to Blood Coagulation

As with many of the other proteases originally considered unique to hemostasis, tissue factor–factor VIIa is pleiotropic, showing activity on cells unrelated to participation in blood coagulation. Notwithstanding the well-known function of tissue factor–factor VIIa in the vascular hemostatic response,[59,63] it is likely that its most important contributions in the interstitial space are unrelated to fibrin formation except in disease conditions, but are related to effects on cellular function. Factor VIIa supports the proliferation of human lung fibroblasts and stimulates the production of ECM components.[79] Wygrecka and coworkers[79] showed that the effect of factor VIIa on human lung fibroblasts was mediated through PAR-2 receptors. The mitogenic effect of factor VIIa on human lung fibroblasts was greatly enhanced by the presence of tissue factor. These investigators also observed that factor Xa had a mitogenic effect on human lung fibroblasts. Tissue factor is also expressed by fibroblasts[80] and the translocation of tissue factor to the cell surface is stimulated by the cleavage of PAR-2 receptors by factor VIIa. Factor VIIa also cleaves PAR-1 receptors but this has no effect on tissue factor translocation. Bachli and coworkers[81] previously observed that factor VIIa did not have any effect on the production of mRNAs for monocyte chemotacticprotein-1 (MCP-1) and interleukin-8 (IL-8) in dermal fibroblasts, while either thrombin or factor Xa could induce the production of mRNA for these proteins. These investigators observed an absence of PAR-2 receptors on dermal fibroblasts, perhaps providing an explanation for the lack of effect of tissue factor on dermal fibroblasts. PAR-1 receptors are present on dermal fibroblasts, providing an explanation for the mitogenic effect of thrombin and factor Xa. However, the concentration of PAR-1 receptors on dermal fibroblasts is lower than that observed with lung fibroblasts; the effect of thrombin or factor X was less on dermal fibroblasts than that of lung fibroblasts with serum-starved cells. Tissue factor–factor VIIa activation of PAR-2 receptors in a mouse model appears to promote obesity by influencing the effect of insulin.[82]

Wang and coworkers[83] showed that factor VIIa binds to tissue factor on human keratinocytes, inducing increased expression of IL-8. Aberg and coworkers[84] presented data showing the binding of factor VIIa to MDA-MB-231 cells inhibited caspase 8 and the extrinsic pathway of apoptosis, independent of interaction with a PAR receptor. Somewhat later, Aberg and Siegbahn[85] reviewed the various pathways for cell activation by factor VIIa binding to tissue factor, which included PAR-1- and PAR-2-dependent pathways. In addition, Aberg and Siegbahn[85] described the activation of PAR-1 and PAR-2 receptors by a membrane bound to a ternary complex of tissue factor–factor VIIa–factor Xa as well as a signaling pathway not involving PAR receptors. This ternary complex has been characterized by physical means,[86,87] and has been implicated in the suppression of apoptosis in a breast cancer cell line by a process not involving PAR receptors.[88] This group has also described the activation of the mTOR pathway by tissue factor–factor VIIa–factor Xa in human breast cancer cells in a process requiring cleavage of PAR-2 but not PAR-1.[89,90] Factor Xa or thrombin can activate cells by cleavage of the PAR-1 receptor.[91–93] Factor Xa, but not thrombin, can modulate cell function by cleavage of the PAR-2 receptor.[94,95] The relative importance of PAR-1, PAR-2, thrombin, and factor Xa in cell activation depends on cell type.[96] This is of considerable importance, as Åberg and Siegbahn[85] emphasized the individuality of monocyte tissue factor expression. These investigators also mentioned the importance of using multiple cell types for making general conclusions.

Our understanding of cell signaling by tissue factor–factor VIIa is further complicated by the biased antagonism of PAR receptors, where different agonists toward a specific PAR receptor would elicit a different response.[97,98] Russo and coworkers[97] pointed out that there are basic differences between PAR receptors and other cell surface receptors. PAR receptors are irreversibly activated by limited proteolysis, while the binding of agonists to most other cell surface receptors is reversible. Furthermore, in the case of PAR-1 receptors on endothelial cells, thrombin activation results in endothelial barrier permeability, while activation by activated protein C stabilizes the endothelial barrier. In the case of tissue factor–factor VIIa, cleavage of PAR-1 results in G_i pathway activation, while thrombin activation of PAR-1 results in G_q pathway activation. The antagonism of G_i and G_q has been observed in other systems.[99]

8.5.3 Factor VII and VIIa in Interstitial Space

Table 8.1 shows that there is likely sufficient factor VII in the interstitial fluid to support the various actions described in the preceding paragraphs. While not directly relevant to the current work, recombinant factor VIIa can pass from the vascular space to the interstitial space and retain activity.[59,100,101] The primary site of synthesis of factor VII is the liver, and there are several studies reporting the extrahepatic synthesis of factor VII in normal and tumor tissues. The synthesis of factor VII by macrophages, smooth muscle cells,[102,103] and colorectal cancer cells has been reported.[104] McGee and coworkers[105] demonstrated the presence of factor VII mRNA in human alveolar macrophages and suggested that expression may be limited by posttranslational processing. There are, then, reasonable data to support the local synthesis of factor VII in the interstitial space, which would be most likely stimulated by inflammation. Basal levels of factor VII would be contributed by extravasation in the absence of inflammation and tumors, recognizing that tumor growth is in fact an inflammatory state.

8.5.4 Tissue Factor–Factor VIIa and Interstitial Pathology

Wendt and coworkers[106] observed an increase in tissue factor in an animal model of hydronephrosis generated by ureteral ligation. This provides a mechanism for the fibrin deposition seen in renal capillaries with hydronephrosis. Hydronephrosis is the swelling of the kidneys when urine flow is obstructed and can result from different factors, including fibrosis. Grandaliano and coworkers[107] suggested that interstitial fibrin deposition has a role in the etiology of chronic allograft nephropathy. Chronic allograft nephropathy can be a consequence of organ transplantation and is a pathological condition characterized by interstitial fibrosis and tubular nephropathy.[108] Fibrosis is defined as the excessive growth of fibrous tissue[109] and is seen in various organs. Interstitial fibrosis is of interest for the current work and is a condition where there is an accumulation of matrix proteins such as collagen and glycosaminoglycans.[110] It is thought that the dysregulation of fibroblasts has a critical role in fibrosis.[111,112]

8.5.4.1 Tissue Factor–Factor VIIa and Tumor Development

Tissue factor–factor VIIa also appears to directly participate in tumor growth and metastasis. Tissue factor is usually first mentioned by authors as a membrane-bound receptor in tumors for factor VIIa responsible for the initiation of blood coagulation.[113–115] While the formation of fibrin driven by the extrinsic system is likely of importance in tumor development,[116,117] the diverse effects of tissue factor–factor VIIa on cells is at least of equal importance. In tumors as in normal tissue, many, if not all, of these effects involve the activation of PAR-2 receptors by tissue factor–factor VIIa.[116] Versteeg and coworkers[117] showed that the coagulant activity of tissue factor–factor VIIa could be distinguished from the effect of tumor cell growth by using specific monoclonal antibodies. One monoclonal antibody inhibited the coagulant activity, while others blocked PAR-2 cleavage and interfered with the interaction of tissue factor with integrins. The importance of the role of tissue factor–factor VIIa in the generation of thrombin,[118] factor Xa,[118] and local fibrin formation[116,117,119,120] is of importance, as local fibrin formation provides a matrix to support angiogenesis.[121]

Koizume and coworkers[122] found factor VII mRNA expression in several breast cancer lines and in some surgical pathology section from ovarian cancer. These investigators also established the presence of γ-glutamyl carboxylase in breast cancer cell lines and ovarian cancer samples. Cells expressing factor VII mRNA were able to support factor X activation. Evidence was provided to support a role for the ectopic expression of factor VII in cancer cells and cell migration. Further work showed that factor Xa was required for cell migration and invasion, perhaps as the ternary complex of tissue factor–factor VIIa–factor Xa, via the PAR-1 receptor. Magnus and coworkers[123] showed that the transformation of glioblastoma multiforme cells by the oncogenic growth factor receptor EGFRvIII resulted in the expression of factor VII; however, exogenous factor VIIa was still required for activation of coagulation or cell signaling. These investigators did show increased expression of tissue factor, PAR-1, and PAR-2.

8.6 INTRINSIC COAGULATION PATHWAY IN INTERSTITIUM

Intrinsic coagulation is a pathway for the formation of thrombin that does not involve participation of tissue factor. As mentioned in Section 8.5, at the time that this mechanism was proposed, the pathway for intrinsic coagulation was considered separate from extrinsic coagulation.[124,125] However, the systems are connected; for example, thrombin can feedback-activate factor XI in a reaction stimulated by the presence of polyanions such as polyphosphate.[126,127] However, what evidence is there for the importance of components of the intrinsic pathway such as factor VIII (Section 8.6.2) in the interstitium? Elevated factor VIII has been found in patients with idiopathic pulmonary fibrosis,[128] which could be related to endothelial cell dysfunction.[129] With the exception of Witte,[23] there is no direct measurement of coagulation factors in interstitial fluid. There are a number of studies on coagulation factors in lymph (Table 8.1). Blomstrand and coworkers[130] showed that the recalcification time for lymph was in the normal range for plasma, suggesting that the intrinsic coagulation system is intact; the one-stage prothrombin time was slightly longer than that for plasma, suggesting an intact extrinsic system. In other work, Fantl and Nelson[13] showed that lymph formed a clot faster in glass tubes than in siliconized tubes, suggesting an intact contact activation system (factor XII–factor XI–prekallikrein–high-molecular-weight kininogen) exists in lymph and, by extension, in interstitial fluid. The data presented in Table 8.1 suggest that there are adequate amounts of factor XII and factor XI in the interstitial space to support contact activation, resulting in factor XIa, which could then activate factor IX.

8.6.1 FACTOR IX

A number of studies have suggested that there is substantial factor IX in the interstitial space (Table 8.1). Factor IX and factor VIII contribute to the formation of a complex that will convert factor X to factor Xa, essentially performing the same function as tissue factor–factor VIIa. Factor IX is of some special interest in that this protein is bound to a basement membrane component in the interstitial space. It has been known for some time that the recovery of factor IX following intravenous infusion is, in general, lower than would be expected.[131] The low recovery of factor IX has been attributed to the binding of extravasated factor IX to collagen IV in the basement membrane.[132] Subsequent work from this group[133] argued that the binding of factor IX to collagen IV represents a storage mechanism for factor IX, which retains activity in the extravascular space. Liles and coworkers[134] showed that either subcutaneous or intramuscular injection of factor IX in a canine hemophilia B model resulted in substantial recovery in the blood; bioavailability was greater with intramuscular injection (83%) than with subcutaneous (64%). A consideration of the various data in Table 8.1 shows factor IX levels in lymph somewhat lower than other vitamin K–dependent factors. Factor IX can also be activated to factor IXa by tissue factor–factor VIIa, a component of the extrinsic system.[135] The sum of the data suggests that there is a stable pool of factor IX in the interstitial space that would be available to function in the activation of factor X.

8.6.2 FACTOR VIII AND VON WILLEBRAND FACTOR

The site of synthesis of factor VIII was the subject of intense debate over 40 years ago,[136–139] and recent work[140,141] has established the endothelial cell as the primary site of synthesis. There is an example of the expression of factor VIII at a local site in the pulmonary bed that may be of significance.[8] There are a wide range of values for factor VIII in lymph (Table 8.1). Witte[63] found lower concentrations of factor VIII and factor V in skin blister fluid than in blood plasma. Presumably, the association of factor VIII with von Willebrand factor in plasma would complicate extravasation.[142] There is also some reason to suggest that factor VIII is subject to degradation in the extracellular space. Fatouros and coworkers[143] showed that a recombinant factor VIII preparation (Factor VIII-SQ) was degraded by extracts from human, monkey, and porcine subcutaneous tissue. Degradation in human tissue (breast tissue) was reduced by the presence of phosphatidylserine/phosphatidylcholine and/ or von Willebrand factor. There is earlier work showing low bioavailability of this factor VIII protein following subcutaneous administration when compared with immunoglobulin.[144–146] Shi and coworkers[147] observed that factor VIII was not taken into the vascular system following subcutaneous administration but was taken following intraperitoneal injection. Peng and coworkers[148] reported that subcutaneous factor VIII was more immunogenic in mice than intravenous factor VIII. Despite the widely varying results, a consideration of the data in Table 8.1 suggests that there is significant factor VIII activity in lymph and is therefore likely in interstitial fluid. The results obtained in the global coagulation assays (recalcification time) are consistent with factor VIII levels above 10%.

It is apparent that vWF is present in lymph or interstitial fluid but not present as high-molecular-weight multimers. Miller and coworkers[18] were unable to detect vWF antigen in peripheral lymph. Le and coworkers[149] found low levels of vWF antigen (<10% of plasma) present as low-molecular-weight multimers in rabbit peripheral lymph. There are a number of studies reporting a relationship between interstitial fibrosis and von Willebrand factor.[128,129,150–156] However, it is not at all clear whether the relationship is causal or a result of endothelial dysfunction secondary to fibrosis. Nakayama and coworkers[129] showed that nitric oxide deficiency in mice (nitric oxide synthase knockout mice) resulted in luminal thrombosis and mesangial deposition of vWF with mesangial matrix expansion. These investigators observed that the baso-lateral secretion of vWF has been observed with activated endothelial cells. Maieron and coworkers[154] suggested that plasma levels of vWF antigen are a biomarker for liver fibrosis. While these authors did not evaluate interstitial levels of vWF, it is not unreasonable to suggest that there would have been increased subendothelial levels of vWF, which could enhance fibrosis.

There would appear to be a relationship between blood coagulation proteins and the development of thrombin in fibrosis.[157,158] The specific role of thrombin in fibrosis is discussed in Section 8.7.5. There may be a role for factor VIII in the develop-ment of thrombosis. Elevated factor VIII levels are observed in idiopathic pulmo-nary fibrosis.[129] While factor VIII is normally associated with vWF, proteolysis can result in dissociation of the complex,[159] resulting in free factor VIII, which may well provide different results in different assay systems.[160] Local synthesis of factor VIII by the pulmonary endothelium has been reported.[8] Basolateral secretion, such as that reported for vWF,[161,162] could result in factor VIII in the interstitium. The contribu-tion of basolateral secretion by endothelial cells and epithelial cells is discussed in Chapter 1 (Section 1.3).

8.7 THROMBIN

The presence of thrombin in the interstitium is inferred from action rather than by physical identification of the protein. Lymph fluid can form a fibrin clot presumably by the same pathways that function in plasma.[12,13] Synovial fluid[163] and follicular fluid[61] can also presumably clot by mechanisms similar to those in blood. Some specific examples of the presence of thrombin in the interstitial space are presented in Sections 8.7.1 and 8.7.5.

8.7.1 FORMATION OF THROMBIN IN INTERSTITIAL SPACE

Unlike factor VIIa, there is no evidence to suggest that thrombin formed in the vas-cular space passes into the interstitium via extravasation. Studies on the clearance of thrombin from the circulation in rabbit[164] and nonhuman primates[165] suggest that thrombin is rapidly bound by antithrombin or α_2-macroglobulin and cleared from the circulation. Visich and coworkers[165] studied the distribution of human throm-bin administered to nonhuman primates either intravenously or subcutaneously and observed that the route of elimination—that is, by formation of a complex with antithrombin—was independent of the route of administration. There was early accumulation of radioactivity (^{125}I) in the thyroid, with later accumulation in the spleen and liver. There is nothing in either of these studies to suggest that thrombin would pass from the vascular system into the interstitial space. There is one study[166] that suggests that thrombin introduced into a canine model system by intravenous injection did pass into the interstitial space and then into the lymph. No direct evidence was presented to show the passage of active thrombin in lymph. The authors also note that it is likely that the marked decrease in fibrinogen in lymph is due to the rapid decrease of plasma fibrinogen.

It would seem reasonable to suggest that thrombin is formed from prothrombin in the interstitium by a mechanism similar to that in circulating blood. It also seems reasonable to assume that, unlike plasma, the rate of thrombin formation is relatively slow and occurs either *in situ* or in the protective environment in which the thrombin is contained, such as the ECM. Bar-Shavit and coworkers[167] demonstrated that thrombin bound to the ECM and retained biological activity, as demonstrated by the clotting of fibrinogen and the activation of platelets. Thrombin bound to the ECM was not inactivated by antithrombin; thrombin bound to the ECM was inhibited by hirudin. Zacharski and coworkers[168] used hirudin followed by an antibody to hirudin to identify enzymatically active thrombin in fixed tissue sections (acetone fixation, followed by methyl benzoate clearing, followed by xylene; the AMeX method).[169] These investigators showed the presence of active thrombin in placenta, rheumatoid synovial tissue, and pulmonary alveolar tissue. The presence of enzymatically active thrombin was also demonstrated in the tumor mass of lung carcinomas, renal cell carcinoma, and malignant melanoma, but not in the stroma. Thrombin was also found in tumor-associated macrophages from adenocarcinoma and squamous cancer of the lung. Friedman and coworkers[170] showed the production of thrombin in injured rat optic nerve and use of a thrombin inhibitor, N-α-(2-naphthylsulphonylglycyl)-4-amidinophenylalanine piperidine acetate, reduced nerve damage.

Given that thrombin is formed *in situ* in the interstitial space, we are presented with the problem of mechanism of formation. We are fortunate in that we have a plethora of good possibilities (Figure 8.2), but there is a paucity of data to support the selection of a given process. The most reasonable mechanism for thrombin formation in the interstitium would involve the "classical" pathways used in the formation of a clot in the vascular system. A "primed" tissue factor pathway[59,63] would not only be useful for hemostasis at specific sites in the circulation[62] but could also serve as an initiator of coagulation in the interstitium. The action of tissue factor in promoting interstitial coagulation is discussed in Section 8.5.1. While it is most likely that tissue factor would be membrane bound, it is possible that there could be "soluble" tissue factor in the interstitium.[171–175] These studies are consistent with the presence of soluble tissue factor in the interstitium, but there are no definitive studies. The various studies on endothelial cells do not distinguish between apical secretion, which would enter the circulation, and basolateral secretion, which would enter the interstitium. There is significant basolateral secretion of a number of proteins, including monocyte inhibitory cytokine-1,[176] IGF-1, and IGFBF-1.[177] Tumor necrosis factor stimulated the secretion of urokinase-like plasminogen activator (uPA) by endothelial cells.[178] In the case of umbilical endothelial cells, secretion was mostly basolateral, while there was marginal polarity with bovine aortic endothelial cells.

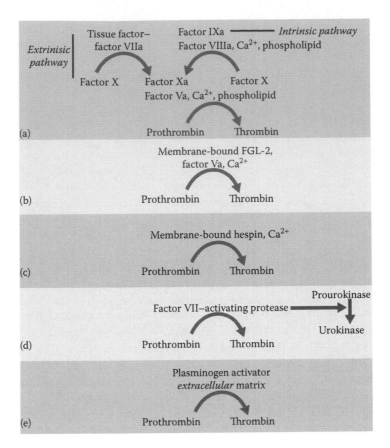

FIGURE 8.2 Possible mechanisms for prothrombin activation in interstitial space. Shown are the several potential mechanism for thrombin formation from prothrombin in the interstitial space. More detail regarding these pathways is presented in the text.

Plasminogen activator inhibitor (PAI)-1 and tissue-type plasminogen activator (tPA) were found in equal quantities on the apical and basolateral sides of umbilical endothelial cells following TNF simulation.

A second possible mechanism for thrombin formation in the interstitium that, on the surface, appears equally plausible, is activation by membrane-bound fibrinogen-like protein-2 (FGL-2; *fgl-2* prothrombinase). FGL-2 is the product of the *fgl-2* gene in cytotoxic T-lymphocytes, which encode a "fibrinogen-like" protein in that it shows homology to the fibrinogen β and γ chains.[179] This gene product was subsequently shown by Parr and coworkers[180] to be identical to murine hepatitis virus–induced prothrombinase activity. Chan and coworkers[181] characterized FGL-2 as serine protease. The recombinant enzyme was inactive until reconstituted in phosphatidylserine:phosphatidylcholine (10:90) vesicles. The activation of prothrombin by purified relipidated enzyme had an absolute requirement for the presence of calcium ions; the activation of prothrombin by *fgl-2* was markedly stimulated by the presence of blood coagulation factor Va, but there was not an absolute dependence on the presence of factor Va. In more recent work, Melnyk and coworkers[182] presented data supporting a role for FGL-2 in rheumatoid arthritis. This work combined with other studies[183,184] showed that the soluble (secreted) form, sFGL-2, bound to the Fcγ receptors on antigen-presenting cells.[184] More recent work has shown that subsets of regulatory T cells (Tregs) secrete FGL-2 resulting in immunosuppression.[185,186]

There is earlier work where as-yet-undefined enzymes converted prothrombin to thrombin. One such example is the work on prothrombin activation by human vascular smooth muscle cells.[187] This activity was inhibited by antibodies to urokinase, tPA, and factor Xa. The nature of the prothrombin activator described by Benzakour and coworkers[187] has not been described and, while it is unlikely that it is FGL-2, it is not impossible. We are unaware of any further work that elucidates the nature of this activity.

Hepsin is a membrane-associated serine protease (type II transmembrane serine protease [TTSP]) identified with cDNA technology in human liver and hepatoma cells.[188] Subsequent work[189] showed that hepsin occurs on a number of different cell types as a membrane-associated enzyme and may promote cell growth.[190] Several years later, the late Walt Kisiel's laboratory[191] showed that hepsin could activate factor VII to factor VIIa, resulting (in the presence of factor X and prothrombin) in the formation of thrombin. A cell line that coexpressed factor VII and hepsin also produced factor VIIa.[192] The expression of hepsin also occurs in renal cell carcinoma.[193] In this study, Zacharski and coworkers[193] used immunohistochemical techniques to demonstrate the presence of hepsin on tumor cell membrane; the presence of hepsin was also demonstrated on the surface of hepatocytes. Hepsin acts on a variety of *in vitro* substrates, but a biological function has not been identified.[194]

Factor VII–activating protease (FSAP) was first identified in prothrombin complex concentrate.[195] This protein was suggested to be identical to a protein previously isolated from plasma that bound hyaluronan.[196,197] FSAP was subsequently reported to be subject to autoactivation and, in addition to activating factor VII, activates single-chain urokinase-type plasminogen activator (scuPA; prourokinase).[198] The autoactivation of the FSAP zymogen protein is promoted by RNA.[199] The effect is dependent on the size of the RNA, with an effective size being 100 nucleotides. Heparin and polyphosphates also stimulate the autoactivation of FSAP.[200] While most of the interest in FSAP has been directed toward the vascular space, there is interest in FSAP activity in the interstitial space.[201–203]

The activation of prothrombin by plasminogen activator in the ECM[204] is another possibility found in the literature for the formation of thrombin in the interstitial space. Benezra and coworkers[204] presented evidence suggesting that either uPA or tPA could activate prothrombin in the presence of subendothelial matrix expressed in culture by bovine corneal endothelial cells. The activation process was slow, as would be expected; the rapid generation of thrombin in the interstitial space would be catastrophic. Friedmann and coworkers[170] cite this work[204] in providing an explanation for the local generation of thrombin in a rodent optic nerve injury model.

Finally, we would be remiss not to mention the cancer procoagulant that was originally described by Stuart Gordon at the University of Colorado in 1975.[205] This paper[205] also describes some early studies that suggested the presence of a coagulant material other than tissue thromboplastin in human tumor tissue. There has been continuing work on this enzyme over the past 40 years.[206] Gordon and coworkers[207] demonstrated the presence of the procoagulant activity primarily in tumor tissue; there was some activity in several control samples. Kee and coworkers[206] also suggested a role for the cancer procoagulant in angiogenesis. The enzyme has a molecular weight of approximately 68 kDa and is inactivated by iodoacetate, mercuric chloride, and oxidation.[208]

There are obviously a number of mechanisms for the generation of thrombin in the interstitial space. Unfortunately, we have no good reason for selecting any of these as a dominant mechanism. Conventional wisdom would focus on tissue factor, and there may well be differences in the tissue distribution of prothrombin activation.[62] However, there is the need to distinguish between cryptic and active tissue factor, as conclusions on the presence of tissue factor in the interstitial space tend to be based on immunohistochemical identification of tissue factor.

8.7.2 FACTORS INFLUENCING ACTIVITY OF THROMBIN IN INTERSTITIAL SPACE

A major question is whether thrombin functions in bulk solution or whether it is bound to the ECM, as suggested by Bar-Shavit and coworkers,[167] or fibrin. Bar-Shavit observed that thrombin bound to the ECM retained activity and was protected from inactivation by antithrombin but not hirudin.[167] These workers also reported that thrombin was most likely bound to dermatan sulfate in the ECM. Hatton[209] also demonstrated the binding of thrombin to dermatan sulfate in rabbit aorta subendothelium. Dermatan sulfate supports the inactivation of thrombin by heparin cofactor II;[210,211] the majority of heparin cofactor II (approximately 70%) is found in the extravascular space.[212,213] One other group[214] reported thrombin bound to the ECM retains enzymatic activity. Salatti and coworkers[214] showed that matrix-bound thrombin could form fibrin from fibrinogen and activate platelets. In a related observation, Hatton and Ross-Ouellet[215] showed that thrombin bound to either sulfopropyl-Sephadex® or heparin-Sepharose® could be inactivated by hirudin, and the hirudin–thrombin complex remained bound to the column. Heparin sulfate proteoglycan is also a component of the ECM, but there is no evidence that heparin sulfate proteoglycan is involved in the binding of thrombin to the ECM. Koo and coworkers[216] demonstrated that heparan sulfate promotes the activation of pro-MMP-2 (progelatinase A) by thrombin. These investigators proposed a mechanism whereby heparan sulfate binds to thrombin, promoting a conformational change. Heparan sulfate also inhibits the degradation of MMP-2 by thrombin. We could find no other studies on conformational changes in the binding of heparan sulfate. There are several studies describing a conformational change in thrombin on binding to heparin[217,218] and on binding to platelet glycoprotein Ibα.[219] Binding of thrombin to sulfated polysaccharides or proteoglycan conjugates does influence enzymatic activity. There are insufficient studies on the binding of thrombin to the ECM to make a judgment on the significance of such sequestration. While thrombin was protected from inactivation by antithrombin, similar information is not available for reaction with heparin cofactor II.

The binding of thrombin to fibrin is somewhat better understood than the binding of thrombin to components of the ECM and may be important in the interstitial space. Although it seems to be assumed that there is fibrin deposition into the interstitial space, there are few papers that directly show the presence of fibrin.[107,220–222] A consideration of these observations suggests that fibrin formation in the interstitium is subsequent to a disease process that would include wound healing. It is important to recognize that fibrinogen bound to components within the ECM[40] may adopt a conformation resembling fibrin.[41]

The binding of thrombin to fibrin has been known for some time, from the work of the late Hymie Nossel and his associates.[223] Somewhat later, it was shown that thrombin bound to fibrin and fibrin fragments retains enzymatic activity.[224–228] Granaliano and coworkers[107] suggested that thrombin bound to fibrin can activate proximal tubular cells, resulting in increased expression of TGF-β and PAI-1. Hogg and coworkers[225] reported that fibrin monomer, heparin, and thrombin could form a ternary complex. These investigators suggested that the formation of this complex is associated with a conformational change in thrombin with alteration in thrombin specificity. It is possible that such a complex could be formed from thrombin, heparan sulfate, and fibrin(ogen) in the ECM. Thrombin bound to fibrin can promote angiogenesis through action on endothelial progenitor cells.[227] Some of these studies[225] suggest that the binding of thrombin results in a change in the specificity of thrombin similar to that observed on binding to thrombomodulin.[228] There is no evidence to support the presence of thrombomodulin in the interstitial space. Jacob and coworkers[62] reported the presence of thrombomodulin on the luminal surface of blood vessels with activated protein C present at venular gaps. Several studies[229,230] report the presence of activated protein C in the alveolar space and show the relationship of decreased levels of activated protein C to the development of interstitial lung disease. There are substantial amounts of protein C in lymph (Table 8.1), and by extension in interstitial fluid, that could be converted to activated protein C by thrombin. Musci and Berliner[231] reported that serotonin and tryptamine could support the activation of protein by thrombin but much less effectively than thrombomodulin; nevertheless, there is a process for the production of activated protein C in the absence of thrombomodulin. Thrombomodulin has been reported to support the activation of MMP-2 (progelatinase A) by thrombin via the participation of protein C.[232] Peckovich and coworkers[232] suggested that activated protein C is responsible for processing the progelatinase activation intermediate generated by MT1-MMP (MMP-14).

8.7.2.1 Effect of Hyaluronan on Thrombin Activity

The effect of hyaluronan, a high-molecular-weight, negatively charged polysaccharide (Chapter 3), on the activity of thrombin in the interstitial space is another area lacking in data. It is estimated that hyaluronan occupies a good portion of the interstitial space and allows access on the basis of charge and molecular size.[233] It is estimated that albumin has access to 60% of the interstitial space.[234] Hyaluronan has been demonstrated to influence fibrin gel structure.[50] The possible effect of hyaluronan on the various biological activities of thrombin remains to be elucidated. Hyaluronan does not inhibit the esterase activity of trypsin.[235]

8.7.3   Substrates for Thrombin in Interstitial Space

Until the work from Sam Rapaport's laboratory in the 1960s on thrombin activation of factor V and factor V in blood coagulation,[236] fibrinogen and platelets were
considered to be the only substrates for thrombin. Over the next 20 years, there were
a number of studies on the effect of thrombin on cells,[237] leading to the work of
Shaun Coughlin and colleagues on protease-activated receptors (PARs) in 1991.[238]
The following decades have seen a great increase in the number of studies on the
effect of thrombin on cells mediated by PARs. It is possible that biological substrates
with a PAR, such as fibroblasts, are more sensitive than fibrinogen to the action of
thrombin in the interstitium. Aronson[239] presented data on this question in 1976, suggesting that factor VIII was 10 times more sensitive than fibrinogen (fibrinopeptide
A release) to the action of thrombin; platelet aggregation was equally as sensitive.
A consideration of recent data on the catalytic efficiency of thrombin to potential
substrates in the interstitium is summarized in Table 8.2. As predicted by Aronson,
factor VIII is the most sensitive physiological substrate. Fibrinogen, PARs, and factor XIII are close to being equal in sensitivity but substantially less sensitive than
factor VIII. Thrombin-activated fibrinolysis inhibitor (TAFI) is similar in sensitivity,
while protein C is less so. The thrombin-catalyzed activation of protein C, TAFI,
scuPA, and factor XIII deserve additional comment. The activation of these proteins
by thrombin requires the presence of a cofactor. In the case of factor XIII, activation
occurs more rapidly with a factor XIII–fibrinogen–fibrin complex.[240] Greenberg and
coworkers[240] reported that soluble fibrin polymer fragments (oligomers) can accelerate the activation of factor XIII by thrombin. The cross-linking of fibrin may be
important in tumor-associated angiogenesis.[121]

8.7.4   Role of Thrombin in Interstitial Fibrosis

There are several potential, interrelated functions for thrombin within the interstitium. The first is the role of thrombin in interstitial fibrosis (fibrotic disease), while
the second is tissue remodeling, which is associated with fibrotic disease and wound
healing. Fibrosis can be defined as the excessive growth of fibrous tissue[109] and is
seen in various organs, with particular interest in renal fibrosis, liver fibrosis, and
pulmonary fibrosis.[241] Interstitial fibrosis is of interest for the current work and is
a condition where there is an accumulation of matrix proteins such as collagen and
glycosaminoglycans.[110] Anstee and coworkers[242] reviewed the role of hypercoagulability in liver fibrogenesis. A review of various data shows that thrombophilia (e.g.,
factor V Leiden), protein C deficiency, and elevated factor VIII levels could contribute to liver fibrogenesis, suggesting a role for thrombin generation.[243] Hewitson
and coworkers[244] demonstrated that thrombin could function as an *in vitro* agonist
for renal fibroblasts. More recent work by Atanelishvili and coworkers[245] showed
that thrombin increased lung fibroblast survival while promoting alveolar epithelial
apoptosis. These investigators suggest these effects are mediated through the expression of CCAAT/enhancer-binding homologous protein (CHOP).
   It is possible that cells such as fibroblasts within the interstitial space are more sensitive to the action of thrombin than the protein substrates (Table 8.2). Thrombin binds

TABLE 8.2

Specificity of Human Thrombin for Various Substrates

Substrate	Km	K_{cat}	K_{cat}/Km	Conditions and Comment	References
ScuPA[a]	7.8 μM	0.30 s^{-1}	3.9×10^4 M^{-1} s^{-1}	20 mM Tris, pH 7.5 with 100 mM NaCl, 3 mM CaCl$_2$, 1 mg/mL BSA, 0.1% Tween 80/37°C	1
ScuPA[a]	0.43 μM	1.2 s^{-1}	2.7×10^6 M^{-1} s^{-1}	20 mM Tris, pH 7.5 with 100 mM NaCl, 3 mM CaCl$_2$, 1 mg/mL BSA, 0.1% Tween 80/37°C + thrombomodulin	1
TAFI[b]	–	–	7.0×10^2 M^{-1} s^{-1}	20 mM HEPES, pH 7.4 with 150 mM NaCl and 0.01% Tween 80/24°C	2
TAFI[b]	0.8 μM	0.74 s^{-1}	0.88×10^6 M^{-1} s^{-1}	20 mM HEPES, pH 7.4 with 150 mM NaCl and 0.01% Tween 80/24°C + thrombomodulin	2
Protein C	1.8 μM	0.009 s^{-1}	5×10^3 M^{-1} s^{-1}	50 mM Tris, pH 7.4 with 100 mM NaCl/37°C	3
Protein C	4.7 μM	0.04 s^{-1}	8×10^3 M^{-1} s^{-1}	50 mM Tris, pH 7.5 with 100 mM NaCl and 0.01% gelatin or 0.01% BSA/20°C	4
Protein C	60 μM	0.02 s^{-1}	3.2×10^2 M^{-1} s^{-1}		5
Protein C	7.6 μM	6.2 s^{-1}	8.2×10^5 M^{-1} s^{-1}	20 mM Tris, pH 7.5 with 100 mM NaCl, 0.1% gelatin and 5 mM CaCl$_2$/37°C + thrombomodulin	6
Protein C	0.1 μM	3.6 s^{-1}	36×10^6 M^{-1} s^{-1}	20 mM Tris, pH 7.5 with 100 mM NaCl, 0.1% gelatin and 5 mM CaCL$_2$/37°C + thrombomodulin and PC/PS (80/20)[c]	6
PAR-1[d]	28 μM	340 s^{-1}	12×10^6 M^{-1} s^{-1}	10 mM Tris, pH 8.0 with 150 mM NaCl/37°C	7
PAR-4[e]	61 μM	17 s^{-1}	0.28×10^6 M^{-1} s^{-1}	10 mM Tris, pH 8.0 with 150 mM NaCl/37°C	7
FGF-2[f]			1.4×10^4 M^{-1} s^{-1}	50 mM Tris, pH 8.0 with 150 mM NaCl/37°C	8
Plasma Fbg, FpA release[g]			5.4×10^6 M^{-1} s^{-1}	50 mM Tris, pH 7.4 with 150 mM NaCl/23°C[h]	9

(Continued)

TABLE 8.2 (CONTINUED)
Specificity of Human Thrombin for Various Substrates

Substrate	Km	K_{cat}	K_{cat}/Km	Conditions and Comment	References
Plasma Fbg, FpB release[i]			$2.8 \times 10^6 \, M^{-1} \, s^{-1}$	50 mM Tris, pH 7.4 with 150 mM NaCl/23°C[h]	9
Human osteopontin	19 μM	0.9 s[-1]	$4.7 \times 10^4 \, M^{-1} \, s^{-1}$ $1.14 \times 10^5 \, M^{-1} \, s^{-1j}$	20 mM HEPES, pH 7.5 with 145 mM NaCl, 5 mM CaCl$_2$ and 0.1% PEG[k] 8000/37°C	10
Formation of F1 from human III			$1.1 \times 10^3 \, M^{-1} \, s^{-1,m}$ $1.2 \times 10^5 \, M^{-1} \, s^{-1,n}$	50 mM HEPES, pH 7.4 with 125 mM NaCl and 0.1% PEG 6000/37°C	11
Human factor V	71 nM	0.23 s[-1]	$3.2 \times 10^6 \, M^{-1} \, s^{-1}$	20 mM Tris, pH 7.4 with 150 mM NaCl/25°C	12
Factor VIII	10.7 nM	5.6 s[-1]	$5.6 \times 10^8 \, M^{-1} \, s^{-1}$	20 mM HEPES, pH 7.2 with 100 mM NaCl, 5 mM CaCl$_2$, 0.01% Tween 20/22°C	13
Factor XIII	84 μM[o]	10 s[-1]	$1.2 \times 10^5 \, M^{-1} \, s^{-1o}$	9.46 mM sodium phosphate, pH 7.4 with 137 mM NaCl, 2.5 mM KCl and 0.1 PEG, 37°C	14
Factor XIII	–	–	$1.4 \times 10^5 \, M^{-1} \, s^{-1}$	40 mM sodium phosphate, pH 7.4 with 84 mM NaCl, 5 mM NaOAc and 0.1% PEG/37°C	15
Factor XIII with fibrin	2.5 μM	29 s[-1]	$12 \times 10^6 \, M^{-1} \, s^{-1}$	40 mM sodium phosphate, pH 7.4 with 84 mM NaCl, 5 mM NaOAc and 0.1% PEG/37°C	15

Note: Data taken from the cited sources.

[a] scuPA; single-chain urokinase-type plasminogen activator.

[b] TAFI; thrombin-activatable fibrinolysis inhibitor.

[c] PC:PS (80:20); a phospholipid vesicle composed of phosphatidylcholine (PC) and phosphatidylserine (PS) with a weight:weight ratio of 80 PC and 20 PS.

[d] PAR-1; protease-activated receptor 1. The ectodomain prepared by recombinant DNA technology in *Escherichia coli* was used as the substrate.

[e] PAR-4; protease-activated receptor 4. The ectodomain prepared by recombinant DNA technology in *E. coli* was used as the substrate.

[f] FbgAα; fibrinogen A alpha chain; peptide contain the scissile Arg–Gly peptide bond.

[g] Plasma Fbg, human plasma fibrinogen (purified); FpA, fibrinopeptide A.

[h] Methods state ambient temperature; 23°C assumed.

[i] Plasma Fbg, human plasma fibrinogen (purified); FpB, fibrinopeptide B.

TABLE 8.2 (CONTINUED)
Specificity of Human Thrombin for Various Substrates

[j] This value was obtained by correcting for substrate/product inhibition.
[k] PEG, poly(ethylene) glycol.
[l] Formation of prothrombin fragment 1 (f1) from prothrombin (II).
[m] With 10 mM $CaCl_2$.
[n] With 1 mM EDTA.
[o] There is some uncertainty in these numbers, reflecting the difficulty in obtaining a reliable Km.

REFERENCES FOR TABLE 8.2

1. de Munk, G.A., Groeneveld, E., and Rijken, D.C., Acceleration of the thrombin inactivation of single chain urokinase-type plasminogen activator (pro-urokinase) by thrombomodulin, *J. Clin. Invest.* 88, 1680–1684, 1991.
2. Schneider, M., Nagashima, M., Knappe, S., et al., Amino acid residues in the P6-P'3 region of thrombin-activable fibrinolysis inhibitor (TAFI) do not determine the thrombomodulin dependence of TAFI activation, *J. Biol. Chem.* 277, 9944–9951, 2002.
3. Amphlett, G.W., Kisiel, W., and Castellino, F.J., Interaction of calcium with bovine plasma protein C, *Biochemistry* 20, 2156–2161, 1981.
4. Le Bonniec, B.F. and Esmon, C.T., Glu-192–Gln substitution in thrombin mimics the catalytic switch induced by thrombomodulin, *Proc. Natl. Acad. Sci. USA* 88, 7371–7375, 1991.
5. Esmon, C.T., Regulation of protein C activation by components of the endothelial cell surface, in *Vascular Endothelium in Hemostasis and Thrombosis*, ed. M. Gimbrone, Jr., pp. 99–119, Churchill Livingstone, London, United Kingdom, 1986.
6. Galvin, J.B., Kurosawa, S., Moore, K., et al., Reconstitution of rabbit thrombomodulin into phospholipid vesicles, *J. Biol. Chem.* 262, 2199–2205, 1987.
7. Nieman, M.T. and Schmaier, A.H., Interaction of thrombin with PAR1 and PAR4 at the thrombin cleavage site, *Biochemistry* 46, 8603–8610, 2007.
8. Totta, P., de Cristofaro, R., Giampietri, C., et al., Thrombin-mediated impairment of fibroblast growth factor-2 activity, *FEBS J.* 276, 3277–3289, 2009.
9. Lord, S.T., Strickland, E., and Jayjock, E., Strategy for recombinant multichain protein synthesis: Fibrinogen B β-chain variants as thrombin substrates, *Biochemistry* 35, 2342–2348, 1996.
10. Myles, T. and Leung, L.L., Thrombin hydrolysis of human osteopontin is dependent on thrombin anion-binding exosites, *J. Biol. Chem.* 283, 17789–17796, 2008.
11. Shi, F., Winzor, D.J., and Jackson, C.M., Temperature dependence of the thrombin-catalyzed proteolysis of prothrombin, *Biophys. Chem.* 110, 1–13. 2004.
12. Monkovic, D.D. and Tracy, P.B., Activation of human factor V by factor Xa and thrombin, *Biochemistry* 29, 1118–1128, 1990.
13. Nogami, K., Zhou, Q., Wakabayashi, H., and Fay, P.J., Thrombin-catalyzed activation of factor VIII with his substituted for Arg^{372} at the P_1 site, *Blood* 105, 4362–4368, 2005.
14. Janus, T.J., Lewis, S.D., Lorand, L., and Shafer, J.A., Promotion of thrombin-catalyzed activation of factor XIII by fibrinogen, *Biochemistry* 22, 6269–6272, 1983.
15. Naski, M.C., Lorand, L., and Shafer, J.A., Characterization of the kinetic pathway for fibrin formation of α-thrombin-catalyzed activation of plasma factor XIII, *Biochemistry* 30, 934–941, 1991.

tightly to fibroblasts[246] and activates fibroblasts by cleavage of PAR-1 receptors.[247] An activation process independent of PAR receptors has also been demonstrated.[248] The binding of thrombin to fibroblasts is not by itself sufficient to activate fibroblasts,[249] but binding does possibly provide proximity to cleavage of the PAR receptor(s).[250] Thrombin activation of epithelial cells is suggested to have a role in the development of fibrosis.[251] Thrombin also induces mitogenesis in smooth muscle cells.[252]

Tissue remodeling occurs with wound healing and with interstitial fibrosis.[253] Fang and coworkers[254] reported that thrombin and cytokines (TNF-α, IL-1β) can cause collagen degradation in a synergistic manner. Cytokines induce the synthesis and secretion of several MMPs in their zymogen forms, which are then activated by thrombin. This action is independent of the stimulation of fibroblasts by thrombin. Sumitomona-Ueda and coworkers[255] showed that heparin cofactor II protected tissue remodeling induced by angiotensin II in a murine model. In addition to the direct activation of MMPs such as MMP-2,[216] thrombin also enhances the expression of MMP_9.[256,257] Both MMP-2 and MMP-9 are involved in tissue remodeling (Chapter 7).

The bulk of the evidence would suggest that thrombin is generated in the interstitial space and contributes to interstitial fibrosis. Subsequently, Favreau and coworkers[258] showed that melagatran (ximelagatran), a thrombin inhibitor,[259,260] prevented chronic graft fibrosis in an *in vitro* porcine kidney model. Bogatkevich and coworkers[261] showed that dabigatran etexilate, another thrombin inhibitor,[262,263] had anti-inflammatory and antifibrotic activity in a murine model of interstitial lung disease.[261] Wygrecka and coworkers[264] have reviewed the potential application of various coagulation inhibitors in interstitial lung disease. The effect of direct thrombin inhibitors on fibrosis is another example of the pleiotropic effects of such drugs.[265]

REFERENCES

1. Mercer, P.F. and Chambers, R.C., Coagulation and coagulation signalling in fibrosis, *Biochim. Biophys. Acta.* 1832, 1018–1027, 2013.
2. Pillai, D.K., Sankoorikal, B.-J.V., Johnson, E., et al., Directional secretomes reflect polarity-specific functions in an *in vitro* model of human bronchial epithelium, *Am. J. Respir. Cell Mol. Biol.* 50, 292–300, 2014.
3. Nakamura, R.M., Spiegelberg, H.L., Lee, S., and Weigle, W.O., Relationship between molecular size and intra- and extravascular distribution of protein antigens, *J. Immunol.* 100, 376–383. 1968.
4. Guadiz, G., Sporn, L.A., Goss, R.A., et al., Polarized secretion of fibrinogen by lung epithelial cells, *Am. J. Respir. Cell. Mol. Biol.* 17, 60–69, 1997.
5. Lozier, J.N., Yankaskas, J.R., Ramsey, W.J., et al., Gut epithelial cells as targets for gene therapy of hemophilia, *Hum. Gene Ther.* 8, 1481–1490, 1997.
6. Shovlin, C.L., Angus, G., Manning, R.A., et al., Endothelial cell processing and alternatively spliced transcripts of factor VIII: Potential implications for coagulation cascades and pulmonary hypertension, *PLoS One* 5(2), e9154, 2010.
7. Liu, N., Ono, T., Suyama, K., et al., Mesangial factor V expression colocalized with fibrin deposition in IgA nephropathy, *Kidney. Int.* 58, 598–606, 2000.
8. Liu, N., Makino, T., Nogaki, F., et al., Coagulation in the mesangial area promotes ECM accumulation through factor V expression in msPGN in rats, *Am. J. Physiol. Renal Physiol.* 287, F612–F620, 2004.

9. Papadimitriou, E., Manolopoulos, V.G., Hayman, G.T., et al., Thrombin modulates vectorial secretion of extracellular matrix proteins in cultured endothelial cells, *Am. J. Physiol.* 272, C1112–C1122, 1997.

10. Jovin, I.S., Willuwelt, A., Taborski, U., et al., Low-density lipoproteins induce the polar secretion of PAI-1 by endothelial cells in culture, *Am. J. Hematol.* 73, 66–68, 2003.

11. Fogh-Andersen, N., Altura, B.M., Altura, B.T., and Siggaard-Andersen, O., Composition of interstitial fluid, *Clin. Chem.* 41, 1522–1525, 1995.

12. Hayem, M.G., Du caillot non rétractil: Suppression de la formation du sérum sanguin dans quelques états pathologiques, *Comp. Rend. Acad. Sci. Paris* 123, 894–896, 1896.

13. Fantl, P. and Nelson, J.F., Coagulation in lymph, *J. Physiol.* 122, 33–37, 1953.

14. Weninger, W., Biro, M., and Jain, R., Leukocyte migration in the interstitial space of non-lymphoid organs, *Nat. Rev. Immunol.* 14, 232–246, 2014.

15. Sibille, Y. and Reynolds, H.Y., Macrophages and polymorphonuclear neutrophils in lung defense and injury, *Am. Rev. Respir. Dis.* 141, 471–501, 1990.

16. Radovanović, J., Korać, A., Koko, V., Nedeljović, M., and Drndarević, N., Diapedesis of thrombocytes from capillary into the intercellular space of interscapular brown adipose tissue and their increase by Ca-Sandoz, *Histol. Histopathol.* 13, 689–695, 1998.

17. Brinkhous, K.M. and Walker, S.A., Prothrombin and fibrinogen in lymph, *Am. J. Physiol.* 132, 666–669, 1941.

18. Miller, G.J., Howarth, D.J., Attfield, J.C., et al., Haemostatic factors in human peripheral afferent lymph, *Thromb. Haemost.* 83, 427–432, 2000.

19. Bell, D.R., Watson, P.D., and Renkin, E.M., Exclusion of plasma proteins in interstitium of tissues from dog hind paw, *Am. J. Physiol.* 239, H532–H538, 1980.

20. Watson, P.D., Bell, D.R., and Renkin, E.M., Early kinetics of large molecule transport between plasma and lymph in dogs, *Am. J. Physiol.* 239, H525–H531, 1980.

21. Sagstad, S.J., Oveland, E., Karlsen, T.V., et al., Age-related changes in rat dermal extracellular matrix composition affect the distribution of plasma proteins as a function of size and charge, *Am. J. Physiol. Heart Circ. Physiol.* 308, H29–H38, 2015.

22. Ohtani, O. and Ohtani, Y., Lymph circulation in the liver, *Anat. Rec. (Hoboken)* 291, 643–652, 2008.

23. Witte, S., Intra- und extravasale Verteilung von Gerinnugsproteinen: Wechselwirkung mit der Gefäswand, *Behring Inst. Mitt.*, 72, 13–28, 1983.

24. vanDeWater, L., Carr, J.M., Aronson, D., and McDonagh, J., Analysis of elevated fibrin(ogen) degradation product levels in patients with liver disease, *Blood* 67, 1468–1473, 1986.

25. Kool, J., Reubsaet, L., Wesseldijk, F., et al., Suction blister fluid as potential body fluid for biomarker proteins, *Proteomics* 7, 3638–3650, 2007.

26. Espelund, U., Søndergaard, K., Bjerring, P., et al., Interstitial fluid contains higher *in vitro* IGF bioactivity than serum: A study utilizing the suction blister technique, *Growth Horm. IGF Res.* 22, 234–239, 2012.

27. Lundberg, J., Rudling, M., and Angelin, B., Interstitial fluid lipoproteins, *Curr. Opin. Lipidol.* 24, 327–331, 2013.

28. Dihanich, M., Kaser, M., Reinhard, E., et al., Prothrombin mRNA is expressed by cells of the nervous system, *Neuron* 6, 575–581, 1991.

29. Arai, T., Miklossy, J., Klegeris, A., et al., Thrombin and prothrombin are expressed by neurons and glial cells and accumulate in neurofibrillary tangles in Alzheimer disease brain, *J. Neuropathol. Exp. Neurol.* 65, 19–25, 2006.

30. Weinstein, J.R., Gold, S.J., Cunningham, D.D., and Gall, C.M., Cellular localization of thrombin receptor mRNA in rat brain: Expression by mesencephalic dopaminergic neurons and codistribution with prothrombin mRNA, *J. Neurosci.* 15, 2906–2919, 1995.

31. Riek-Burchardt, M., Striggow, F., Henrich-Noack, P., Reiser, G., and Reymann, K.G., Increase in prothrombin-mRNA after global cerebral ischemia in rats, with constant expression of protease nexin-1 and protease-activated receptors, *Neurosci. Lett.* 329, 181–184, 2002.

32. Sokolova, E. and Reiser, G., Prothrombin/thrombin and thrombin receptors PAR-1 and PAR-4 in the brain: Localization, expression and participation in neurodegenerative diseases, *Thromb. Haemost.* 100, 576–581, 2008.

33. Lewczuk, P., Reiber, H., and Ehrenreich, H., Prothrombin in normal human cerebrospinal fluid originates from the blood, *Neurochem. Res.* 23, 1027–1030, 1998.

34. Gingrich, M.B. and Traynelis, S.E.F., Serine proteases and brain damage: Is there a link?, *Trends Neurosci.* 23, 399–407, 2000.

35. Clark, R.A., Horsburgh, C.R., Hoffman, A.A., et al., Fibronectin deposition in delayed-type hypersensitivity: Reactions of normals and a patient with afibrinogenemia, *J. Clin. Invest.* 74, 1011–1016, 1984.

36. Atkins, P.C., von Allmen, C., Moskovitz, A., et al., Fibrin formation during ongoing cutaneous allergic reactions: Comparison of responses to antigen and codeine, *J. Allergy Clin. Immunol.* 91, 956–960, 1993.

37. Follin, P., Skin chamber technique for study of *in vivo* exudated human neutrophils, *J. Immunol. Methods* 232, 55–65, 1999.

38. Siméon, A., Monier, F., Emonard, H., et al., Expression and activation of matrix metalloproteinases in wounds: Modulation by the tripeptide–copper complex glycyl-L-histidyl-L-lysine-Cu^{2+}, *J. Invest. Dermatol.* 112, 957–964, 1999.

39. Alexander, J.W. and Alexander, N.S., The influence of route of administration on wound fluid concentration of prophylactic antibiotics, *J. Trauma* 16, 488–495, 1976.

40. Simpson-Haidaris, P.J. and Rybarczyk, B., Tumors and fibrinogen: The role of fibrinogen as an extracellular matrix protein, *Ann. N.Y. Acad. Sci.* 936, 406–425, 2001.

41. Zamarron, C., Ginsberg, M.H., and Plow, E.F., Monoclonal antibodies specific for a conformationally altered state of fibrinogen, *Thromb. Haemost.* 64, 41–46, 1990.

42. Sahni, A., Simpson-Haidaris, P.J., Sahni, S.K., et al., Fibrinogen synthesized by cancer cells augments the proliferative effect of fibroblast growth factor-2 (FGF-2), *J. Thromb. Haemost.* 6, 176–183, 2008.

43. Rybarczyk, B.J., Lawrence, S.O., and Simpson-Haidaris, P.J., Matrix-fibrinogen enhances would closure by increasing both cell proliferation and migration, *Blood* 102, 4035–4043, 2003.

44. Boyles, P.W., Ferguson, J.H., and Muehlke, P.H., Mechanisms involved in fibrin formation, *J. Gen. Physiol.* 34, 493–513, 1951.

45. Fenton, J.W., II and Fasco, M.J., Polyethylene glycol 6,000 enhancement of the clotting of fibrinogen solutions in visual and mechanical assays, *Thromb. Res.* 4, 809–817, 1974.

46. Olesen, E.S., Effect of acid polysaccharides on the fibrinolytic system in guinea-pig serum, *Acta Pharmacol. Toxicol. (Copenh.)* 15, 307–315, 1959.

47. Bergqvist, D. and Arfors, K.E., Effect of dextran and hyaluronic acid on the development of postoperative peritoneal adhesions in experimental animals, *Eur. Surg. Res.* 9, 321–325, 1977.

48. LeBoeuf, R.D., Raja, R.H., Fuller, G.M., and Weigel, P.H., Human fibrinogen specifically binds hyaluronic acid, *J. Biol. Chem.* 261, 12588–12592, 1986.

49. Van Damme, M.P., Moss, J.M., Murphy, W.H., and Preston, B.N., Binding of hyaluronan to lysozyme at various pHs and salt concentrations, *Biochem. Int.* 24, 605–613, 1991.

50. LeBoeuf, R.D., Gregg, R.R., Weigel, P.H., and Fuller, G.M., Effects of hyaluronic acid and other glycosaminoglycans on fibrin polymer formation, *Biochemistry* 26, 6052–6057, 1987.

51. Rinanudo, M., Rheological investigation on hyaluronan–fibrinogen interaction, *Int. J. Biol. Macromol.* 43, 444–450, 2008.
52. Wight, T.N. and Potter-Perigo, S., The extracellular matrix: An active or passive player in fibrosis?, *Am. J. Physiol. Gastrointest. Liver Physiol.* 301, G950–G955, 2011.
53. Svee, K., White, J., Vaillant, P., et al., Acute lung injury fibroblast migration and invasion of a fibrin matrix is mediated by CD44, *J. Clin. Invest.* 98, 1713–1727, 1996.
54. Raman, P.S., Alves, C.S., Wirtz, D., and Konstantopoulos, K., Distinct kinetic and molecular requirements govern CD44 binding to hyaluronan versus fibrin(ogen), *Biophys. J.* 103, 415–423, 2012.
55. Sullan, R.M., Churnside, A.B., Nguyen, D.C., Bull, M.S., and Perkins, T.T., Atomic force microscopy with sub-picoNewton force stability for biological applications, *Methods* 60, 131–141, 2013.
56. Lin, J., Deng, H., Jin, L., et al., Design, synthesis, and biological evaluation of peptidomimetic inhibitors of factor XIa as novel anticoagulants, *J. Med. Chem.* 49, 7781–7791, 2006.
57. Silverberg, S.A., Nemerson, Y., and Zur, M., Kinetics of the activation of bovine coagulation factor X by components of the extrinsic pathway: Kinetic behavior of two-chain factor VII in the presence and absence of tissue factor, *J. Biol. Chem.* 252, 8481–8488, 1977.
58. Kirchhofer, D., Eigenbrot, C., Lipari, M.T., et al., The tissue factor region that interacts with factor Xa in the activation of factor VII, *Biochemistry* 40, 675–682, 2001.
59. Gopalakrishnan, R., Hedner, U., Clark, C., et al., rFVIIa transported from the blood stream into issues is functionally active, *J. Thromb. Haemost.* 8, 2318–2321, 2010.
60. McBane, R.D., Miller, R.S., Hassinger, N.L., et al., Tissue prothrombin: Universal distribution in smooth muscle, *Arterioscler. Thromb. Vasc. Biol.* 17, 2430–2436, 1997.
61. Gentry, P.A., Plante, L., Schroeder, M.O., et al., Human ovarian follicular fluid has functional systems for the generation and modulation of thrombin, *Fertil. Steril.* 73, 848–854, 2000.
62. Jacob, M., Chappell, D., Stoeckelhuber, M., et al., Perspectives in microvascular fluid handling: Does the distribution of coagulation factors in human myocardium comply with plasma extravasation in the venular coronary segments? *J. Vasc. Res.* 48, 219–226, 2011.
63. Hoffman, M., Colina, C.M., McDonald, A.G., et al., Tissue factor around dermal vessels has bound factor VII in the absence of injury, *J. Thromb. Haemost.* 5, 1403–1408, 2007.
64. Maugeri, N. and Manfredi, A.A., Tissue factor expressed by neutrophils: Another piece in the vascular inflammation puzzle, *Semin. Thromb. Hemost.* 41, 728–736, 2015.
65. Laurent, M., Joimel, U., Varin, R., et al., Comparative study of the effect of rivaroxaban and fondaparinux on monocyte's coagulant activity and cytokine release, *Exp. Hematol. Oncol.* 3:30, 2014.
66. Gonzalez-Gronow, M., Selim, M.A., Papalas, J., and Pizzo, S.V., GRP78: A multifunctional receptor on the cell surface, *Antioxid. Redox Signal.* 11, 2299–2306, 2009.
67. Bhattacharjee, G., Ahamed, J., Pedersen, B., et al., Regulation of tissue factor–mediated initiation of the coagulation cascade by cell surface grp78, *Arterioscler. Thromb. Vasc. Biol.* 25, 1737–1743, 2005.
68. Pozza, L.M. and Austin, R.C., Getting a GRP on tissue factor activation, *Arterioscler. Thromb. Vasc. Biol.* 25, 1529–1531, 2005.
69. Al-Hashimi, A.A., Caldwell, J., Gonzalez-Gronow, M., et al., Binding of anti-GRP78 autoantibodies to cell surface GRP78 increases tissue factor procoagulant activity via the release of calcium from endoplasmic reticulum stores, *J. Biol. Chem.* 285, 28912–28923, 2010.

70. Maynard, J.B., Dreyer, B.E., Stemerman, M.B., and Pitlick, F.A., Tissue-factor coagulant activity of cultured human endothelial and smooth muscle cells and fibroblasts, *Blood* 50, 387–396, 1977.

71. Rickles, F.R., Hair, G.A., Zeff, R.A., et al., Tissue factor expression in human leukocytes and tumor cells, *Thromb. Haemost.* 74, 391–395, 1995.

72. Carson, S.D., Manifestation of cryptic fibroblast tissue factor occurs at detergent concentrations which dissolve the plasma membrane, *Blood Coagul. Fibrinolysis* 7, 303–313, 1996.

73. Kothari, H., Pendurthi, U.R., and Rao, L.V., Analysis of tissue factor expression in various cell model systems: Cryptic vs. active, *J. Thromb. Haemost.* 11, 1353–1363, 2013.

74. Chen, V.M., Ahamed, J., Versteeg, H.H., et al., Evidence for activation of tissue factor by an allosteric disulfide bond, *Biochemistry* 45, 12020–12028, 2006.

75. Langer, F. and Ruf, W., Synergies of phosphatidylserine and protein disulfide isomerase in tissue factor activation, *Thromb. Haemost.* 111, 590–597, 2014.

76. Egorina, E.M., Sovershaev, M.A., and Hansen, J.B., The role of tissue factor in systemic inflammatory response syndrome, *Blood Coagul. Fibrinolysis* 22, 451–456, 2011.

77. Ahamed, J., Versteeg, H.H., Kerver, M., et al., Disulfide isomerization switches tissue factor from coagulation to signaling, *Proc. Natl. Acad. Sci. USA* 103, 13932–13927, 2006.

78. Camerer, E. and Trejo, J., Cryptic messages: Is noncoagulant tissue factor reserved for cell signaling? *Proc. Natl. Acad. Sci. USA* 103, 14259–14260, 2006.

79. Wygrecka, M., Kwapiszewska, G., Jablonska, E., et al., Role of protease-activated receptor-2 in idiopathic pulmonary fibrosis, *Am. J. Respir. Crit. Care Med.* 183, 1703–1714, 2011.

80. Mandal, S.K., Pendurthi, U.R., and Rao, L.V., Tissue factor trafficking in fibroblasts: Involvement of protease-activated receptor-mediated cell signaling, *Blood* 110, 161–170, 2007.

81. Bachli, E.B., Pech, C.M., Johnson, K.M., et al., Factor Xa and thrombin, but not factor VIIa, elicit specific cellular responses in dermal fibroblasts, *J. Thromb. Haemost.* 1, 1935–1944, 2003.

82. Badeanlou, L., Fuller-Freguia, C., Yang, G., et al., Tissue factor–protease-activated receptor 2 signaling promotes diet-induced obesity and adipose inflammation, *Nat. Med.* 17, 1490–1497, 2011.

83. Wang, X., Gjernes, E., and Prydz, H., Factor VIIa induces tissue factor-dependent upregulation of interleukin-8 in a human keratinocyte line, *J. Biol. Chem.* 277, 23620–23626, 2002.

84. Åberg, M., Johnell, M., Wickström, M., and Siegbahn, A., Tissue factor/FVIIa prevents the extrinsic pathway of apoptosis by regulation of the tumor-suppressor death-associated protein kinase 1 (DAPK1), *Thromb. Res.* 127, 141–148, 2011.

85. Åberg, M. and Siegbahn, A., Tissue factor non-coagulant signaling: Molecular mechanisms and biological consequences with a focus on cell migration and apoptosis, *J. Thromb. Haem.* 11, 817–825, 2013.

86. Norledge, B.V., Petrovan, R.J., Ruf, W., and Olson, A.J., The tissue factor/factor VIIa/factor Xa complex: A model built by docking and site-directed mutagenesis, *Proteins* 53, 640–648, 2003.

87. Lee, C.J., Chandrasekaran, V., Wu, S., et al., Recent estimates of the structure of the factor VIIa (FVIIa)/tissue factor (TF) and factor Xa (FXa) ternary complex, *Thromb. Res.* 125(Suppl. 1), S7–S10, 2010.

88. Jiang, X., Guo, Y.L., and Bromberg, M.E., Formation of tissue factor–factor VIIa–factor Xa complex prevents apoptosis in human breast cancer cells, *Thromb. Haemost.* 96, 196–201, 2006.

89. Jiang, X., Bailly, M.A., Panetti, T.S., et al., Formation of tissue factor–factor VIIa–factor Xa complex promotes cellular signaling and migration of human breast cancer cells, *J. Thromb. Haemost.* 2, 93–101, 2004.

90. Jiang, X., Zhu, S., Panetti, T.S., and Bromberg, M.E., Formation of tissue factor–factor VIIa–factor Xa complex induces activation of the mTOR pathway which regulates migration of human breast cancer cells, *Thromb. Haemost.* 100, 127–133, 2008.

91. Blanc-Brude, O.P., Archer, F., Leoni, P., et al., Factor Xa stimulates fibroblast procollagen production, proliferation, and calcium signaling via PAR1 activation, *Exp. Cell Res.* 304, 16–27, 2005.

92. Schuepbach, R.A. and Riewald, M., Coagulation factor Xa cleaves protease-activated receptor-1 and mediates signaling dependent on binding to the endothelial protein C receptor-1, *J. Thromb. Haemost.* 8, 379–388, 2010.

93. Bastiaans, J., van Meurs, J.C., van Holten-Neelen, C., et al., Factor Xa and thrombin stimulate proinflammatory and profibrotic mediator production by retinal pigment epithelial cells: A role in vitreoretinal disorders? *Graefes Arch. Clin. Exp. Ophthalmol.* 251, 1723–1733, 2013.

94. Daubie, V., De Decker, R., Nicaise, C., and Pochet, R., Osteosarcoma cell–calcium signaling through tissue factor–factor VIIa complex and factor Xa, *FEBS Lett.* 581, 2611–2615, 2007.

95. Bukowska, A., Zacharias, I., Weinert, S., et al., Coagulation factor Xa induces an inflammatory signalling by activation of protease-activated receptors in human atrial tissue, *Eur. J. Pharmacol.* 718, 114–123, 2013.

96. Camerer, E., Kataoka, H., Kahn, M., et al., Genetic evidence that protease-activated receptors mediate factor Xa signaling in endothelial cells, *J. Biol. Chem.* 277, 16081–16087, 2002.

97. Russo, A., Soh, U.J., and Trejo, J., Protease display biased agonism at protease-activated receptors: Location matters! *Mol. Interv.* 9, 87–96, 2009.

98. Canto, I., Soh, U.J.K., and Trejo, J., Allosteric modulation of protease-activated receptor signaling, *Mini-Rev. Med. Chem.* 12, 804–811, 2012.

99. Malin, S.A. and Molliver, D.C., Gi- and Gq-coupled ADP (P2Y) receptors act in opposition to modulate nociceptive signaling and inflammatory pain behavior, *Mol. Pain* 6(21), 2010.

100. Gopalakrishnan, R., Hedner, U., Ghosh, S., et al., Bio-distribution of pharmacologically administered recombinant factor VIIa (rFVIIa), *J. Thromb. Haemost.* 8, 301–310, 2010.

101. Ahonen, J., The role of recombinant activated factor VII in obstetric hemorrhage, *Curr. Opin. Anesthesiol.* 25, 309–314, 2012.

102. Wilcox, J.N., Noguchi, S., Casanova, J.R., and Rasmussen, M.E., Extrahepatic synthesis of FVII in human atheroma and smooth muscle cells *in vitro*, *Ann. N.Y. Acad. Sci.* 947, 433–438, 2001.

103. Wilcox, J.N., Noguchi, S., and Casanova, J., Extrahepatic synthesis of factor VII in human atherosclerotic vessels, *Arterioscler. Thromb. Vasc. Biol.* 23, 136–141, 2003.

104. Tang, J.Q., Fan, Q., Wu, W.H., et al., Extrahepatic synthesis of coagulation factor VII by colorectal cancer cells promotes tumor invasion and metastasis, *Chin. Med. J.* 123, 3559–3565, 2010.

105. McGee, M.P., Wallin, R., Devlin, R., and Rothsberger, H., Identification of mRNA coding for factor VII protein in human alveolar macrophages: Coagulant expression may be limited due to deficient postribosomal processing, *Thromb. Haemost.* 61, 170–174, 1989.

106. Wendt, T., Zhang, Y.M., Bierhaus, A., et al., Tissue factor expression in an animal model of hydronephrosis, *Nephrol. Dial. Transplant* 10, 1820–1828, 1995.

107. Grandaliano, G., Di Paolo, S., Manno, R., et al., Protease-activated receptor 1 and plasminogen activator inhibitor 1 expression in chronic allograft nephropathy, *Transplantation* 72, 1437–1443, 2001.
108. Campistol, J.M., Boletis, I.N., Dantal, J., et al., Chronic allograft nephropathy: A clinical syndrome; Early detection and the potential role of proliferation signal inhibitors, *Clin. Transplant.* 23, 769–777, 2009.
109. *Oxford English Dictionary*, Oxford University Press, Oxford, United Kingdom, 2014. http://www.oed.com.
110. Eddy, A.A., Molecular insights into renal interstitial fibrosis, *J. Am. Soc. Nephrol.* 7, 2495–2508, 1996.
111. Yamashita, M., Yamauchi, K., Chiba, R., et al., The definition of fibrogenic processes in fibroblastic foci of idiopathic pulmonary fibrosis based on morphometric quantification of extracellular matrices, *Human Pathol.* 40, 1278–1287, 2009.
112. Thannickal, V.J., Toews, G.B., and Phan, S.H., Role and origin of the fibroblast in the pathogenesis of interstitial lung disease, in *Interstitial Lung Disease*, 5th edn., eds. M.I. Schwarz and T.E. King, Jr., Chapter 17, pp. 395–406, People's Medical Publishing House, Shelton, CO, 2011.
113. Siddiue, F.A., Aminkhosravi, A., Amaya, M., et al., Purification and properties of human melanoma cell tissue factor, *Clin. Appl. Thromb. Hemost.* 7, 289–295, 2001.
114. Chand, H.S. and Kisiel, W., Quantitative real-time reverse transcription polymerase reaction analysis of a novel tissue factor splice variant in select human solid tumors, *J. Thromb. Haemost.* 5, 640–641, 2007.
115. Henriquez, S., Calderon, C., Quezada, M., et al., Progesterone utilizes pools of tissue factor to increase coagulation and invasion and these effects are inhibited by TFPI, *J. Cell. Physiol.* 226, 3278–3285, 2013.
116. Ruf, W., Yokota, N., and Schaffner, F., Tissue factor in cancer progression and angiogenesis, *Thromb. Res.* 125(Suppl. 2), S36–S38, 2010.
117. Versteeg, H.H., Schäffner, F., Kerver, M., et al., Inhibition of tissue factor signaling suppresses tumor growth, *Blood* 111, 190–199, 2008.
118. Versteeg, H.H., Emerging insights in the role of tissue factor in cancer, *Curr. Gen.* 6, 372–382, 2005.
119. Boccaccio, C. and Medico, E., Cancer and blood coagulation, *Cell. Mol. Life Sci.* 63, 1024–1027, 2006.
120. Yapijakis, C., Bramos, A., Nixon, A.M., et al., The interplay between hemostasis and malignancy: The oral cancer paradigm, *Anticancer Res.* 32, 1791–1800, 2012.
121. Fernandez, P.M., Patierno, S.R., and Rickles, F.R., Tissue factor and fibrin in tumor angiogenesis, *Semin. Thromb. Hemost.* 30, 31–44, 2004.
122. Koizuma, S., Jin, M.S., Miyagi, E., et al., Activation of cancer cell migration and invasion by ectopic synthesis of coagulation factor VII, *Cancer Res.* 66, 9453–9460, 2006.
123. Magnus, N., Garnier, D., and Rak, J., Oncogenic epidermal growth factor receptor up-regulates multiple elements of the tissue factor signaling pathway in human glioma cells, *Blood* 116, 815–818, 2010.
124. Davie, E.W. and Ratnoff, O.D., Waterfall sequence for intrinsic blood clotting, *Science* 145, 1310–1312, 1964.
125. MacFarlane, R.G., An enzyme cascade in the blood clotting mechanism, and its function as a biochemical amplifier, *Nature* 202, 498–499, 1964.
126. Morrissey, J.H., Choi, S.H., and Smith, S.A., Polyphosphate: An ancient molecule that links platelets, coagulation, and inflammation, *Blood* 119, 5972–5979, 2012.
127. Geng, Y., Verhamme, I.M., Smith, S.B., et al., The dimeric structure of factor XI and zymogen activation, *Blood* 121, 3962–3969, 2013.

128. Magro, C.M., Allen, J., Pope-Harmon, A., et al., The role of microvascular injury in the evolution of idiopathic pulmonary fibrosis, *Am. J. Clin. Pathol.* 119, 556–567, 2003.
129. Magro, C.M., Waldman, W.J., Knight, D.A., et al., Idiopathic pulmonary fibrosis related to endothelial injury and antiendothelial cell antibodies, *Hum. Immunol.* 67, 284–297, 2006.
130. Blomstrand, B., Nilsson, I.M., and Dahlbäck, O., Coagulation studies on human thoracic duct lymph, *Scand. J. Clin. Lab. Invest.* 15, 248–254, 1963.
131. Poon, M.-C., Pharmacokinetics of factors IX, recombinant factor VII and factor XIII, *Haemophilia* 12(suppl. 4), 61–69, 2006.
132. Wolberg, A.S., Stafford, D.W., and Eric, D.A., Human factor IX binds to specific sites on the collagenous domain of collagen IV, *J. Biol. Chem.* 272, 16717–16720, 1997.
133. Feng, D., Stafford, K.A., Broze, G.J., and Stafford, D.W., Evidence of clinically significant extravascular stores of factor IX, *J. Thromb. Haemost.* 11, 2176–2178, 2013.
134. Liles, D., Landen, C.N., Monroe, D.M., et al., Extravascular administration of factor I: Potential for replacement therapy of canine and human hemophilia B, *Thromb. Haemost.* 77, 944–948, 1997.
135. Jesty, J. and Morrison, S.A., The activation of factor IX by tissue factor–factor VII in a bovine plasma system lacking factor X, *Thromb. Res.* 32, 171–181, 1983.
136. Dodds, W.J., Hepatic influence on splenic synthesis and release of coagulation activities, *Science* 166, 882–883, 1969.
137. Norman, J.C., Lambilliotte, J.P., Kojima, Y., and Sise, H.S., Antihemophilic factor release by perfused liver and spleen: Relationship to hemophilia, *Science* 158, 1060–1061, 1967.
138. Webster, W.P., Zukoski, C.F., Hutchin, P., et al., Plasma factor VIII synthesis and control as revealed by canine organ transplantation, *Am. J. Physiol.* 220, 1147–1154, 1971.
139. Barrow, E.M. and Graham, J.B., Kidney antihemophilic factor: Partial purification and some properties, *Biochemistry* 7, 3917–3925, 1968.
140. Jacquemin, M., Neyrinck, A., Hermanns, M.I., et al., FVIII production by human lung microvascular endothelial cells, *Blood* 108, 515–517, 2006.
141. Fahs, S.A., Hille, M.T., Shi, Q., et al., A conditional knockout mouse model reveals endothelial cells as the principal and possibly exclusive source of plasma factor VIII, *Blood* 123, 3706–3713, 2014.
142. Thomson, C., Forbes, C.D., and Prentice, C.R., Evidence for a qualitative defect in factor-VIII-related antigen in von Willebrand's disease, *Lancet* 303(7858), 594–596, 1974.
143. Fatouros, A., Liden, Y., and Sjöstrom, B., Recombinant factor VIII SQ: Stability of VIII:C in homogenates from porcine, monkey, and human subcutaneous tissue, *J. Pharm. Pharmacol.* 52, 797–805, 2000.
144. Smith, G.N., Griffiths, B., Mollison, D., and Mollison, P.L., Uptake of IgG after intramuscular and subcutaneous injection, *Lancet* 299(7762), 1208–1212, 1972.
145. Waniewski, J., Gardulf, A., and Hammarström, L., Bioavailability of gamma-globulin after subcutaneous infusions in patients with common variable immunodeficiency, *J. Clin. Immunol.* 14, 90–97, 1994.
146. Goodrick, J., Kumpel, B., Pamphilon, D., et al., Plasma half-lives and bioavailability of human monoclonal RhD antibodies BRAD-3 and BRAD-5 following intramuscular injection into RH D-negative volunteers, *Clin. Exp. Immunol.* 98, 17–20, 1994.
147. Shi, Q., Kuether, E.L., Schroeder, J.A., et al., Intravascular recovery of vWF and FVIII following intraperitoneal injection and differences from intravenous and subcutaneous injection in mice, *Haemophilia* 18, 639–646, 2012.
148. Peng, A., Gaitonde, P., Kosloski, M.P., et al., Effect of route of administration of human recombinant factor VIII on its immunogenicity in hemophilia a mice, *J. Pharm. Sci.* 98, 4480–4484, 2009.

149. Le, D.T., Borgs, P., Toneff, T.W., et al., Hemostatic factors in rabbit limb lymph: Relationship to mechanisms regulating extravascular coagulation, *Am. J. Physiol.* 274, H769–H776, 1998.

150. Kasper, M., Schöbl, R., Haroske, G., et al., Distribution of von Willebrand factor in capillary endothelial cells of rat lungs with pulmonary fibrosis, *Exp. Toxicol. Pathol.* 48, 283–288, 1996.

151. Kobayashi, H., Horikoshi, K., Yamataka, A., et al., Hyaluronic acid: A specific prognostic indicator of hepatic damage in biliary atresia, *J. Pediatr. Surg.* 34, 1791–1794, 1999.

152. Bowyer, S.L., Ragsdale, C.G., and Sullivan, D.B., Factor VIII related antigen and childhood rheumatic diseases, *J. Rheumatol.* 16, 1093–1097, 1989.

153. Maieron, A., Salzi, P., Peck-Radosavljevic, M., et al., Von Willebrand factor as a new marker for non-invasive assessment of liver fibrosis and cirrhosis in patients with chronic hepatic C, *Aliment. Pharmacol. Ther.* 39, 331–338, 2014.

154. Geggel, R.L., Carvalho, A.C., Hoyer, L.W., and Reid, L.M., Von Willebrand factor abnormalities in pulmonary hypertension, *Am. Rev. Respir. Dis.* 135, 294–299, 1987.

155. Nakayama, T., Sato, W., Yoshimura, A., et al., Endothelial von Willebrand factor release due to eNOS deficiency predisposes to thrombotic microangiopathy in mouse aging kidney, *Am. J. Pathol.* 176, 2198–2208, 2010.

156. Hernández-Romero, D., Lahoz, Á., Roldan, V., et al., Von Willebrand factor is associated with atrial fibrillation development in ischaemic patients after cardiac surgery, *Europace* pii, euv354, 2015.

157. de Ridder, G.G., Lundblad, R.L., and Pizzo, S.V., Actions of thrombin in the interstitium, *J. Thromb. Haemost.* 14, 40–47, 2016.

158. Amerci, A., Kurachi, S., Sueishi, K., et al., Myocardial fibrosis in mice with overexpression of human blood coagulation factor IX, *Blood* 101, 1871–1873, 2003.

159. Lollar, P., The association of factor VIII with von Willebrand factor, *Mayo Clin. Proc.* 66, 524–534, 1991.

160. Lundblad, R.L., Kingdon, H.S., Mann, K.G., and White, G.C., Issues with the assay of factor VIII activity in plasma and factor VIII concentrates, *Thromb. Haemost.* 84, 942–948, 2000.

161. Sporn, L.A., Marder, V.J., and Wagner, D.D., Differing polarity of the constitutive and regulated secretory pathways for von Willebrand factor in endothelial cells, *J. Cell. Biol.* 108, 1283–1289, 1989.

162. van Buul-Wortelboer, M.F., Brinkman, H.J., Reinders, J.B., et al., Polar secretion of von Willebrand factor by endothelial cells, *Biochim. Biophys. Acta* 1011, 129–133, 1989.

163. Chang, P., Aronson, D.L., Borenstein, D.G., and Kessler, C.M., Coagulant proteins and thrombin generation in synovial fluid: A model for extravascular coagulation, *Am. J. Hematol.* 50, 79–83, 1995.

164. Vogel, C.N., Kingdon, H.S., and Lundblad, R.L., Correlation of *in vivo* and *in vitro* inhibition of thrombin by plasma inhibitors, *J. Lab. Clin. Med.* 93, 661–673, 1979.

165. Visich, J.E., Byrnes-Blake, K.A., Lewis, K.B., et al., Bioavailability and relative tissue distribution of [125I]-recombinant human thrombin following intravenous or subcutaneous administration to non-human primates, *J. Thromb. Haemost.* 4, 1962–1968, 2006.

166. Leandoer, L. and Niléhn, J.E., Effect of intravenous injection of stypven or thrombin on coagulation and fibrinolysis of blood and lymph in dogs, *Acta Chir. Scand.* 135, 7–13, 1969.

167. Bar-Shavit, R., Eldor, A., and Vlodavsky, I., Binding of thrombin to subendothelial matrix: Protection and expression of functional properties, *J. Clin. Invest.* 84, 1096–1104, 1989.

168. Zacharski, L.R., Memoil, V.A., Morain, W.D., et al., Cellular localization of enzymatically active thrombin in intact human tissues by hirudin binding, *Thromb. Haemost.* 73, 793–797, 1995.

169. Sato, X., Mukai, K., Watanabe, S., et al., The AMeX method: A simplified technique of tissue processing and paraffin embedding with improved preservation of antigens for immunostaining, *Am. J. Pathol.* 125, 431–435, 1986.

170. Friedmann, I., Yoles, E., and Schwartz, M., Thrombin attenuation is neuroprotective in the injured rat optic nerve, *J. Neurosurg.* 76, 641–649, 2001.

171. Schlaepfer, W.W. and Freeman, L.A., Calcium-dependent degradation of mammalian neurofilaments by soluble tissue factor(s) from rat spinal cord, *Neuroscience* 5, 2305–2314, 1980.

172. Szotowski, B., Antoniak, S., Poller, W., et al., Procoagulant soluble tissue factor is released from endothelial cells in response to inflammatory cytokines, *Circ. Res.* 96, 1233–1239, 2005.

173. Ott, I., Soluble tissue factor emerges from inflammation, *Circ. Res.* 96, 1217–1218, 2005.

174. Khan, M.M., Hattori, T., Niewiarowski, S., et al., Truncated and microparticle-free soluble tissue factor bound to peripheral monocytes preferentially activated factor VII, *Thromb. Haemost.* 95, 462–468, 2006.

175. Determann, R.M., Millo, J.L., Garrard, C.S., and Schultz, M.J., Bronchoalveolar levels of plasminogen activator inhibitor-1 and soluble tissue factor are sensitive specific markers of pulmonary inflammation, *Intensive Care Med.* 32, 946–947, 2006.

176. Jurczyluk, J., Brown, D., and Stanley, K.K., Polarized secretion of cytokines in primary human microvascular endothelial cells is not dependent on N-linked glycosylation, *Cell Biol. Int.* 27, 997–1003, 2003.

177. Taylor, W.R., Nerem, R.M., and Alexander, R.W., Polarized secretion of IGF-1 and IGF-1 binding protein activity by cultured aortic endothelial cells, *J. Cell. Physiol.* 154, 139–142, 1993.

178. van Hinsbergh, V.W., van den Berg, E.A., Fiers, W., and Dooijewaard, G., Tumor necrosis factor induces the production of urokinase-type plasminogen activator by human endothelial cells, *Blood* 75, 1991–1998, 1990.

179. Koyama, T., Hall, L.R., Haseer, W.G., et al., Structure of a cytotoxic T-lymphocyte-specific gene shows a strong homology to fibrinogen β and γ-chains, *Proc. Natl. Acad. Sci. USA* 84, 1609–1613, 1987.

180. Parr, R.L., Fung, L., Reneker, J., et al., Association of mouse fibrinogen-like protein with murine hepatitis virus-induced prothrombinase activity, *J. Virol.* 69, 5033–5038, 1995.

181. Chan, C.W.Y., Chan, M.W.C., Liu, M., et al., Kinetic analysis of a unique direct prothrombinase, *fgl2*, and identification of a serine residue critical for prothrombinase activity, *J. Immunol.* 168, 5170–5177, 2002.

182. Melnyk, M.C., Shalev, I., Zhang, J., et al., The prothrombinase activity of FGL2 contributes to the pathogenesis of experimental arthritis, *Scand. J. Rheumatol.* 40, 269–270, 2011.

183. Shalev, I., Liu, H., Koscik, C., et al., Targeted deletion of *fgl2* leads to impaired regulatory T cell activity and development of autoimmune glomerulonephritis, *J. Immunol.* 180, 249–260, 2008.

184. Liu, H., Shalev, I., Manuel, J., et al., The FGL2-FcγRIIB pathways: A novel mechanism leading to immunosuppression, *Eur. J. Immunol.* 38, 3114–3126, 2008.

185. Liu, H., Yang, P.S., Zhu, T., et al., Characterization of fibrinogen-like protein 2 (FGL2): Monomeric FGL2 has enhanced immunosuppressive activity in comparison to oligomeric FGL2, *Int. J. Biochem. Cell Biol.* 45, 408–418, 2013.

186. Joller, N., Lozano, E., Burkett, P.R., et al., Treg cells expressing the coinhibitory molecule TIGIT selectively inhibit proinflammatory Th1 and Th17 cell responses, *Immunity* 40, 569–581, 2014.

187. Benzakour, O., Kanthou, C., Lupu, F., et al., Prothrombin cleavage by human vascular smooth muscle cells: A potential alternative pathway to the coagulation cascade, *J. Cell. Biochem.* 59, 514–528, 1995.

188. Leytus, S.P., Loeb, K.R., Hagen, F.S., et al., A novel trypsin-like serine protease (hepsin) with a putative transmembrane domain expressed by human liver and hepatoma cells, *Biochemistry* 27, 1067–1074, 1988.

189. Tsuji, A., Torres-Rosado, A., Arai, T., et al., Hepsin, a cell membrane-associated protease: Characterization, tissue distribution, and gene localization, *J. Biol. Chem.* 266, 16948–16953, 1991.

190. Torres-Rosado, A., O'Shea, K.S., Tsuji, A., et al., Hepsin, a putative cell-surface serine protease, is required for mammalian cell growth, *Proc. Natl. Acad. Sci. USA* 90, 7181–7185, 1993.

191. Kazama, Y., Hamamoto, T., Foster, D.C., and Kisiel, W., Hepsin, a putative membrane-associated serine protease, activates human factor VII and initiates a pathway of blood coagulation on the cell surface leading to thrombin formation, *J. Biol. Chem.* 270, 66–72, 1995.

192. Halabian, R., Roudkenar, M.H., Esmaeili, N.S., et al., Establishment of a cell line expressing recombinant factor VII and its subsequent conversion to active form FVIIa through hepsin by genetic engineering method, *Vox Sang.* 96, 309–315, 2009.

193. Zacharaski, L.R., Ornstein, D.L., Memoli, V.A., et al., Expression of the factor VII activating protease, hepsin, in situ in renal cell carcinoma, *Thromb. Haemost.* 79, 876–877, 1998.

194. Wu, Q. and Peng, J. Hepsin, in *Handbook of Proteolytic Enzymes*, eds. N.D. Rawlings and G.S. Salveson, Chapter 652, pp. 2985–2989, Academic Press/Elsevier, Amsterdam, the Netherlands, 2013.

195. Römisch, J., Feussner, A., Vermöhlen, S., and Stöhr, H.A., A protease isolated from human plasma activating factor VII independent of tissue factor, *Blood Coagul. Fibrinolysis* 10, 471–479, 1999.

196. Choi-Miura, N.-H., Tobe, T., Sumiya, J.-I., et al., Purification and characterization of a novel hyaluronan-binding protein (PHBP) from human plasma: It has three EGF, a kringle and a serine protease domain, similar to hepatocyte growth factor activator, *J. Biochem.* 119, 1157–1165, 1996.

197. Sumiya, J., Asakawa, S., Tobe, T., et al., Isolation and characterization of the plasma hyaluronan-binding protein (PHBP) gene (HABP2), *J. Biochem.* 122, 983–990, 1997.

198. Kannemeier, C., Feussner, A., Stöhr, H.-A., et al., Factor VII and single-chain plasminogen activator activating protease: Activation and autoactivation of the proenzyme, *Eur. J. Biochem.* 268, 3789–3796, 2001.

199. Nakazawa, F., Kannemeier, C., Shibamiya, A., et al., Extracellular RNA is a natural cofactor for the (auto-)activation of factor VII-activating protease (FSAP), *Biochem. J.* 385, 831–838, 2005.

200. Muhl, L., Galuska, S.P., Oörni, K., et al., High negative charge-to-size ratio in polyphosphates and heparin regulates factor VII-activating protease, *FEBS J.* 276, 4828–4839, 2009.

201. Kannemeier, C., Al-Fakhri, N., Preissner, K.T., and Kanse, S.M., Factor VII-activating protease (FSAP) inhibits growth factor-mediated cell proliferation and migration of vascular smooth muscle cells, *FASEB J.* 18, 728–730, 2004.

202. Wygrecka, M., Markart, P., Fink, L., et al., Raised protein levels and altered cellular expression of factor VII activating protease (FSAP) in the lungs of patients with acute respiratory distress syndrome (ARDS), *Thorax* 62, 880–888, 2007.

203. Parahuleva, M.S., Ball, N., Parviz, B., et al., Factor seven activating protease (FSAP) expression in human placenta and its role in trophoblast migration, *Eur. J. Obstet. Gynecol. Reprod. Biol.* 167, 34–40, 2013.

204. Benezra, M., Vlodavsky, I., and Bar-Shavit, R., Prothrombin conversion to thrombin by plasminogen activator residing in the subendothelial extracellular matrix, *Semin. Thromb. Hemost.* 19, 405–411, 1993.

205. Gordon, S.G., Franks, J.J., and Lewis, B., Cancer procoagulant A: A factor X activating procoagulant from malignant tissue, *Thromb. Res.* 6, 127–137, 1975.
206. Kee, N.L., Naudé, R.J., Blatch, G.L., and Frost, C.L., The effect of cancer procoagulant on expression of metastatic and angiogenic markers in breast cancer and embryonic stem cell lines, *Biol. Chem.* 393, 113–121, 2012.
207. Gordon, S.G., Franks, J.J., and Lewis, B.J., Comparison of procoagulant activities in extracts of normal and malignant human tissue, *J. Natl. Cancer Inst.* 62, 773–776, 1979.
208. Gordon, S.G., Hasiba, U., Cross, B.A., et al., Cysteine proteinase procoagulant from amnion-chorion, *Blood* 66, 1261–1265, 1985.
209. Hatton, M.W., Evidence for thrombin binding to dermatan sulfate sites in the rabbit aorta subendothelium *in vitro*, *Blood Coagul. Fibrinolysis* 4, 927–933, 1993.
210. Tollefsen, D.M., Pestka, C.A., and Monafo, W.J., Activation of heparin cofactor II by dermatan sulfate, *J. Biol. Chem.* 258, 6713–6716, 1983.
211. Rau, J.C., Mitchell, J.W., Fortenberry, Y.M., and Church, F.C., Heparin cofactor II: Discovery, properties, and role in controlling vascular homeostasis, *Semin. Thromb. Hemost.* 37, 339–348, 2011.
212. Whinna, H.C., Choi, H.U., Rosenberg, L.C., and Church, F.C., Interaction of heparin cofactor II with biglycan and decorin, *J. Biol. Chem.* 268, 3920–3924, 1993.
213. Sumitomo-Ueda, Y., Aihara, K., Ise, T., et al., Heparin cofactor II protects against angiotensin II-induced cardiac remodeling via attenuation of oxidative stress in mice, *Hypertension* 56, 430–436, 2010.
214. Salatti, J.A., Fenton, J., II., Anton, P., and Sakariassen, K.S., α-Thrombin bound to extracellular endothelial matrix induces pronounced fibrin deposition and platelet thrombus growth in flowing non-anticoagulated human blood, *Blood Coagul. Fibrinolysis* 5, 561–566, 1994.
215. Hatton, M.W. and Ross-Ouellet, B., Radiolabeled r-hirudin as a measure of thrombin activity at, or within, the rabbit aorta wall *in vitro* and *in vivo*, *Thromb. Haemost.* 71, 499–506, 1994.
216. Koo, B.-H., Han, J.H., Yeom, Y.I., et al., Thrombin-dependent MMP-2 activity is regulated by heparan sulfate, *J. Biol. Chem.* 285, 41270–41279, 2010.
217. Semenova, O.A. and Strukova, S.M., Ultraviolet difference spectroscopy study of α- and βγ-thrombin binding to heparin, *Biokhimiia* 45, 2225–2232, 1980.
218. Guillin, M.C., Bezeaud, A., Bouton, M.C., and Jandrot-Perrus, M., Thrombin specificity, *Thromb. Haemost.* 74, 129–133, 1995.
219. Li, C.Q., Vindigni, A., Sadler, J.E., and Wardel, M.R., Platelet glycoprotein Ibα binds to thrombin anion-binding exosite II inducing allosteric changes in the activity of thrombin, *J. Biol. Chem.* 276, 6161–6168, 2001.
220. Takada, H., Kishimoto, C., Hiraoka, Y., et al., Captopril suppresses interstitial fibrin deposition in coxsackievirus B3 myocarditis, *Am. J. Physiol.* 272, H211–H219, 1997.
221. Durham, S.K., Mezza, L.E., and Imamura, T., Pulmonary endothelial and alveolar epithelial lesions induced by O,O,S-trimethyl phosphorothioate in rats, *J. Pathol.* 155, 247–257, 1988.
222. Dvorak, A.M., Costa, J.J., Monahan-Earley, R.A., et al., Ultrastructural analysis of human skin biopsy specimens from patients receiving recombinant human stem cell factor: Subcutaneous injection of rhSCF induces dermal mast cell degranulation and granulocyte recruitment at the injection site, *J. Allergy Clin. Immunol.* 101, 793–806, 1998.
223. Liu, C.Y., Nossel, H.L., and Kaplan, K.L., The binding of thrombin by fibrin, *J. Biol. Chem.* 254, 10421–10425, 1979.
224. Francis, C.W., Markham., R.E., Jr., Barlow, G.H., et al., Thrombin activity of fibrin thrombi and soluble plasmic derivatives, *J. Lab. Clin. Med.* 102, 220–230, 1983.

225. Hogg, P.J., Jackson, C.M., Labanowski, J.K., and Bock, P.E., Binding of fibrin monomer and heparin to thrombin in a ternary complex alters the environment of the thrombin catalytic site, reduces affinity for hirudin, and inhibits cleavage of fibrinogen, *J. Biol. Chem.* 271, 26088–26095, 1996.

226. Kaminski, M. and McDonagh, J., Inhibited thrombins: Interactions with fibrinogen and fibrin, *Biochem. J.* 242, 881–887, 1987.

227. Smadja, D.M., Basire, A., Amelot, A., et al., Thrombin bound to a fibrin clot confers angiogenic and haemostatic properties on endothelial progenitor cells, *J. Cell. Mol. Med.* 12, 975–986, 2008.

228. Lovely, R.S., Moaddel, M., and Farrell, D.H., Fibrinogen γ chain binds thrombin exosite II, *J. Thromb. Haemost.* 1, 124–131, 2003.

229. Kobayashi, H., Gabazza, E.C., Taguchi, O., et al., Protein C anticoagulant system in patients with interstitial lung disease, *Am. J. Respir. Crit. Care Med.* 157, 1850–1854, 1998.

230. Yasui, H., Gabazza, E.C., Taguchi, O., et al., Decreased protein C activation is associated with abnormal collagen turnover in the intraalveolar space of patients with interstitial lung disease, *Clin. Appl. Thromb. Hemost.* 6, 202–205, 2000.

231. Musci, G. and Berliner, L.J., Ligands which effect human protein C activation by thrombin, *J. Biol. Chem.* 262, 13889–13891, 1987.

232. Pekovich, S.R., Bock, P.E., and Hoover, R.L., Thrombin-thrombomodulin activation of protein C facilitates the activation of progelatinase A, *FEBS Lett.* 494, 129–132, 2001.

233. Wiig, H. and Tenstad, O., Interstitial exclusion of positively and negatively charged IgG in rat skin and muscle, *Am. J. Physiol. Heart Circ. Physiol.* 280, H1505–H1512, 2001.

234. Wiig, H., Gyenge, C., Iversen, P.O., et al., The role of the extracellular matrix in tissue distribution of macromolecules in normal and pathological tissues: Potential therapeutic consequences, *Microcirculation* 15, 283–296, 2008.

235. Jacobson, B., Dorfman, T., Basu, P.K., and Hasany, S.M., Inhibition of vascular endothelial cell growth factor and trypsin by vitreous, *Exp. Eye Res.* 41, 581–595, 1985.

236. Rapaport, S.I., Schiffman, S., Patch, M.J., and Ames, S.B., The importance of activation of antihemophilic globulin and proaccelerin by traces of thrombin in the generation of intrinsic prothrombinase activity, *Blood* 21, 221–236, 1963.

237. Lundblad, R.L., Fenton, J.W., II, and Mann, K.G., eds., *Chemistry and Biology of Thrombin*, Ann Arbor Science, Ann Arbor, MI, 1977.

238. Vu, T.K., Hung, D.T., Wheaton, V.I., and Coughin, S.R., Molecular cloning of a functional thrombin receptor reveals a novel proteolytic mechanism of receptor activation, *Cell* 64, 1057–1068, 1991.

239. Aronson, D.L., Comparison of the actions of thrombin and the thrombin-like venom enzymes ancrod and batroxobin, *Thromb. Haemost.* 36, 9–13, 1976.

240. Greenberg, C.S., Achyuthan, K.E., Rajagopalan, S., and Pizzo, S.V., Characterization of the fibrin polymer structure that accelerates thrombin cleavage of plasma factor XIII, *Arch. Biochem. Biophys.* 262, 142–148, 1988.

241. Albeiroti, S., Soroosh, A., and de la Motte, C.A., Hyaluronan's role in fibrosis: A pathogenic factor or a passive player?, *Biomed. Res. Int.* 2015:790203, 2015.

242. Anstee, Q.M., Dhar, A., and Thursz, M.R., The role of hypercoagulability in liver fibrogenesis, *Clin. Res. Hepatol. Gastroenterol.* 35, 526–533, 2011.

243. Tripodi, A., Anstee, Q.M., Sogaard, K.K., et al., Hypercoagulability in cirrhosis: Causes and consequences, *J. Thromb. Haemost.* 9, 1713–1723, 2011.

244. Hewitson, T.D., Martic, M., Kelynack, K.J., et al., Thrombin is a pro-fibrotic factor for rat renal fibroblasts *in vitro*, *Nephron Exp. Nephrol.* 101, e42–e49, 2005.

245. Atanelishvili, I., Liang, J., Akter, T., et al., Thrombin increases lung fibroblasts survival while promoting alveolar epithelial cell apoptosis via the endoplasmic reticulum stress marker CCAAT enhancer–binding homologous protein, *Am. J. Respir. Cell Mol. Biol.* 50, 893–902, 2014.

246. Carney, D.H. and Cunningham, D.D., Role of specific cell surface receptors in thrombin-stimulated cell division, *Cell* 15, 1341–1349, 1978.
247. Chambers, R.C., Dabbagh, K., McAnulty, R.J., et al., Thrombin stimulates fibroblast procollagen production via proteolytic activation of protease-activated receptor 1, *Biochem. J.* 333, 121–127, 1998.
248. Ortiz-Stern, A., Deng, X., Smoktunowicz, N., et al., PAR-1-dependent and PAR-independent pro-inflammatory signaling in human lung fibroblasts exposed to thrombin, *J. Cell. Physiol.* 227, 3575–3584, 2012.
249. Van Obberghen-Schilling, E. and Pouysségur, J., Affinity labeling of high affinity α-thrombin binding sites on the surface of hamster fibroblasts, *Biochim. Biophys. Acta* 847, 335–343, 1985.
250. Lechtenberg, B.C., Freund, S.M., and Huntington, J.A., GpIbα interacts exclusively with exosite II of thrombin, *J. Mol. Biol.* 426, 881–893, 2014.
251. Wygrecka, M., Didiasova, M., Berscheid, S., et al., Protease-activated receptors (PAR)-1 and -3 drive epithelial-mesenchymal transition of alveolar epithelial cells: Potential role in lung fibrosis, *Thromb. Haemost.* 110, 295–307, 2013.
252. Bachhuber, B.G., Sarembock, I.J., Gimple, L.W., et al., Thrombin-induced mitogenesis in cultured aortic smooth muscle cells requires prolonged thrombin exposure, *Am. J. Physiol.* 268, C1141–1147, 1995.
253. Clarke, D.L., Carruthers, A.M., Mustelin, T., and Murray, L.A., Matrix regulation of idiopathic pulmonary fibrosis: The role of enzymes, *Fibrogenesis Tissue Repair* 6(1), 20, 2013.
254. Fang, Q., Liu, X., Al-Mugotir, M., et al., Thrombin and TNF-α/IL-1β synergistically induce fibroblast-mediated collagen gel degradation, *Am. J. Respir. Cell Mol. Biol.* 35, 714–721, 2006.
255. Sumitomo-Udea, Y., Aihara, K., Ise, T., et al., Heparin cofactor II protects against angiotensin II–induced cardiac remodeling via attenuation of oxidative stress in mice, *Hypertension* 56, 430–436, 2010.
256. Chang, C.-J., Hsu, L.-A., Ko, Y.-H., et al., Thrombin regulates matrix metalloproteinase-9 expression in human monocytes, *Biochem. Biophys. Res. Commun.* 385, 241–246, 2009.
257. Mogami, H., Keller, P.W., Shi, H., and Word, R.A., Effect of thrombin on human amnion mesenchymal cells, mouse fetal membranes, and preterm birth, *J. Biol. Chem.* 289, 13295–13307, 2014.
258. Favreau, F., Thuillier, R., Cau, J., et al., Anti-thrombin therapy during warm ischemia and cold preservation prevents chronic kidney graft fibrosis in a DCD model, *Am. J. Transplant.* 10, 30–39, 2010.
259. Eriksson, H., Eriksson, U.G., Frison, L., et al., Pharmacokinetics and pharmacodynamics of melagatran, a novel synthetic LMW thrombin inhibitor, in patients with acute DVT, *Thromb. Haemost.* 81, 358–363, 1999.
260. Hopfner, R., Ximelagatran (AstraZeneca), *Curr. Opin. Investig. Drugs* 3, 246–251, 2002.
261. Bogatkevich, G.S., Ludwicka-Bradley, A., Nietert, P.J., et al., Antiinflammatory and antifibrotic effects of the oral direct thrombin inhibitor dabigatran etexilate in a murine model of interstitial lung disease, *Arthritis Rheum.* 63, 1416–1425, 2011.
262. Sanford, M. and Plosker, G.L., Dabigatran etexilate, *Drugs* 68, 1699–1709, 2008.
263. van Ryn, J., Stangier, J., Haertter, S., et al., Dabigatran etexilate: A novel, reversible, oral direct thrombin inhibitor; Interpretation of coagulation assays and reversal of anticoagulant activity, *Thromb. Haemost.* 103, 1116–1127, 2010.
264. Wygrecka, M., Jablonska, E., Guenther, A., et al., Current view on alveolar coagulation and fibrinolysis in acute inflammatory and chronic interstitial lung disease, *Thromb. Haemost.* 99, 494–501, 2008.
265. Schneider, D.J., Potential contribution of pleiotropic effects of direct anticoagulants to clinical benefits, *Drug Develop. Res.* 74, 472–477, 2013.

9 Protease Inhibitors in the Interstitial Space

9.1 PROTEOLYTIC REGULATION IN INTERSTITIAL SPACE

Proteolysis is an active process in the interstitial space. Activities range from digestive, as in the remodeling of tissues by the various matrix metalloproteinases (MMPs), to regulatory, as demonstrated in the action of enzymes such as thrombin, hepsin, and matriptase in the control of physiological processes. The activity of these various enzymes is controlled by the expression of activity, such as the surface expression of MMP-14 and other membrane-type matrix metalloproteinases (MT-MMPs), by the conversion of zymogen forms into active enzymes, such as the activation of prostasin by matriptase, and by inactivation with protein proteinase inhibitors, such as serine proteinase inhibitors (serpins).

This chapter is focused on a consideration of protease inhibitors that may regulate proteolysis in the interstitial space. It is acknowledged that there are few real data to support the activity of serpins in the interstitial space, and while some of the protease inhibitors may have important functions in the interstitial space, other inhibitors may not be significant. Several protease inhibitors are pleiotropic and their "off-label" activities may be more important than their canonical functions as protease inhibitors. These off-label activities may depend on a conformational change in the inhibitor, resulting in a stable conformer. Some protease inhibitors considered to be of importance in the interstitial space are shown in Table 9.1.

We acknowledge that the coverage of protease inhibitors in this section is limited. Some inhibitors, most notably tissue inhibitors of metalloproteinases (TIMPs), are discussed in Chapters 4 and 7. As discussed in Chapter 4, there are several mechanisms for the control of proteases in the interstitial space and it is our sense that protein protease inhibitors may be a minor part of the overall control process.

9.2 ANTITHROMBIN

Antithrombin (serpinC1) is considered to be the most important inhibitor of thrombin and other coagulation proteases in the circulation. As with other serpins, antithrombin is a metastable protein that assumes a more stable conformation on the binding of a target protease. Antithrombin was originally described as antithrombin III to distinguish the protein from other thrombin regulatory factors, such as antithrombin I (the binding of thrombin) and antithrombin II (heparin cofactor II). The rate of reaction of antithrombin with thrombin and other coagulation proteases is enhanced by the presence of heparin *in vitro*, while *in vivo* acceleration is provided by heparan sulfate on the luminal surface. The mechanism for rate enhancement with heparin differs depending on the proteases. Heparin appears to orient thrombin

TABLE 9.1
Protease Inhibitors of Importance in Interstitial Space

Inhibitor	Target Proteinase	Reference
α$_1$-Antitrypsin (alpha-1 proteinase inhibitor)	α$_1$-Antitrypsin is a serine protease inhibitor (serpin), best known for its role in the control of neutrophil elastase in the pulmonary interstitial space.[1,2] Native α$_1$-antitrypsin is associated with immune modulating effects.[3] α$_1$-Antitrypsin can assume a latent conformation, but the assumption of the latent conformation does not confer any new biological activities.	1–3
α$_2$-Macroglobulin	α$_2$-Macroglobulin is a broad-spectrum protease inhibitor. It is a large protein composed of two or four 180 kDa subunits and differs from serpins in that inhibition is based on entrapping the protease after cleavage of a bait region.[4] The action of proteases on the bait region or reaction with surrogate methylamine results in the conformational change of α$_2$-macroglobulin, which entraps the protein; this is also described as *activation*, which causes a change in the binding properties of the protein.[6] Both native and activated α$_2$-macroglobulin bind cytokines and cells.[6]	4–6
Antithrombin and latent antithrombin	The most significant inhibitor of coagulation proteases in the interstitial space. Activity is enhanced by binding to heparan sulfate proteoglycans in the ECM.[7] Latent antithrombin, which has reduced ability to inhibit thrombin, has potent antiangiogenic activity depending on the heparin-binding site and possibly involves interaction with perlecan in the BM.[8] While the reaction with thrombin can be inferred, evidence is only available for inhibition of matriptase.[9]	7–9
Heparin cofactor II	Heparin cofactor II is considered to be the major extravascular inhibitor of thrombin[10] but has seen more recent investigation into its effects on cell function.[11–13]	10–13
Hepatocyte growth factor activator inhibitor type 1 (HAI-1)	HAI-1 is a Kunitz-type membrane-bound serine protease inhibitor[14] that can inhibit several interstitial proteases including hepsin, HGF activator, and matriptase.[15] HAI-1 contains two Kunitz domains.[16] HAI-1 ectodomain is shed into the extracellular/pericellular space in two forms, one with one Kunitz domain and one with two Kunitz domains.[15]	14–16
Pigment epithelium–derived factor (PEDF)	Sequence homology supports PEDF as a member of the serpin gene family but lacks the canonical sequence necessary for protease inhibition.[17] PEDF has antiangiogenic and antitumor effects.[18] PEDF does not inhibit the catalytic activity of membrane type-1 matrix metalloproteinase (MT1-MMP; MMP-14), but does downregulate the surface expression of the enzyme.[19]	17–19
Plasminogen activator inhibitor 1 (PAI-1)	PAI-1 is the primary inhibitor of uPA and tPA.[20] PAI-1 also interacts with cells via interaction with vitronectin[20] as well as LPR-1.[21] As with other serpins, PAI-1 can assume a latent conformation but without unique biological activity.[22]	20–22

TABLE 9.1 (CONTINUED)
Protease Inhibitors of Importance in Interstitial Space

Inhibitor	Target Proteinase	Reference
Protease nexin 1	Protease nexin 1 may be the most potent inhibitor of thrombin.[10] Protease nexin 1 is a cell surface protein found on fibroblasts[23,24] and other cells such as vascular smooth muscle and endothelial cells. The reaction of protease nexin 1 with thrombin is accelerated by heparan sulfate proteoglycan.[25]	10,23–25
Protease nexin 2	Protease nexin 2 is the secreted form of amyloid precursor protein, which contains a Kunitz domain, providing the ability to be a potent inhibitor of serine proteases, including factor Xia and trypsin.[26] The secreted amyloid precursor proteins are secreted by a number of cell types, including platelets.[26] The Kunitz domain may be cleaved by mesotrypsin, resulting in a loss of the ability to inhibit proteases.[27]	26,27
Tissue inhibitors of metalloproteinases (TIMPs)	There are four TIMPs, 1–4, which were originally described as *inhibitors of matrix metalloproteinases* but have also been shown to inhibit ADAM and ADAMTS proteases.[28] TIMPS are relatively small proteins with a molecular mass in the range of 20–23 kDa. TIMPs are considered to function in the regulation of the degradation of the ECM; the specific function of an individual TIMP depends on tissue.[29] TIMPs form a stoichiometric complex with MMPs, with K_i constants in the nanomolar to micromolar range.[30] TIMPs may also form complexes with proenzymes and may play a role in activation of the proenzyme.[31]	28–31

REFERENCES TO TABLE 9.1

1. Ohlsson, K., Fryksmark, U., Ohlsson, M., and Tegner, H., Interaction of granulocyte proteases with inhibitors in pulmonary diseases, *Adv. Exp. Med. Biol.* 167, 299–312, 1984.
2. Garratt, L.W., Sutanto, E.N., Ling, K.M., et al., Alpha1-antitrypsin mitigates the inhibition of airway epithelial cell repair by neutrophil elastase, *Am. J. Respir. Cell Mol. Biol.* 54, 341–349, 2016.
3. Ehlers, M.R., Immune-modulating effects of alpha-1 antitrypsin, *Biol. Chem.* 395, 1187–1193, 2014.
4. Barrett, A.J. and Starkey, P.M., The interaction of α_2-macroglobulin with proteinases: Characteristics and specificity of the reaction and a hypothesis concerning its molecular mechanisms, *Ann. N.Y. Acad. Sci.* 133, 709–724, 1973.
5. Gonias, S.L., Reynolds, J.A., and Pizzo, S.V., Physical properties of human α_2-macroglobulin following reaction with methylamine and trypsin, *Biochim. Biophys. Acta* 705, 306–314, 1982.
6. Hart, J.E. and Pizzo, S.V., α_2-Macroglobullin, in *Thrombosis and Hemostasis: Basic Principles and Clinical Practice*, 5th edn., eds. R.W. Colman, V.J. Marder, A.N. Clowes, J.N. George, and S.Z. Goldhaber, Chapter 21, pp. 395–421, Lippincott, Williams & Wilkins, Philadelphia, PA, 2006.

7. Mertens, G., Cassiman, J.J., Van den Berghe, H., Vermylen, J., and David, G., Cell surface heparan sulfate proteoglycans from human vascular endothelial cells: Core protein characterization and antithrombin III binding properties, *J. Biol. Chem.* 267, 20435–20443, 1992.

8. Zhang, W., Swanson, R., Izaquirre, G., et al., The heparin-binding site of antithrombin is crucial for antiangiogenic activity, *Blood* 106, 1621–1628 2005.

9. Chen, Y.W., Xu, Z., Baksh, A.N., et al., Antithrombin regulates matriptase activity involved in plasmin generation, syndecan shedding, and HGF activation in keratinocytes, *PLoS One* 8(5), e62826, 2013.

10. Huntington, J.A., Thrombin inhibition by the serpins, *J. Thromb. Haemost.* 11(Suppl. 1), 254–264, 2013.

11. Ikeda, Y., Aihara, K., Yoshida, S., et al., Heparin cofactor II, a serine protease inhibitor, promotes angiogenesis via activation of the AMP-activated protein kinase-endothelial nitric oxide synthase signaling pathway, *J. Biol. Chem.* 287, 34256–34263, 2012.

12. Kalle, M., Papareddy, P., Kasetty, G., et al., A peptide of heparin cofactor II inhibits endotoxin-mediated shock and invasive *Pseudomonas aeruginosa* infection, *PLoS One* 9(7), e102577, 2014.

13. Liao, W.Y., Ho, C.C., Hou., H.H., et al., Heparin co-factor II enhances cell motility and promotes metastasis in non-small cell lung cancer, *J. Pathol.* 235, 50–64, 2015.

14. Kataoka, H., Suganuma, T., Shimomura, T., et al., Distribution of hepatocyte growth factor activator inhibitor type 1 (HAI-1) in human tissues: Cellular surface localization of HAI-1 in simple columnar epithelium and its modulated expression in injured and regenerative tissues, *J. Histochem. Cytochem.* 47, 673–682, 1999.

15. Kato, M., Hashimoto, T., Shimomura, T., et al., Hepatocyte growth factor activator inhibitor type 1 inhibits protease activity and proteolytic activation of human airway trypsin-like protease, *J. Biochem.* 151, 179–187, 2012.

16. Denda, K., Shimomura, T., Kawaguchi, T., et al., Functional characterization of Kunitz domains in hepatocyte growth factor activator inhibitor type 1, *J. Biol. Chem.* 277, 14053–14059, 2002.

17. Steele, F.R., Chader, G.J., Johnson, L.V., and Tombran-Tink, J., Pigment epithelium-derived factor: Neurotropic activity and identification as a member of the serine protease gene family, *Proc. Natl. Acad. Sci. USA* 90, 1526–1530, 1993.

18. Ladhani, O., Sánchez-Martinez, C., Orgaz, J.L., Jimenez, B., and Volpert, O.V., Pigment epithelium-derived factor blocks tumor extravasation by suppressing amoeboid morphology and mesenchymal proteolysis, *Neoplasia* 13, 633–642, 2011.

19. Alcantara, M.B. and Dass, C.R., Pigment epithelium-derived factor as a natural matrix metalloproteinase inhibitor: A comparison with classic matrix metalloproteinase inhibitors used for cancer treatment, *J. Pharm. Pharmacol.* 66, 895–902, 2014.

20. Wind, T., Hansen, M., Jensen, J.K., and Andreasen, P.A., The molecular basis for anti-proteolytic and non-proteolytic functions of plasminogen activator inhibitor type-1: Roles of the reactive centre loop, the shutter region, the flexible joint region and the small serpin fragment, *Biol. Chem.* 383, 21–36, 2002.

21. Koziova, N., Jensen, J.K., Chi, T.F., Samoylenko, A., and Kietzmann, T., PAI-1 modulates cell migration in a LRP1-dependent manner via β-catenin and ERK1/2, *Thromb. Haemost.* 113, 988–998, 2015.

22. Sprang, S.R., The latent tendencies of PAI-1, *Trends Biochem. Sci.* 17, 49–50, 1992.

23. Wagner, S.L., Lau, A.L., and Cunningham, D.D., Binding of protease nexin-1 to the fibroblast surface alters its target proteinase specificity, *J. Biol. Chem.* 264, 611–615, 1989.

24. Francois, D., Venisse, L., Marchal-Somme, J., et al., Increased expression of protease nexin-1 in fibroblasts during idiopathic pulmonary fibrosis regulates thrombin activity and fibronectin expression, *Lab. Invest.* 94, 1237–1246, 2014.

25. Hiramoto, S.A. and Cunningham, D.D., Effects of fibroblasts and endothelial cells on inactivation of target proteases by protease nexin-1, heparin cofactor II, and C1-inhibitor, *J. Cell. Biochem.* 36, 199–207, 1988.
26. Navaneetham, D., Sinha, D., and Walsh, P.N., Mechanisms and specificity of factor Xia and trypsin inhibition by protease nexin 2 and basic pancreatic trypsin inhibitor, *J. Biochem.* 148, 467–479, 2010.
27. Salamen, M.A., Robinson, J.L., Navaneetham, D., et al., The amyloid precursor protein protease nexin 2 Kunitz inhibitor is a highly specific substrate of mesotrypsin, *J. Biol. Chem.* 285, 1939–1949, 2010.
28. Brew, K. and Nagase, H., The tissue inhibitors of metalloproteinases (TIMPs): An ancient family with structural and functional diversity, *Biochim. Biophys. Acta* 1803, 55–71, 2010.
29. Arpino, V., Brock, M., and Gill, S.E., The role of TIMPs in regulation of extracellular matrix proteolysis, *Matrix Biol.* 44–46, 247–254, 2015.
30. Olson, M.W., Gervasi, D.C., Mobashery, S., and Fridman, R., Kinetic analysis of the binding of human matrix metalloproteinase-2 and -9 to tissue inhibitor of metalloproteinase (TIMP)-1 and TIMP-2, *J. Biol. Chem.* 272, 29975–29983, 1997.
31. Overall, C.M., Tam, E., McQuibban, G.A., et al., Domain interactions in the gelatinase A TIMP-2 MT1-MMP activation complex: The ectodomain of the 44-kDa form of membrane type-1 matrix metalloproteinase does not modulate gelatinase A activation, *J. Biol. Chem.* 275, 39497–39506, 2000.

and antithrombin, while causing a conformational change in the reaction with factor Xa. In the case of heparan sulfate proteoglycan, which is bound to the cell surface, antithrombin is bound to heparin sulfate proteoglycan, where it reacts with the target protease. Heparan sulfate proteoglycan is also found on the subluminal membrane and, in the case of the epidermal basement membrane (BM), the heparan sulfate chains are integrated with the collagen IV matrix.[1] The rate of reaction of antithrombin with thrombin can also be enhanced by other sulfated proteoglycans such as dermatan sulfate and chondroitin sulfate, both of which are found in the extracellular matrix (ECM). However, dermatan sulfate and chondroitin sulfate are more effective in enhancing the rate of inactivation of thrombin by heparin cofactor II. Biglycan and decorin, two smaller dermatan sulfate–containing proteoglycans present in the ECM, also accelerate the inactivation of thrombin by heparin cofactor II.[2] The combination of heparin cofactor II and biglycan or decorin provides a thromboresistant surface. Biglycan or decorin do not stimulate the inactivation of thrombin by antithrombin. Thrombin enhances biglycan synthesis by cardiac fibroblasts.[3] Both dermatan sulfate and chondroitin sulfate are important in the binding of growth factors and neurotropic factors.[4] Both low- and high-molecular-weight dextran sulfate accelerate the activation of plasminogen by either tissue plasminogen activator (tPA) or urokinase-type plasminogen activator (uPA).[5]

Antithrombin has been found in kidney with the use of immunohistochemical techniques.[6,7] It was not possible to demonstrate the presence of interstitial antithrombin, but there was considerable reactivity in proximal tubule epithelial cells. Immunofluorescence techniques demonstrated the presence of antithrombin on the BM consistent with the binding of antithrombin to heparan sulfate proteoglycan, which is present in the BM.[6] Xu and Slayter[7] found immunoreactive antithrombin in variable amounts in the subluminal (subendothelial) space of various tissues. The highest concentration was found in kidney, with lesser amounts in other tissues. Antithrombin appears to be associated with the basal lamina. Pretreatment of tissue sections with heparanase resulted in the loss of immunoreactive antithrombin. Antithrombin binds to heparan sulfate proteoglycans with nanomolar avidity. In addition to providing a thromboresistant surface, the binding of antithrombin to heparan sulfate proteoglycan provides a storage mechanism for antithrombin.

Heparan sulfate proteoglycan is present in the BM. Giradin and coworkers[8] used fluorescent-labeled antithrombin to demonstrate the presence of heparan sulfate proteoglycan in glomerular BM. They observed that antithrombin binds to heparan sulfate proteoglycan with loss of the heparin-binding site. These investigators also suggested that the presence of antithrombin bound to heparan sulfate proteoglycan provides a thromboresistant surface for plasma proteins passing through the glomerular endothelium.

While antithrombin passes rapidly from the vascular bed into the interstitial space,[9] basolateral secretion of antithrombin in MDCK cells has been observed.[10] Vogel and coworkers observed that there were equivalent amounts of antithrombin and plasminogen activator inhibitor (PAI)-1 in apical and basolateral secretion. This differed from other serpins such as α_1-antitrypsin, which exhibit predominant apical secretion. In subsequent work, Vogel and coworkers[11] showed that replacement of the amino-terminal sequence of antithrombin with that from α_1-antitrypsin resulted in predominantly apical secretion of the mutant protein.

Hedin and Hahn[9] showed that 75% of the antithrombin in infused plasma was present in the extravascular space within 8 hours of administration. There is more extravasation of antithrombin in some clinical situations,[12] which can result in acquired antithrombin deficiency.[13] The concentration of antithrombin in interstitial fluid, based on immunological measurements in lymph, is approximately 60% of that in plasma.[14] This is based on immunoassay and may not be representative of the level of functional antithrombin. Much of the antithrombin may be bound with the ECM and not available for assay in solution; it is recognized that the antithrombin bound to heparan sulfate proteoglycan may be the functional anticoagulant in the interstitial space. Chang and coworkers[15] have reported that hyaluronic acid inhibits the activity of antithrombin in the presence of calcium ions and ferric ions. These investigators also observed that chondroitin sulfate A, B, and C also inhibited the inactivation of thrombin by antithrombin but to a lesser extent than hyaluronic acid.

While best known for the inhibition of coagulation proteases, antithrombin does inhibit other proteases, such as soluble matriptase. Matriptase is a class-II transmembrane serine protease and a member of the MEROPS peptidase family. Matriptase is thought to be involved in the maintenance of epithelial barrier function. Matriptase is derived from a membrane-bound single-chain zymogen form, which is converted into a two-chain active enzyme by a process of transactivation involving the interaction of two zymogen forms, leading to proteolysis beyond the prodomain.[16,17] Transproteolysis is also suggested to be involved in the release of the two-chain matriptase from the cell surface.[17] Platelet-derived growth factor D (PDGF-D) induces extracellular acidification, enhancing the matriptase activation of release from the cell surface.[18] Matriptase bound to the cell surface has been suggested to be the initiating factor in functional cascades in epithelial cells.[19] Ovaere and coworkers[19] suggest that matriptase activates prostasin, which in turn activates the epithelial Na+ channel, initiating an intracellular process resulting in the formation of filaggrin from profilaggrin. Filaggrin binds to keratin in the process of cornification.[20] The activity of membrane-bound matriptase in the activation of prostasin is regulated by hepatocyte growth factor activator inhibitor (HAI)-1.[21,22] HAI-1 is a membrane-bound serine proteinase inhibitor containing two Kunitz domains, which are vital to the inhibition of matriptase, trypsin, hepsin, and other proteases.[23] Matriptase also activates epidermal prokallikrein in a process that may be important in skin pathology.[24,25] Chou and coworkers[26] showed that soluble matriptase is inhibited by antithrombin in a reaction that is stimulated by the presence of heparin. Tseng and coworkers[27] had previously demonstrated the presence of a matriptase–antithrombin complex in human milk. Antithrombin appears to have a role in the modulation of matriptase activity in plasminogen activation, syndecan shedding, and hepatocyte growth factor (HGF) activation in the pericellular space around keratinocytes. Soluble matriptase also processes platelet-derived growth factor C.[28]

It has been known for some time that factor IX is bound to collagen IV in the BM.[29] More recent work demonstrates that antithrombin bound to heparan sulfate proteoglycan colocalizes with factor IX in the BM.[30]

Surprisingly, there is little work on the pleiotropic function of antithrombin in the interstitial space. Presumably, the anticoagulant function provides for homeostasis in the interstitial space and the lymphatics. Loss of this anticoagulant function may result in fibrosis. We could not find any studies addressing the effect of antithrombin deficiency and fibrotic disease. The use of dabigatran etexilate, a synthetic thrombin inhibitor, has an antifibrotic effect in a murine model.[31]

Totzke and coworkers[32] have shown that antithrombin influences the regulated release of tumor necrosis factor (TNF)-α and IL-1β from vascular smooth muscle cells. At supranormal concentrations (540 U/mL), antithrombin inhibited the lipopolysaccharide (LPS)-induced synthesis of TNF-α and IL-1β in vascular smooth muscle cells, while at lower concentrations (0.5, 1.0 U/mL), a modest stimulation of TNF-α synthesis was observed with an LPS challenge. Similar results were obtained with Trp[49]-antithrombin, a modified antithrombin that does not bind to glycosaminoglycans.[33,34] These results suggest that antithrombin has an anti-inflammatory effect unrelated to its anticoagulant activity. This group[35] also showed that antithrombin stimulates regulated (inducible) nitric oxide synthase expression in vascular smooth muscle cells in the presence of IL-1β or LPS in combination with interferon-γ. Antithrombin inhibits LPS-induced TNF-α production by monocytes.[36] Roemisch and coworkers[37] have presented a review of the nonanticoagulant actions of antithrombin, including anti-inflammatory activity unrelated to the inhibition of coagulation proteases.

9.3 LATENT ANTITHROMBIN

Antithrombin is a metastable protein that, while stable, can transition to a more stable form upon perturbation. In its function as an anticoagulant, a more stable state is achieved on binding a target protease such as thrombin. Antithrombin can also be found in a latent form that is stable and lacks anticoagulant activity.[38] Carrell and coworkers[38] produced a latent form of antithrombin by treatment with 0.9 M guanidine hydrochloride; this form of antithrombin showed reduced affinity for heparin and was inactive as an anticoagulant. Subsequent work by Wardell and coworkers[39] demonstrated the presence of a latent antithrombin in crystallization studies under mild conditions (18% PEG-4000). Subsequently, latent antithrombin has been found in commercial antithrombin concentrates obtained from human plasma.[40] Other studies have shown low levels of latent antithrombin in blood, perhaps reflecting rapid clearance, as observed for enzyme–serpin complexes.[41] Latent antithrombin has also been shown to be present in a recombinant DNA preparation.[42]

Latent antithrombin appeared to be an interesting laboratory observation until 1999, when work from Folkman's laboratory at Harvard University[43] showed that latent antithrombin had antiangiogenic activity. Antithrombin that had been subjected to proteolysis (cleaved antithrombin) also inhibited angiogenesis. Subsequent work from Folkman's laboratory showed that both latent antithrombin and cleaved latent antithrombin could be produced from systemically available antithrombin.[44] Subsequent work by Larsson and coworkers[45] showed that latent antithrombin inhibited fibroblast growth factor (FGF)-stimulated angiogenesis in a chick embryo system. These investigators also showed that latent antithrombin could induce apoptosis in endothelial cells by disrupting cell–matrix interactions. Other work[46] showed that latent antithrombin (antiangiogenic antithrombin) inhibited the expression of perlecan, a heparan sulfate proteoglycan, on endothelial cells. Zhang and coworkers[47] showed that latent and native antithrombin had differential binding characteristics to heparan sulfate proteoglycan. O'Reilly[48] has reviewed antiangiogenic antithrombin. It is suggested that latent antithrombin, either binding directly to endothelial cells or via binding to perlecan, reduces the ability of basic fibroblast growth factor (bFGF) or vascular endothelial growth factor (VEGF) to stimulate angiogenesis. Latent antithrombin inhibits the growth of neuroblastoma and lung carcinoma tumors.[49] A prelatent form of antithrombin has been described[50] that is suggested to have enhanced antiangiogenic activity. Latent antithrombin is described as *denatured* or *partially denatured* antithrombin; the terms *conformer* or *conformationally altered* would be preferable.

Somewhat, if not completely, ignored in the discussion of latent antithrombin is that its activity is most likely manifested in the interstitial space. Latent antithrombin is said to influence the expression of perlecan by endothelial cells.[46] Perlecan is a component of the BM of endothelial cells. There is considerable antithrombin in the interstitial space that is thought to be bound to heparan sulfate proteoglycans in the BM, providing a thromboresistant surface (see Section 9.2). However, this is assuming that such can be extrapolated from measurements in lymph. Miller and coworkers[51] measured immunologically reactive antithrombin in human peripheral lymph; the concentration of antithrombin antigen in lymph was 65% that of plasma. Li and coworkers[52] found there was a higher concentration of immunologically reactive antithrombin in peripheral rabbit lymph than that of biologically active antithrombin; the difference in concentrations is statistically significant. These investigators also found low levels of factor Xa–antithrombin complex. It is possible to speculate that the difference between antigenically active antithrombin and biologically active antithrombin reflects the presence of latent antithrombin in peripheral lymph, and that lymph is the source of latent antithrombin in the circulation. It has been suggested that there is steady-state formation of latent antithrombin in plasma[53] and that latent antithrombin is cleared at the same rate as the native protein.[53,54] Corral and coworkers[54] have reported that the clearance of a polymeric form of antithrombin slowed that either native or latent antithrombin.

It is possible to suggest that the low levels of latent antithrombin in the circulation are formed in the interstitial space and pass into the lymphatics and hence to the vascular bed. It is possible to further speculate that the transition from native antithrombin to latent antithrombin reflects its interaction with hyaluronan. In this model, there would be substantial amounts of latent antithrombin in the interstitial space. If the foregoing hypothesis is correct, there will be substantial amounts of latent antithrombin in the interstitial space in contact with BM heparan sulfate proteoglycan, which would block angiogenesis.

9.4   PLASMINOGEN ACTIVATOR INHIBITOR 1

PAI-1 (serpinE1) is a primary inhibitor of uPA and tPA in the interstitial space (Chapter 5); it is another serpin that assumes a latent conformation similar to that of antithrombin.[55–58] However, unlike latent antithrombin, latent PAI-1 does not have biological activity that is not seen with the native protein.[59] Kamikbubo and coworkers[59] showed that all forms of PAI-1, native, latent, and cleaved, are able to activate Janus kinase (JAK) and cell migration by binding to the low-density lipoprotein receptor–related protein (LPR). Binding of PAI-1 to vitronectin suppresses the effect on JAK and cell migration. The binding of PAI-1 to vitronectin suppresses the transition to the latent form.[60] Binding of PAI-1 to vitronectin enhances the ability of PAI-1 to inhibit thrombin[61] and is associated with antiadhesive qualities.[62] Latent PAI-1 does not form a complex with vitronectin.[63] The pleiotropic effects of PAI-1 have been reviewed by Lijnen.[64]

9.5 α_1-ANTITRYPSIN

α_1-Antitrypsin (serpinA1) is the serpin with the highest concentration in the circulation. It is also present in the interstitial space, inferred from measurements in lymph;[30] differing from antithrombin and PAI-1, secretion of α_1-antitrypsin is apical, precluding significant basolateral secretion. Basolateral secretion of α_1-antitrypsin was observed after the transfection of human respiratory epithelial cells with α_1-antiproteinase cDNA.[65]

A survey of the literature failed to show measurements of α_1-antitrypsin other than that reported by Miller.[51] α_1-Antitrypsin and inhibitor complexes have been measured in other extravascular fluids such as synovial fluid.[66] α_1-Antitrypsin is also referred to as α_1-*proteinase inhibitor* to reflect its likely primary function in the inhibition of other proteases, most notably neutrophil elastase. The aerosol application of α_1-antitrypsin into the lung results in its transfer from the epithelial surface into the pulmonary interstititum.[67,68] α_1-Antitrypsin inhibits matriptase, a membrane-bound serine proteinase.[69] Oxidized α_1-antitrypsin does not inactivate matriptase. α_1-Antitrypsin forms a latent conformation by incubation at high temperature (67°C) for 12 hours;[70] the latent conformation is no longer active as an inhibitor. Latent α_1-antitrypsin is also present in therapeutic concentrates of α_1-antitrypsin.[71]

Separate from its role in protease inactivation, α_1-antitrypsin might be important in regulating the activity of cells in the interstitial space. It is not clear whether latent α_1-antitrypsin is active or whether the activity is unique to the native protein or other derivative forms (Table 9.2). Katooka and coworkers[72] reviewed the pleiotropic activities of α_1-antitrypsin.

9.6   HEPARIN COFACTOR II

Heparin cofactor II (originally described as antithrombin II)[73] is considered to be the major extracellular inhibitor of thrombin. The bulk of heparin cofactor II is found in the extracellular space, but there is little direct evidence to suggest a critical role in the inhibition of thrombin in the interstitial space. It can be assumed that heparin cofactor II is bound to heparin sulfate proteoglycans in the ECM. ECM proteoglycans such as dermatan sulfate are important in enhancing the rate of reaction of heparin cofactor II with thrombin and other target proteases.[74,75] However, recent work has demonstrated that heparin cofactor II is degraded upon binding to the heparan sulfate proteoglycan.[76] Antithrombin and pigment epithelium–derived factor were also degraded by heparan sulfate proteoglycans. While dextran sulfate also degraded heparin cofactor II, other glycosaminoglycans were ineffective, including hyaluronan, a major constituent of the interstitial space. The reaction of heparan sulfate proteoglycan with heparin cofactor II and other proteins was performed at pH 8.5 at 55°C, so the physiological significance could be questioned. However, if heparin factor II is bound to a heparan sulfate proteoglycan in the BM, removal from bulk solution could enhance the rate of degradation. The degraded heparin cofactor II lost the ability to inhibit thrombin, but derivative activities were not examined. As with other proteases, heparin cofactor II and its derivative fragments have activities other than the inhibition of proteases. It is assumed that these various activities will be largely confined to the interstitial space. Some of these activities are listed in Table 9.3.

9.7 α_2-MACROGLOBULIN

The presence of α_2-macroglobulin in interstitial fluid has been documented by other investigators.[77–79] The concentration of α_2-macroglobulin in interstitial fluid is approximately 20% that of plasma, with the concentration elevated during inflammation.[78] The size of α_2-macroglobulin[80] presents challenges to extravasation, but there are a number of sites of synthesis including fibroblasts and macrophages.[81] There is significant synthesis of α_2-macroglobulin in astrocytes,[82–85] providing an extravascular source of synthesis within the brain. While α_2-macroglobulin is a protease inhibitor with broad specificity, it seems likely that it is an inhibitor secondary to serpins in functional importance. α_2-Macroglobulin would appear to be far more important as a transporter of cytokines and growth factors[86,87] and there are differences in binding specificity between native α_2-macroglobulin and *activated* α_2-macroglobulin.[88] Activated α_2-macroglobulin refers to a form that has been cleaved in the bait region,

TABLE 9.2
Pleiotropic Activities for α_1-Antitrypsin

Cell	Effect	Reference
Human primary monocytes	α_1-Antitrypsin oxidized with N-chlorosuccinimide (active-site methionine) activates monocytes, as shown by an upregulation of reactive oxygen species production, inducing the release of monocyte chemotactic protein (MCP)-1 and proinflammatory cytokines.[1] C-36 peptide, a C-terminal fragment of α_1-antitrypsin comprising residues 359 to 394, has been shown to stimulate human monocytes in a manner similar to LPS activation.[1a]	1,2
Fibroblast	α_1-Antitrypsin stimulates procollagen production in fibroblasts. α_1-Antitrypsin also stimulates fibroblast proliferation in a process independent of the procollagen production. It is suggested that stimulation of fibroblasts by α_1-antitrypsin is important in tissue repair by ECM production. It is also suggested that α_1-antitrypsin stimulation of fibroblasts might be involved in the development of liver fibrosis.	3
Neutrophils	C-36, a peptide derived from α_1-antitrypsin by proteolysis of the Met–Ser peptide bond at the reactive site, has been shown to produce a proinflammatory response in neutrophils, including neutrophil chemotaxis, adhesion, degranulation, and reactive oxygen (superoxide) production. Native α_1-antitrypsin does not elicit a proinflammatory response in neutrophils.[3] Earlier work had shown that α_1-antitrypsins degraded by macrophage elastase[4] and the complex of α_1-antitrypsin with human leukocyte elastase[5] were potent chemoattractants for neutrophils. In both cases, the activity was due to a 4.2 kDa peptide derived from cleavage in the vicinity of Met^{358}. However, while the free peptide has activity, the peptide remains bound to the parent α_1-antitrypsin under physiological conditions.	4–6

REFERENCES TO TABLE 9.2

1. Moraga, F. and Janciauskiene, S., Activation of primary human monocytes by the oxidized form of α_1-antitrypsin, *J. Biol. Chem.* 275, 7693–7700, 2000.
2. Subramaniyam, D., Glader, P., von Wachenfeldt, K., et al., C-36 peptide, a degradation product of α_1-antitrypsin, modulates human monocyte activation through LPS signaling pathways, *Int. J. Biochem. Cell Biol.* 38, 563–575, 2006.
3. Dabbagh, K., Laurent, G.J., Shock, A., et al., Alpha-1-antitrypsin stimulates fibroblast proliferation and procollagen production and activates classical MAP kinase signaling pathways, *J. Cell Physiol.* 186, 73–81, 2001.
4. Janciauskiene, S., Zeluyte, I., Jansson, L., and Stevens, T., Divergent effects of α_1-antitrypsin, *Biochem. Biophys. Res. Commun.* 315, 288–296, 2004.
5. Banda, M.J., Rice, A.G., Griffin, G.L., and Senior, R.M., α_1-proteinase inhibitor is a neutrophil chemoattractant after proteolytic inactivation by macrophage elastase, *J. Biol. Chem.* 263, 4481–4484, 1988.
6. Banda, M.J. Rice, A.G., Griffin, G.L., and Senior, R.M., The inhibitory complex of human α_1-proteinase inhibitor and leukocyte elastase is a neutrophil chemoattractant, *J. Exp. Med.* 167, 1608–1615, 1988.

TABLE 9.3

Pleiotropic Activities of Heparin Cofactor II

Cell/Tissue/System	Biological Response	Reference
Nonsmall cell lung cancer	Heparin cofactor enhances cancer cell migration through PI3K, which can be blocked by heparin. The effect of heparin cofactor II on tumor cells is independent of thrombin.[1]	1
Antibacterial activity	Heparin cofactor II has been shown to have antimicrobial activity after proteolytic digestion with neutrophil elastase.[2] The activity has been localized to a 28-peptide sequence (KYE-28) comprising helix D of heparin cofactor II.[3] The peptide has been shown to have antibacterial activity against both gram-negative and gram-positive bacteria.	2,3
Blockage of LPS activation of immune cells	The KYE-28 peptide derived from heparin cofactor II[3] has been shown to inhibit LPS stimulation by decreasing NF-κB/AP-1 activation. Another peptide (GKS-26) derived from the A helix of heparin cofactor II has also been shown to modulate LPS stimulation.	3,4
Angiogenesis	Studies in a murine model system suggest that heparin cofactor II stimulates angiogenesis via an AMP-activated protein kinase and endothelial nitric oxidase system. Other investigators[6] have suggested a role for heparin cofactor II in vascular remodeling.	5,6
Monocytes and wound healing	Heparin cofactor II is associated with monocytes to provide for inhibition of thrombin. Distribution of heparin cofactor II is different from that of antithrombin.	7
Fibroblasts	Dermatan sulfate on the surface of fibroblasts accelerates the inactivation of thrombin by heparin cofactor II.	8
Vascular smooth muscle cells	Dermatan sulfate on the surface of fibroblasts accelerates the inactivation of thrombin by heparin cofactor II.	8
Neutrophils	Chemotactic peptides derived from the proteolysis of heparin cofactor II by cathepsin or elastase.	9–11

REFERENCES TO TABLE 9.3

1. Liao, W.Y., Ho, C.C., Hou, H.H., et al., Heparin co-factor II enhances cell motility and promotes metastasis in non-small cell lung cancer, *J. Pathol.* 235, 50–64, 2015.
2. Kalle, M., Papareddy, P., Kasetty, G., et al., Proteolytic activation transforms heparin cofactor II into a host defense molecule, *J. Immunol.* 190, 6303–6310, 2013.
3. Kalle, M., Papareddy, P., Kasetty, G., et al., A peptide of heparin cofactor II inhibits endotoxin-mediated shock and invasive *Pseudomonas aeruginosa* infection, *PLoS One* 9(7), e102577, 2014.
4. Papareddy, P., Kalle, M., Singh, S., et al., An antimicrobial helix A–derived peptide of heparin cofactor II blocks endotoxin responses *in vivo*, *Biochim. Biophys. Acta* 1838, 1225–1234, 2014.
5. Ikeda, Y., Aihara, K., Yoshida, S., et al., Heparin cofactor II, a serine protease inhibitor, promotes angiogenesis via activation of the AMP-activated protein kinase–endothelial nitric-oxide synthase signaling pathway, *J. Biol. Chem.* 287, 34256–24263, 2012.

6. Aihara, K., Heparin cofactor II attenuates vascular remodeling in humans and mice, *Circ. J.* 74, 1518–1523, 2010.

7. Hoffman, M., Loh, K.L., Bond, V.K., et al., Localization of heparin cofactor II in injured human skin: A potential role in wound healing, *Exp. Mol. Pathol.* 75, 109–118, 2003.

8. McGuire, E.A. and Tollesfen, D.M., Activation of heparin cofactor II by fibroblasts and vascular smooth muscle cells, *J. Biol. Chem.* 262, 169–175, 1987.

9. Hoffman, M., Pratt, C.W., Corbin, L.W., and Church, F.C., Characteristics of the chemotactic activity of heparin cofactor II proteolysis products, *J. Leukoc. Biol.* 48, 156–162, 1990.

10. Church, F.C., Pratt, C.W., and Hoffman, M., Leukocyte chemoattractant peptides from the serpin heparin cofactor II, *J. Biol. Chem.* 266, 704–709, 1991.

11. Hoffman, M., Faulkner, K.A., Iannone, M.A., and Church, F.C., The effects of heparin cofactor II-derived chemotaxins on neutrophil active conformation and cyclic AMP levels, *Biochim. Biophys. Acta* 1095, 78–82, 1991.

yielding a conformationally altered form of α_2-macroglobulin[89] with altered binding characteristics.[90–96]

9.8   TISSUE INHIBITORS OF METALLOPROTEINASES

The presence of an endogenous inhibitor of collagenase was suggested in 1975 by Bauer and coworkers,[97] and the term *tissue inhibitor of metalloproteinase* appears to have been introduced by Cawston and coworkers[98] in 1981. There are now four TIMPs: TIMP-1, TIMP-2, TIMP-3, and TIMP-4.[99] Originally described as inhibitors of MMPs (Chapter 7) such as collagenase[97] and elastase,[100] these small proteins have also been shown to inhibit ADAM and ADAMTS proteases (Chapter 4).[99,101] The primary function of TIMPs is thought to be the regulation of the ECM.[101–103] TIMPs bind to MMPs and other metalloproteinases with high affinity but little selectivity,[104–108] forming a stoichiometric complex.[99,109–111] TIMPs can bind to the proenzyme or zymogen forms of MMPs.[109,111] In the case of pro-MMP-2, binding of TIMP-2 yields a biomolecular complex that promotes activation of pro-MMP-2 by MMP-14.[107,112] However, the interaction of TIMPs with metalloproteinases is complex; TIMP-2 promotes the activation of pro-MMP-2, while TIMP-3 appears to inhibit it[107,113] or has no effect on the activation of pro-MMP by MMP-14.[114] TIMP-3 has been reported to enhance the activation of pro-MMP-2 by MMP-16 (MT3-MMP) but not by MMP-14.[115] TIMPs are also pleiotropic in that the binding of TIMP-2 to MMP-14 has been shown to activate the AKT pathway by a process unrelated to the proteolytic activity of MMP-14.[116]

REFERENCES

1. Behrens, D.T., Villone, D., Koch, M, et al., The epidermal basement membrane is a composite of separate laminin or collagen IV–containing networks connected by aggregate perlecan but not by nidogens, *J. Biol. Chem.* 287, 18700–18709, 2012.

2. Whinna, H.C., Choi, H.C., Rosenberg, L.C., and Church, F.C., Interaction of heparin cofactor II with biglycan and decorin, *J. Biol. Chem.* 268, 3920–3924, 1993.

3. Tiede, K., Melchior-Becker, A., and Fischer, J.W., Transcriptional and protranscriptional regulation of biglycan in cardiac fibroblasts, *Basic Res. Cardiol.* 105, 99–105, 2010.

4. Nandini, C.D., Itoh, N., and Sugahara, K., Novel 70-kDa chondroitin sulfate/dermatan sulfate hybrid chains with a unique heterogeneous sulfation pattern from shark skin, which exhibits neuritogenic and binding activities for growth factors and neurotropic factors, *J. Biol. Chem.* 280, 4058–4069, 2005.

5. Castañon, M.M., Gamba, C., and Kordich, L.C., Insight into the profibrinolytic activity of dermatan sulfate: Effect on the activation of plasminogen mediated by tissue and urinary plasminogen activator, *Thromb. Res.* 120, 745–752, 2007.

6. Torry, R.J., Labarrere, C.A., Nelson, D., Pantaleo, A., and Faulk, W.P., Localization and characterization of antithrombin in human kidneys, *J. Histochem. Cytochem.* 47, 313–322, 1999.

7. Xu, Y. and Slayter, H.S., Immunocytochemical localization of endogenous antithrombin III in the vasculature or rat tissues reveals localization of anticoagulantly active heparan sulfate proteoglycan, *J. Histochem. Cytochem.* 42, 1365–1376, 1994.

8. Giradin, E.P., Hajmohammedi, S., Birmele, B. et al., Synthesis of anticoagulantly active heparan sulfate proteoglycan by glomerular epithelial cells involves multiple 3-O-sulfotransferase isoforms and a limiting precursor pool, *J. Biol. Chem.* 280, 38059–38070, 2005.

9. Hedin, A. and Hahn, P.G., Volume expansion and plasma protein clearance during intravenous infusion of 5% albumin and autologous plasma, *Clin. Sci. (London)* 108, 117–124. 2004.

10. Vogel, L.K. and Larsen, J.E., Apical and non-polarized secretion of serpins from MDCK cells, *FEBS Lett.* 473, 297–302, 2000.

11. Vogel, L.K., Sahkri, S., Sjostrom, H., Noren, O., and Spiess, M., Secretion of antithrombin is converted from nonpolarized to apical by exchanging its amino terminus from that of apically secreted family members, *J. Biol. Chem.* 277, 13883–13888, 2002.

12. Morikawa, M., Yamada, T., Yamada, T., et al., Evidence of the escape of antithrombin from the blood into the interstitial space in pregnant women, *J. Perinat. Med.* 38, 613–615, 2010.

13. Omaghi, S., Barnhart, K.T., Frieling, J., Streisand, J., and Padias, M.J., Clinical syndromes associated with acquired antithrombin deficiency via microvascular leakage and the related risk of thrombosis, *Thromb. Res.* 133, 972–984, 2014.

14. Miller, G.J., Howarth, D.J., Attfield, J.C., et al., Haemostatic factors in human peripheral afferent lymph, *Thromb. Haemost.* 83, 427–432, 2000.

15. Chang, X., Yamada, R., and Yamamoto, K., Inhibition of antithrombin by hyaluronic acid may be involved in the pathogenesis of rheumatoid arthritis, *Arthritis Res. Ther.* 7, R268–R273, 2005.

16. Oberst, M.D, Williams, C.A., Dickson, R.B., Johnson, M.D., and Lin, C.Y., The activation of matriptase requires its noncatalytic domains, serine protease domain, and its cognate inhibitor, *J. Biol. Chem.* 278, 26773–26779, 2003.

17. Stirnberg, M., Mauer, E., Horstmeyer, A., et al., Proteolytic processing of the serine protease matriptase-2: Identification of the cleavage sites required for its autocatalytic release from the cell surface, *Biochem. J.* 430, 87–95, 2010.

18. Najy, A.J., Dyson, G., Jena, B.P., Lin, C.Y., and Kim, H.C., Matriptase activation and shedding through PDGF-D-mediated extracellular acidosis, *Am. J. Physiol. Cell. Physiol.* 310, C293–304, 2016.

19. Ovaere, P., Lippens, S., Vandenabella, P., and Declercq, W., The emerging role of serine protease cascades in the epidermis, *Trends Biochem. Sci.* 34, 453–463, 2009.

20. Candi, E., Schmidt, R., and Melino, G., The cornified envelope: A model of cell death in the skin, *Nat. Rev. Mol. Cell Biol.* 5, 328–340, 2005.

21. Chen, Y.W., Wang, J.K., Chou, F.P., et al., Regulation of the matriptase-prostasin cell surface proteolytic cascade by hepatocyte growth factor inhibitor-1 during epidermal differentiation, *J. Biol. Chem.* 285, 31755–31762, 2010.

22. Miller, G.S. and Lisk, K., The matriptase–prostasin cascade in epithelial development and pathology, *Cell Tissue Res.* 351, 245–253, 2013.

23. Miyata, S., Fukushima, T, Kohama, K., et al., Roles of Kunitz domains in the anti-invasive effect of hepatocyte growth factor activator inhibitor type-1 in human glioblastoma cells, *Hum. Cell* 20, 100–106, 2007.

24. Sales, K.U., Masedunskas, A., Bey, A.L., et al., Matriptase initiates activation of epidermal pro-kallikrein and disease onset in a mouse model of Netherton syndrome, *Nat. Genet.* 42, 676–683, 2010.

25. Ishida-Yamamoto, A. and Igawa, S., The biology and regulation of corneodesmosomes, *Cell Tissue Res.* 360, 477–482, 2015.

26. Chou, F.P., Xu, H., Lee, M.S., et al., Matriptase is inhibited by extravascular antithrombin in epithelial cells but not in most carcinoma cells, *Am. J. Physiol. Cell Physiol.* 301, C1093–1103, 2011.

27. Tseng, I.C., Chou, F.P., and Su, S.F., Purification from human mile of matriptase complexes with secreted serpins: Mechanism for inhibition of matriptase other than HAI-1, *Am. J. Physiol. Cell Physiol.* 295, C423–C431, 2008.

28. Hurst, N.J., Jr., Najy, A.J., Utach, C.V., Movilla, L., and Kim, H.R., Platelet-derived growth factor-C (PDGF-C) activation by serine proteases: Implications for breast cancer progression, *Biochem. J.* 441, 909–918, 2012.

29. Wolberg, A.S., Stafford, D.W., and Erie, D.A., Human factor IX binds to specific sites on collagen IV, *J. Biol. Chem.* 272, 16717–16720, 1997.

30. Westmark, P.R., Tarantana, P., and Sheehan, J.P., Selective disruption of heparin and antithrombin-mediated regulation of human factor IX, *J. Thromb. Haemost.* 13, 1053–1063, 2015.

31. Bogatkevich, G.S., Ludwicka-Bradley, A., Nietert, P.J., et al., Antiinflammatory and antifibrotic effects of the oral direct thrombin inhibitor dabigatran etexilate in a murine model of interstitial lung disease, *Arthritis Rheum.* 63, 1416–1425, 2011.

32. Totzke, G., Schobersberger, W., Schloesser, M., Czechowski, M., and Hoffman, G., Effects of antithrombin III on tumor necrosis factor-alpha and interleukin 1-beta synthesis in vascular smooth muscle cells, *J. Interferon Cytokine Res.* 21, 1063–1069, 2001.

33. Blackburn, M.N., Smith, R.L., Carson, J., and Sibley, C.C., The heparin-binding site of antithrombin III: Identification of a critical tryptophan in the amino acid sequence, *J. Biol. Chem.* 259, 939–941, 1984.

34. Monien, B.H., Krishnaswamy, C., Olson, S.T., and Desai, U.R., Importance of tryptophan 49 of antithrombin in heparin binding and conformational activation, *Biochemistry* 44, 11660–11668, 2005.

35. Totzke, G., Smolny, M., Siebel, M., et al., Antithrombin III enhances inducible nitric oxide synthase expression in vascular smooth muscle cells, *Cell. Immunol.* 208, 1–8, 2001.

36. Komura, H., Uchiba, M., Mizuchi, Y., et al., Antithrombin inhibits lipopolysaccharide-induced tumor necrosis factor-alpha production by monocytes *in vitro* through inhibition of Egr-1 expression, *J. Thromb. Haemost.* 6, 499–507, 2008.

37. Roemisch, J., Gray, E., Hoffmann, J.N., and Wiedermann, C.J., Antithrombin: A new look at the actions of a serine protease inhibitor, *Blood Coagul. Fibrinolysis* 13, 657–670, 2002.

38. Carrell, R.W., Evans, D.L., and Stein, P.E., Mobile reactive centre of serpins and the control of thrombosis, *Nature* 353, 576–578, 1991.

39. Wardell, M.R., Abrahams, J.P., Bruce, D., Skinner, R., and Leslie, A.G., Crystallization and preliminary X-ray diffraction analysis of two conformations of intact human antithrombin, *J. Mol. Biol.* 234, 1253–1258, 1993.

40. Chang, W.S. and Harper, P.L., Commercial antithrombin concentrate contains inactive L-forms for antithrombin, *Thromb. Haemost.*77, 323–328, 1997.

41. Corral, J., Rivera, J., Martinez, C., et al., Detection of conformational transformation of antithrombin in blood with cross immunoelectrophoresis: New application for a classical method, *J. Lab. Clin. Med.* 142, 298–305, 2003.

42. Mochizuki, S., Miyano, K., Kondo, M., et al., Purification and characterization of recombinant human antithrombin containing prelatent form in Chinese hamster ovary cells, *Protein Expr. Purif.* 41, 323–331, 2005.

43. O'Reilly, M.S., Pirie-Shepherd, S., Lane, W.S., and Folkman, J., Antiangiogenic activity of the cleaved conformation of the serpin antithrombin, *Science* 285, 1926–1928, 1999.

44. Kisker, O., Onizuka, S., Banyard, J., et al., Generation of multiple angiogenesis inhibitors by human pancreatic cancer, *Cancer Res.* 61, 7298–7304, 2001.

45. Larsson, H., Sjöblom, T., Dixelius, J., et al., Antiangiogenic effects of latent antithrombin through perturbed cell–matrix interactions and apoptosis of endothelial cells, *Cancer Res.* 60, 6723–6729, 2000.

46. Zhang, W., Chuang, Y.J., Swanson, R., et al., Antiangiogenic antithrombin downregulates the expression of the proangiogenic heparan sulfate proteoglycan, perlecan, in endothelial cells, *Blood* 103, 1185–1191, 2004.

47. Zhang, W., Swanson, R., Xiong, Y., Richard, B., and Olson, S.T., Antiangiogenic antithrombin blocks the heparan sulfate–dependent binding of proangiogenic antithrombin to their endothelial cell receptors: Evidence for differential binding of antiangiogenic and anticoagulant forms of antithrombin to proangiogenic heparan sulfate domains, *J. Biol. Chem.* 281, 37302–37310, 2006.

48. O'Reilly, M.S., Antiangiogenic antithrombin, *Semin. Thromb. Haemost.* 33, 660–666, 2007.

49. Azhar, A., Singh, P., Rashid, Q., et al., Antiangiogenic function of antithrombin is dependent on its conformational variation: Implications for other serpins, *Protein Pept. Lett.* 20, 403–411, 2013.

50. Richard, B., Swanson, R., Schedin-Weiss, S., et al., Characterization of the conformational alterations, reduced anticoagulant activity, and enhanced antiangiogenic activity of prelatent antithrombin, *J. Biol. Chem.* 283, 14417–14429, 2008.

51. Miller, G.J., Howarth, D.J., Attfield, J.C., et al., Haemostatic factors in human peripheral afferent lymph, *Thromb. Haemost.* 83, 427–432, 2000.

52. Li, D.T., Borga, P., Toneff, T.W., Witte, M.H., and Rapaport, S.I., Hemostatic factors in rabbit limb lymph: Relationship to mechanisms regulating extravascular coagulation, *Am. J. Physiol.* 274, H769–H776, 1998.

53. Mushunje, A., Evans, G., Brennan, S.O., Carrell, R.W., and Zhou. A., Latent antithrombin and its detection, formation and turnover in the circulation, *J. Thromb. Haemost.* 2, 2170–2177, 2004.

54. Corral, J., Rivera, J., Guerrero, J.A., et al., Latent and polymeric antithrombin: Clearance and potential thrombotic risk, *Exp. Biol. Med. (Maywood)*, 232, 219–226, 2007.

55. Wardell, M.R., Chang, W.S., Bruce, D., et al., Preparative induction and characterization of L-antithrombin: A structural homologue of latent PAI-1, *Biochemistry* 36, 13133–13142, 1997.

56. Gils, A., Vleuels, N., Tobback, K., Knockaert, I., and Declerk, P.J., Characterization of PAI-1 mutants containing the P13 to P10 region of ovalbumin or antithrombin III: Evidence that the P13 residue contributes significantly to the active to substrate transition, *Biochim. Biophys. Acta* 1387, 291–297, 1998.

57. Wind, T., Jensen, J.K., Dupont, D.M., Kulig, P., and Andreasen, P.A., Mutational analysis of PAI-1, *Eur. J. Biochem.* 270, 1680–1688, 2003.
58. Dunstone, M.A. and Whisstock, J.C., Crystallography of serpins and serpin complexes, *Methods Enzymol.* 501, 63–87, 2011.
59. Kamikbubo, Y., Neels, J.G., and Degryse, B., Vitronectin inhibits PAI-1-induced signaling and chemotaxis by blocking PAI-1 binding to low-density lipoprotein receptor-related protein, *Int. J. Biochem. Cell Biol.* 41, 578–585, 2009.
60. Jensen, S., Kirkegaard, T., Pedersen, K.E., et al., The role of β-strand 5A of plasminogen activator inhibitors-1 in regulation of its latency transition and inhibitory activity by vitronectin, *Biochim. Biophys. Acta* 1597, 301–310, 2002.
61. Rezaie, A.R., Role of exosites 1 and 2 in thrombin reaction with PAI-1 in the absence and presence of cofactors, *Biochemistry* 38, 14592–14599, 1999.
62. Ngo, T.H., Hoylaerts, M.F., Knockaert, I., Brouwers, E., and Declerck, P.J., Identification of a target site in PAI-1 that allows neutralization of its inhibitor properties concomitant with an allosteric up-regulation of its antiadhesive properties, *J. Biol. Chem.* 276, 26243–26248, 2001.
63. Sigurdardóttir, O. and Wiman, B., Complex formation between plasminogen activator inhibitor 1 and vitronectin in purified systems and in plasma, *Biochim. Biophys. Acta* 1035, 56–61, 1990.
64. Lijnen, H.R., Pleiotropic functions of PAI-1, *J. Thromb. Haemost.* 3, 35–45, 2005.
65. Siegfried, W., Rosenfeld, M., Stier, L., et al., Polarity of secretion of alpha-1-antitrypsin by human respiratory epithelial cells after adenoviral transfer of a human alpha-1-antitrypsin cDNA, *Am. J. Respir. Cell Mol. Biol.* 12, 379–384, 1995.
66. Abbink, J.J., Kamp, A.M., Swaak, A.J., and Hack, C.E., Production of monoclonal antibodies against inactivated alpha-1-antitrypsin: Cross-reactivity with complexed alpha-1-antitrypsin and application in an assay to determine inactivated and complexed alpha-1-antitrypsin in biological fluids, *J. Immunol. Methods* 143, 197–208, 1991.
67. Hubbard, R.C., McElvaney, N.G., Sellers, S.E., et al., Recombinant DNA-produced alpha-1-antitrypsin administered by aerosol augments lower respiratory tract antineutrophil elastase defenses in individuals with alpha-1-antitrypsin, *J. Clin. Invest.* 84, 1349–1354, 1989.
68. Siekmeier, R., Lung deposition of inhaled alpha-1-antitrypsin (alpha-1-PI): Problems and experience of alpha-1-PI inhalation therapy in patients with hereditary alpha-1-PI deficiency and cystic fibrosis, *Eur. J. Med. Res.* 15(Suppl. 2), 164–174, 2010.
69. Janciauskiene, S., Nita, I., Subramaniyam, D., et al., Alpha1-antitrypsin inhibits the activity of the matriptase catalytic domain *in vitro*, *Am. J. Respir. Cell Mol. Biol.* 39, 631–637, 2008.
70. Lomas, D.A., Elliott, P.R., Chang, W.S., Wardell, M.R., and Carrell, R.W., Preparation and characterization of latent alpha-1-antitrypsin, *J. Biol. Chem.* 270, 5282–5288, 1995.
71. Lomas, D.A., Elliott, P.R., and Carrell, R.W., Commercial plasma alpha1-antitrypsin (Prolastin) contains a conformationally inactive, latent component, *Eur. Respir. J.* 10, 672–675, 1997.
72. Kataoka, H., Itoh, H., and Koona, M., Emerging multifunctional aspects of cellular serine proteinase inhibitors in tumor progression and tissue regeneration, *Pathol. Int.* 52, 89–102, 2002.
73. Biggs, R. and Denson, K.W.E., Natural and pathological inhibitors of blood coagulation, in *Blood Coagulation, Haemostasis and Thrombosis*, ed. R. Biggs, Chapter 7, pp. 133–158, Blackwell Scientific, Oxford, United Kingdom, 1972.
74. Tollefsen, D.M., Pestkas, C.A., and Monafo, W.I., Activation of heparin cofactor II by dermatan sulfate, *J. Biol. Chem.* 258, 6713–6716, 1983.

75. Yamagishi, R., Niwa, M., Kondo, S., Sakuragawa, N., and Koide, T., Purification and biological property of heparin cofactor II: Activation of heparin cofactor II and antithrombin III by dextran sulfate and various glycosaminoglycans, *Thromb. Res.* 36, 633–642, 1984.
76. Saito, A., Heparin cofactor II is degraded by heparan sulfate and dextran sulfate, *Biochem. Biophys. Res. Commun.* 457, 585–588, 2015.
77. Worm, A.-M., Exchange of macromolecules between plasma and skin interstitium in extensive skin disease, *J. Invest. Dermatol.* 76, 489–492, 1981.
78. Haaverstad, R., Romslo, I., and Myhre, H.O., The concentration of high molecular weight compounds in interstitial tissue fluid: A study in patients with post-reconstructive leg oedema, *Eur. J. Vasc. Endovasc. Surg.* 13, 355–360, 1997.
79. Svedman, C., Yu, B.B., Ryan, T.J., and Svensson, H., Plasma proteins in a standardized skin mini-erosion (I): Permeability changes as a function of time, *BMC Dermatol.* 2, 4, 2002.
80. Sottrup-Jensen, L., α-Macroglobulins: Structure, shape, and mechanism of proteinase complex formation, *J. Biol. Chem.* 264, 11539–11542, 1989.
81. Hart, J.E. and Pizzo, S.V., α₂-Macroglobulin, in *Thrombosis and Hemostasis: Basic Principles and Clinical Practice*, 5th edn., eds. R.W. Colman, V.J. Marder, A.N. Clowes, J.N. George, and S.Z. Goldhaber, Chapter 21, pp. 395–407, Lippincott, Williams & Wilkins, Philadelphia, PA, 2006.
82. Kowarik, M.C., Dzieciatkowska, M., Wemlinger, S., et al., The cerebrospinal fluid immunoglobulin transcriptome and proteome in neuromyelitis optica reveals central nervous system-specific B cell populations, *J. Neuroinflammation* 12, 19, 2015.
83. Gerbicke-Haerter, P.J., Bauer, J., Brenner, A., et al., Alpha 2-macroglobulin synthesis in an astrocyte subpopulation, *J. Neurochem.* 49, 1139–1145, 1987.
84. Bauer, J., Gerbicke-Haerter, P.J., Ganter, U., et al., Astrocytes synthesize and secrete alpha 2-macroglobulin synthesis in rat liver and brain, *Adv. Exp. Med. Biol.* 240, 199–205, 1988.
85. Fabrizi, C., Colasanti, M., Persichini, T., et al., Interferon gamma up-regulates α₂-macroglobulin expression in human astrocytoma cells, *J. Neuroimmunol.* 53, 31–37, 1994.
86. Borth, W., α₂-Macroglobulin, a multifunctional binding protein with targeting characteristics, *FASEB. J.* 6, 335–3353, 1992.
87. Feige, J.J., Negoescu, A., Keramides, M., Souchelnitskiy, S. and Chambaz, E.M., α₂-Macroglobulin: A binding protein for transforming growth factor-β and various cytokines, *Horm. Res.* 45, 227–232, 1996.
88. LaMarca, J., Wollenberg, G.K., Gonias, S.L., and Hayes, M.A., Cytokine binding and clearance properties of proteinase-activated α₂-macroglobulin, *Lab. Invest.* 65, 3–14, 1991.
89. Kaczowka, S.J., Madding, L.S., Epting, K.L, et al., Probing the stability of native and activated forms of α₂-macroglobulin, *Int. J. Biol. Macromol.* 42, 62–67, 2008.
90. Webb, D.J., Atkins, T.L., Crookston, K.P., et al., Transforming growth factor β isoform 2-specific high affinity binding to native α₂-macroglobulin: Chimeras identify a sequence that determines affinity for native not activated α₂-macroglobulin, *J. Biol. Chem.* 229, 30402–30406, 1994.
91. Webb, D.J. and Gonias, S.L., A modified human α₂-macroglobulin derivative that binds tumor necrosis factor-α and interleukin-1β with high affinity *in vitro* and reverses lipopolysaccharide toxicity *in vivo* in mice, *Lab. Invest.* 78, 939–948, 1998.
92. Bhatacharjee, G., Asplin, I.R., Wu, S.M., Gawdi, G., and Pizzo, S.V., The conformation-dependent interaction of α₂-macroglobulin/growth factor binding, *J. Biol. Chem.* 275, 26806–26811, 2000.
93. Misra, U.K., Deedwania, R., and Pizzo, S.V., Binding of activated α₂-macroglobulin to its cell surface receptor GRP78 in 1-LN prostate cancers cells regulates PAK-2-dependent activation of LIMK, *J. Biol. Chem.* 280, 26278–26286, 2005.

94. French, K., Yerbury, J.J., and Wilson, M.R., Protease activation of α_2-macroglobulin modulates chaperone-like action with broad specificity, *Biochemistry* 47, 1176–1185, 2008.

95. Wyatt, A.R., Constantinescu, P., Ecroyd, H., et al., Protease-activated α_2-macroglobulin can inhibit amyloid formation via two distinct mechanisms, *FEBS Lett.* 587, 398–403, 2013.

96. Misra, U.K. and Pizzo, S.V., Activated α_2-macroglobuln binding to cell surface GRP78 induces T-loop phosphorylation of Akt1 and PDK1 in association with Raptor, *PLoS One* 9(2), e88373, 2014.

97. Bauer, E.A., Stricklin, G.P., Jeffrey, J.J., and Eisen, A.Z., Collagenase production by human skin fibroblasts, *Biochem. Biophys. Res. Commun.* 64, 232–340, 1975.

98. Cawston, T.E., Galloway, W.A., Mercer, E., Murphy, G., and Reynolds, J.J., Purification of rabbit bone inhibitor of collagenase, *Biochem. J.* 195, 159–165, 1981.

99. Brew, K. and Nagase, H., The tissue inhibitors of metalloproteases (TIMPs): An ancient family with structural and functional diversity, *Biochim. Biophys. Acta* 1803, 55–71, 2010.

100. Albin, R.J., Senior, R.M., Welgus, H.G., Connolly, N.L., and Campbell, E.J., Human alveolar macrophages secrete an inhibitor of metalloproteinase elastase, *Am. Rev. Respir. Dis.* 135, 1281–1285, 1987.

101. Arpino, V., Brock, M., and Gill, S.E., The role of TIMPs in regulation of extracellular matrix proteolysis, *Matrix Biol.* 44–46, 247–254, 2015.

102. Edwards, D.R., Beaudry, P.P., Laing, T.D., et al., The roles of tissue inhibitors of metalloproteinases in tissue remodeling and cell growth, *Int. J. Obes. Relat. Metab. Disord.* 20(Suppl. 3), S9–S15, 1996.

103. Gomez, D.E., Alonso, D.F., Yoshiji, H., and Thorgeirsson, U.P., Tissue inhibitors of metalloproteinases: Structure, regulation and biological functions, *Eur. J. Cell Biol.* 74, 111–122, 1997.

104. Troeberg, L., Tanaka, M., Wait, T., et al., *E. coli* expression of TIMP-4 and comparative kinetic studies with TIMP-1 and TIMP-2: Insights into the interactions of TIMPs and matrix metalloproteinase 2 (gelatinase A), *Biochemistry* 41, 15025–15035, 2002.

105. Nagase, H. and Brew, K., Designing TIMP (tissue inhibitor of metalloproteinases) variants that are selective metalloproteinase inhibitors, *Biochem. Soc. Symp.* 70, 201–212, 2003.

106. Higashi, S., Hirose, T., Takeuchi, T., and Miyazaki, K., Molecular design of a highly selective and strong protein inhibitor against matrix metalloproteinase-2 (MMP-2), *J. Biol. Chem.* 288, 9066–9076, 2013.

107. Wang, Z., Famulski, K., Lee, J., et al., TIMP2 and TIMP3 have divergent roles in early renal tubulointerstitial injury, *Kidney Int.* 85, 82–93, 2014.

108. Newby, A.C., Metalloproteinases promote plaque rupture and myocardial infarction: A persuasive concept waiting for clinical translation, *Matrix Biol.* 44–46, 157–166, 2015.

109. Emmert-Buck, M.R., Emonard, H.P., Corcoran, M.L., et al., Cell-surface binding of TIMP-2 and pro-MMP-2/TIMP-2 complex, *FEBS Lett.* 364, 28–32, 1995.

110. Nagase, H., Suzuki, K., Cawston, T.E., and Brew, K., Involvement of a region near valine-69 of tissue inhibitor of metalloproteinase (TIMP)-1 in the interaction with matrix metalloproteinase 3 (stromelysin 1), *Biochem. J.* 325, 163–167, 1997.

111. Ardi, V.C., Kupriyanova, T.A., Deryugina, E.I., and Quigley, J.P., Human neutrophils uniquely release TIMP-free MMP-9 to provide a potent catalytic stimulator of angiogenesis, *Proc. Natl. Acad. Sci. USA* 104, 20262–20267, 2007.

112. Wang, Z., Juttermann, R., and Soloway, P.D., TIMP-2 is required for efficient activation of proMMP-2 *in vivo*, *J. Biol. Chem.* 275, 26411–26415, 2000.

113. English, J.L., Kassiri, Z., Koskivirta, I., et al., Individual *Timp* deficiencies differentially impact Pro-MMP-2 activation, *J. Biol. Chem.* 281, 10337–10346, 2006.

114. Butler, G.S., Aptel, S.S., Willenbrock, F., and Murphy, G., Human tissue inhibitor of metalloproteinases 3 interacts with both the N- and C-terminal domains of gelatinases A and B, *J. Biol. Chem.* 274, 10846–1985, 1999.
115. Zhao, H., Bernardo, M.M., Osenkowski, P., et al., Differential inhibition of membrane type 3 (MT3)-matrix metalloproteinase and MT1-MMP by tissue inhibitor of metalloproteinase (TIMP)-2 and TIMP-3 regulates pro-MMP-2 activation, *J. Biol. Chem.* 279, 8592–8601, 2004.
116. Valacca, C., Tassone, E., and Mignatti, P., TIMP-2 interaction with MT1-MMP activates the AKT pathway and protects tumor cells from apoptosis, *PLoS One* 10(9), e0136797, 2015.

Index

Printed and bound by CPI Group (UK) Ltd, Croydon, CR0 4YY

24/10/2024

01778281-0007